# The Tarascon Internal Medicine & Critical Care Pocketbook, 3rd Edition

# Tarascon Internal Medicine & Critical Care Pocketbook

## 3rd edition

## James S. Winshall, M.D.

*Assistant Professor of Medicine, Harvard Medical School*
*Division of General Medicine, Brigham & Women's Hospital*
*Boston, Massachusetts, USA*

## Robert J. Lederman, M.D.

*Investigator, Cardiovascular Branch*
*National Heart, Lung and Blood Institute*
*National Institutes of Health, Bethesda, Maryland, USA*

*This book was co-authored by Robert J. Lederman in his private capacity. The views expressed in the book do not necessarily represent the views of the NIH, DHHS, nor the United States.*

*"It's not how much you know, it's how fast you can find the answer."* ®

**Artwork:** *Examination of a Leper* by Hans von Gersdorff, Strasbourg, 1540. Courtesy of the National Library of Medicine, Images from the History of Medicine.

# Editorial Board

## A Note from the Authors

The *IMCCP* is intended as a "head of the bed" reference for a variety of internal medicine emergencies. While the 3rd edition has been expanded and updated, we have continued to include only a selection of life-threatening or less-common clinical problems (OK already, we added something about diabetes). To use this book effectively, please take a few minutes to familiarize yourself with its structure and contents.

Many users have sent in comments since the publication of the first edition; we are grateful for their input. If you find an error or wish to make a suggestion, please let us know (e-mail: editor@tarascon.com). Otherwise, a pox on you!

The authors would like to acknowledge the helpful comments and suggestions from the following individuals: Dan Briggs; Tony Furnary; Eli Gelfand; Laura Michaelis; Kris Mogensen; Malcolm Robinson; Paul Sax; Dan Solomon; Pratiksha Somaia; Andy Wagner; Marshall Wolf; and Rich Zane.

Dedicated to my incredibly understanding family and to the BWH house staff (JSW) and to Bunny & the Snaurus (RJL).

Order form on last page

For TARASCON BOOKS/SOFTWARE, VISIT **WWW.TARASCON.COM**
**Tarascon Pocket Pharmacopoeia®**
  • Classic Shirt-Pocket Edition
  • Deluxe Labcoat Pocket Edition
  • PDA software for Palm OS ® or Pocket PC ®
**Other Tarascon Pocketbooks**
  • Tarascon Internal Medicine & Critical Care Pocketbook
  • Tarascon Primary Care Pocketbook
  • Tarascon Pediatric Emergency Pocketbook (& PDA software)
  • Tarascon Adult Emergency Pocketbook
  • Tarascon Pocket Orthopaedica ®
  • How to be a Truly Excellent Junior Medical Student

# Abbreviations

↓: decrease, low
↑: increase, high
Δ: change
Ab: antibody
ABG: arterial blood gas
ACE: angiotensin converting enzyme
ACLS: advanced cardiac life support
ACS: acute coronary syndrome
ADH: antidiuretic hormone
AF or A-fib: atrial fibrillation
Ag: antigen
AI: aortic insufficiency
ALT: alanine aminotransferase
AML: acute myelogenous leukemia
Amp: ampule
ANA: antinuclear antibody
aPTT: activated partial thromboplastin time
ARDS: adult respiratory distress syndrome
ARF: acute renal failure
AS: aortic stenosis
ASD: atrial septal defect
AST: aspartate aminotransferase
ATN: acute tubular necrosis
AV: atrioventricular
AVB: atrioventricular block
AVM: arteriovenous malformation
AWMI: anterior wall myocardial infarction
BBB: bundle branch block
BLS: basic life support
BMT: bone marrow transplant
BP: Blood pressure
Ca: calcium
CABG: coronary artery bypass graft
CAD: coronary artery disease
CAPD: continuous ambulatory peritoneal dialysis
CAVH/D: continuous arteriovenous hemofiltration/dialysis

CCS: Canadian angina class
CHF: congestive heart failure
CLL: chronic lymphocytic leukemia
CMV: cytomegalovirus
CNS: central nervous system
CO: carbon monoxide
COPD: chronic obstructive pulmonary disease
CPR: cardiopulmonary resuscitation
Cr: creatinine
CrCL: creatinine clearance
CSF: cerebrospinal fluid
CT: computed tomography
CXR: chest radiograph
d: day
D5W: dextrose 5% in water
D50: dextrose 50% in water
DA: dopamine
DBP: diastolic BP
DIC: disseminated intravascular coagulation
DKA: diabetic ketoacidosis
dL: deciliter
DVT: deep vein thrombosis
DM: diabetes mellitus
Dz: disease
EBV: Epstein-Barr virus
ECG: electrocardiogram
EEG: electroencephalogram
EP: electrophysiology testing
ERCP: endoscopic retrograde cholangio-pancreatography
ESRD: end-stage renal disease
EtOH: ethanol
FENa: fractional excretion of sodium
$FEV_1$: forced expiratory volume in 1 second
$F_iO_2$: inspired oxygen fraction
FFP: fresh frozen plasma
FVC: forced vital capacity
G6PD: glucose-6-phosphate dehydrogenase
GFR: glomerular filtration rate
GI: gastrointestinal
gm: gram
gtts: drops

GVHD: graft vs. host disease
h or hr: hour
Hb: hemoglobin
HBsAb/Ag: hepatitis B surface Ab, Antigen
HBV: hepatitis B virus
HCV: hepatitis C virus
$HCO_3$: bicarbonate
HELLP: hemolytic anemia, elevated liver enzymes and low platelets
HIT: heparin-induced thrombocytopenia
H&P: history & physical exam
HR: heart rate
HSV: herpes simplex virus
HTN: hypertension
HUS: hemolytic-uremic syndrome
IABP: intraaortic balloon counterpulsation pump
ICD: implantable cardiac defibrillator
IE: infective endocarditis
IM: intramuscular
IMV: intermittent mandatory ventilation
IU: international units
IV: intravenous
IVC: inferior vena cava
IVDU: intravenous drug user
IVIG: intravenous immunoglobulin
IVP: intravenous push
IWMI: inferior wall myocardial infarction
JVP: jugular vein pressure
K: potassium
L: left, liter
LA: left atrium
LAO: left anterior oblique
LBBB: left bundle branch block
LDH: lactate dehydrogenase
LMWH: low molecular weight heparin
LN: lymph node
LV: left ventricle
LVEDP: left ventricular end-diastolic pressure

LVH: left ventricular hypertrophy
MAOI: monoamine oxidase inhibitor
MetHb: methemoglobin
Mg: magnesium
MI: myocardial infarction
min: minutes
MS: mitral stenosis
$M_VO_2$: myocardial oxygen consumption
MVP: mitral valve prolapse
Na: sodium
NE: norepinephrine
Nml: normal
NS: normal (0.9%) saline
NSAID: nonsteroidal antiinflammatory drug
NSR: normal sinus rhythm
NSTEMI: non-ST elevation myocardial infarction
NTG: nitroglycerin
N/V/D: nausea, vomiting, diarrhea
$O_2$sat: arterial oxygen saturation
PA: pulmonary artery, posteroanterior
PAD: PA diastolic pressure, Peripheral artery disease
$P_aCO_2$: arterial partial pressure of carbon dioxide
PAgram: pulmonary arteriogram
$P_aO_2$: arterial partial pressure of oxygen
$P_AO_2$: alveolar partial pressure of oxygen
PCA: procainamide
PCI: percutaneous coronary intervention
PCN: penicillin
PCP: *Pneumocystis carinii* pneumonia
PCR: polymerase chain reaction
PCWP: pulmonary capillary wedge pressure
PDA: patent ductus arteriosus
PE: pulmonary embolism
PEEP: positive end-expiratory pressure
PFT: pulmonary function test

PMN: polymorphonuclear leukocyte
PNGT: via nasogastric tube
PO: orally
PRBC: packed RBCs
PSA: prostate specific antigen
PSVT: paroxysmal supraventricular tachycardia
Pt: patient
PT: prothrombin time
PTCA: percutaneous transluminal coronary angioplasty
PTU: propylthiouracil
PUD: peptic ulcer disease
PVR: pulmonary vascular resistance
R: right
RA: right atrium
RAO: right anterior oblique
RBBB: right bundle branch block
RBC: red blood cell
RCT: randomized controlled trial
R/O: rule out
RSV: respiratory syncytial virus
RTA: renal tubular acidosis
RV: right ventricle
RVEDP: right ventricular end-diastolic pressure
Rx: therapy
SA: sinoatrial
SAH: subarachnoid hemorrhage
$S_aO_2$: arterial oxygen saturation
SBP: systolic blood pressure; spontaneous bacterial peritonitis
SC: subcutaneous
SIADH: syndrome of inappropriate ADH secretion
SLE: systemic lupus erythematosus
SNRT: sinus node recovery time
s/p: status post
STEMI: ST elevation myocardial infarction
SVC: superior vena cava

SVR: systemic vascular resistance
SVT: supraventricular tachycardia
Sx: symptoms
$T\frac{1}{2}$: half-life
TB: tuberculosis
TCA: tricyclic antidepressant
Td: tetanus-diphtheria vaccine
TEE: transesophageal echocardiography
TN: true negative
Tn: troponin
TP: true positive
TPN: total parenteral nutrition
TTKG: trans-tubular potassium gradient
TTP: thrombotic thrombocytopenia purpura
U: Unit
UGI: upper gastrointestinal
US: ultrasound
VC: vital capacity
VF: ventricular fibrillation
V/Q: ventilation/perfusion
VSD: ventricular septal defect
VT: ventricular tachycardia
vWF: von Willebrand factor
VZV: varicella-zoster virus
WBC: white blood cell
WPW: Wolff-Parkinson-White syndrome
XRT: radiation therapy

# Handy Formulas

## Acid-Base Rules of Thumb[1]

| | | Acidosis | Alkalosis |
|---|---|---|---|
| **Respiratory** | Acute | $\Delta pH = -0.008 \times \Delta PaCO_2$ <br> $\Delta [HCO_3^-] = 0.1 \times \Delta PaCO_2 \ (\pm 3)$ | $\Delta pH = 0.008 \times \Delta PaCO_2$ <br> $\Delta [HCO_3^-] = -0.2 \times \Delta PaCO_2$ <br> (usually not to less than 18mEq/L) |
| | Chronic | $P_aCO_2 = 2.4 \times [HCO_3^-] - 22$ <br> $\Delta [HCO_3^-] = 0.35 \times \Delta PaCO_2 \ (\pm 4)$ | $\Delta [HCO_3^-] = -0.4 \times \Delta PaCO_2$ <br> (usually not to less than 18 mEq/L) |
| **Metabolic** | | $P_aCO_2 = 1.5 \times [HCO_3^-] + 8 \pm 2$ <br> $P_aCO_2 \cong$ last two digits of pH <br> $\Delta P_aCO_2 = 1.2 \times \Delta [HCO_3^-]$ | $P_aCO_2 = 0.9 \times [HCO_3^-] + 9 \pm 2$ <br> $\Delta P_aCO_2 = 0.6 \times \Delta [HCO_3^-]$ |

## Acid-Base Map [2]

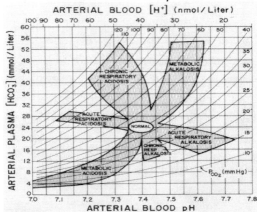

1   Schrier RW. *Renal and Electrolyte Disorders*. 5th ed. Philadelphia: Lippincott-Raven; 1997.  Rose BD, Post TW. *Clinical Physiology of Acid-Base and Electrolyte Disorders*. 5th ed. New York: McGraw-Hill, Medical Pub. Division; 2001.
2   Reprinted with permission from Brenner BM, Rector FC. *Brenner and Rector's The Kidney*. 6th ed. Figure 21-9. Philadelphia: Elsevier, 2000.

# *Other Renal Equations*

mmol/L = mg/dL × 10 ÷ molecular weight

mEq/L = mmol/L × valence

mOsm/kg = mmol/L × n (where $n$ is number of dissociable particles per molecule)

$$\text{Calculated Osmolarity} = 2 \times Na(mEq/L) + \frac{BUN(mg/dL)}{2.8} + \frac{Glucose(mg/dL)}{18} + \frac{EtOH(mg/dL)}{4.6}$$

$$+ \frac{Isopropanol\,(mg/dL)}{6} + \frac{methanol}{3.2} + \frac{ethylene\ glycol}{6.2} \quad \text{(Normal 275 - 290 mOsm/kg)}$$

Osmolar gap = Measured osmolarity - calculated osmolarity (normal < 10 mOsm/kg)

Anion Gap        = [Na] - [Cl] - [HCO₃]

Urinary anion gap      = [Na] + [K] - Cl - HCO₃ (may ignore HCO₃ if pH < 6.5)

$$\text{Free water deficit} = 0.4 \times \text{lean body wt} \times \left\{ \frac{\text{plasma [Na +]}}{140} - 1 \right\}$$

$$\text{Creatinine Clearance} = \frac{U_{Cr} \times V}{P_{Cr}} = \frac{\text{[Urine creatinine (mg/dL)]} \times \text{[Urine volume (ml/day)]}}{\text{[Plasma creatinine (mg/dL)]} \times 1440\ min/day}$$

$$\text{Creatinine Clearance} \approx \frac{140 - \text{Age (yrs)}}{\text{Serum creatinine (mg/dL)} \times 72} \times \text{weight (kg)} \ (\times 0.85 \text{ If woman})$$

Creatinine Clearance (MDRD estimation)=

$170 \times [Cr] \times \text{Age (yrs)}^{-0.18} \times [0.762 \text{ if female}] \times [1.18 \text{ if black}] \times [BUN]^{-0.17} \times [Alb]^{0.32}$

$$\text{Fractional Excretion of Sodium (FE}_{Na}) = \frac{\text{[Urine Na]} \times \text{[Plasma Cr]}}{\text{[Urine Cr]} \times \text{[Plasma Na]}}$$

Trans-tubular K⁺ gradient (TTKG) = $(U_K \times P_{Osm}) \div (P_K \times U_{Osm})$

## Rules of thumb:

Estimated 24-hr urinary protein excretion (g/day) ≈ spot urine prot/creat ratio

Potassium and pH:     [K⁺] increases 0.6 mEq/L for each pH drop of 0.1

Sodium and glucose:    [Na⁺] decreased 1.6 mEq/L per 100 mg/dl increase in glucose

Calcium and albumin:    [Ca⁺⁺] decreases 0.8 mg/dl for each 1.0 g/dl ↓ in albumin

# Pharmacology Equations

Elimination constant : $K_{el} = \ln \dfrac{[peak]}{[trough]} \div (Time_{peak} - Time_{trough})$

Clearance: $Cl = V_d \times K_{el}$

Half-life: $T_{1/2} = 0.693 \div K_{el} = 0.693 \times V_d \div Cl$

Loading dose $= V_d \times [target\ peak]$

Dosing interval $= \dfrac{1}{K_{el}} \times \dfrac{[desired\ peak]}{[desired\ trough]} + infusion\ time$

Ideal body weight (male) $=$ 50 kg + (2.3 kg per inch over 5 feet)

Ideal body weight (female) $=$ 45 kg + (2.3 kg per inch over 5 feet)

# Hemodynamic Equations

Blood pressure: $MAP = \dfrac{Systolic\ BP\ +\ (2\ \times\ Diastolic\ BP)}{3} = DBP + \dfrac{SBP - DBP}{3}$

Fick Cardiac Output :

$CO = \dfrac{O_2\ Consumption}{(Arterial - Venous)\ O_2\ Content} = \dfrac{10 \times V_{O2}(ml/min/m^2)}{Hb\ (gm/dL) \times 1.39 \times (Arterial\ O_2\ Sat\% - Venous\ O_2\ Sat\%)}$

Cardiac Index : $CI = \dfrac{CO}{BSA}$ (Normal 2.5 - 4.2L/min/m$^2$)

Stroke Volume : $SV = \dfrac{CO}{HR}$

Pulmonary vascular resistance (PVR) $= \dfrac{80 \times [Mean\ PA\ pressure\ -\ mean\ PCWP]}{Cardiac\ output\ (L/min)}$

Systemic vascular resistance (SVR) $= \dfrac{80 \times [MAP\ (mmHg)\ -\ RA\ pressure\ (mmHg)]}{Cardiac\ output\ (L/min)}$

Body surface area (BSA) in $m^2$ = height(cm)$^{0.718}$ × weight (kg)$^{0.43}$ × 74.5

$= \sqrt{height\ (cm) \times weight\ (kg) \div 3600}$

# Pulmonary Equations

Tidal Volume :
$$V_T = (V_{dead\ space} + V_{alveolar\ space}) = V_D + V_A$$

Minute Ventilation :
$$V_E = \frac{0.863 \times V_{CO_2(ml/min)}}{P_{aCO_2} \times (1 - \frac{V_D}{V_T})} \quad \text{(Normal 4 - 6 L/min)}$$

Bohr Dead Space :
$$\frac{V_D}{V_T} = \frac{P_{ACO_2} - P_{expired\ CO_2}}{P_{ACO_2}} \quad \text{(Normal 0.2 - 0.3)}$$

Physiologic Dead Space:
$$\frac{V_D}{V_T} = \frac{P_aCO_2 - P_{expired\ CO_2}}{P_aCO_2}$$

Static Compliance =
$$\frac{V_T}{P_{plateau} - P_{end\ expiration}} \quad \text{(Normal > 60 mL / cm H2O)}$$

LaPlace law of surface tension:
$$\text{Pressure} = \frac{2 \times \text{Tension}}{\text{Radius}}$$

Alveolar O2 estimate:
$$P_{AO_2} = FiO_2 \times [p\text{Atmospheric} - p\text{H}_2\text{O}] - \frac{pCO_2}{\text{Resp Quotient}}$$

$$= FiO_2 \times [760 - 47\ mm\ Hg] - \frac{pCO_2}{0.8}$$

Alveolar - arterial O2 gradient = $P_{AO_2} - P_{aO_2} \approx 2.5 + 0.21 \times$ Age (yrs) upright

PaO2 upright $\approx 104.2 - 0.27 \times$ Age (yrs)

PaO2 supine $\approx 103.5 - 0.42 \times$ Age (yrs)

PaCO2 $= K \times \dfrac{CO_2\ \text{Production}}{\text{Alveolar Ventilation}} = 0.863 \times \dfrac{V_{CO_2}}{V_A}$

Shunt Fraction :
$$\frac{Q_s}{Q_t} = \frac{(A - aDO_2)\ x\ 0.0031}{(A - aDO_2)\ x\ 0.0031 + C_aO_2 - C_vO_2}$$

$C_aO_2$ = Arterial $O_2$ content
$C_vO_2$ = Mixed venous $O_2$ content (from PA catheter)
$C_xO_2$ = [1.39 x Hb (g/dl) x ($O_2$sat %)] + [0.0031 x $P_xO_2$]
A-aDO2 = Alveolar - arterial oxygen difference (mmHg)

# Hemodynamic Values [3]

| Pressure Parameter | Normal (mmHg) |
|---|---|
| Right atrium (RA) | |
| mean | 0 – 8 |
| "a"-wave | 2 – 10 |
| "v"-wave | 2 – 10 |
| Right ventricle (RV) | |
| systolic | 15 – 30 |
| diastolic | 0 – 8 |
| Pulmonary artery (PA) | |
| systolic | 15 – 30 |
| diastolic | 3 – 12 |
| mean | 9 – 16 |
| PA wedge | |
| mean | 1 – 10 |
| "a"-wave | 3 – 15 |
| "v"-wave | 3 – 12 |

| Parameter | Normal Value |
|---|---|
| Cardiac output | 4.0 – 6.0 L/min |
| Cardiac index | 2.6 – 4.2 L/min/m$^2$ |
| Systemic vascular resistance (SVR) | 1130 ± 178 dyne/sec/cm$^{-5}$ |
| Pulmonary vascular resistance (PVR) | 67 ± 23 dyne/sec/cm$^{-5}$ |
| $O_2$ consumption | 110 – 150 mL/min/m$^2$ |
| Arterial-venous $O_2$ difference (AVDO$_2$) | 3.0 – 4.5 mL/dL |

# SI Lab Value Converter [4]

| Lab Value | US Unit | SI Unit | Factor* | Lab Value | US Unit | SI Unit | Factor* |
|---|---|---|---|---|---|---|---|
| **Chemistry** | | | | **Blood Gas** | | | |
| ALT, AST | U/L | μkat/L | 0.0167 | PaCO$_2$ | mmHg | kPa | 0.133 |
| Alk phos | U/L | μkat/L | 0.0167 | PaO$_2$ | mmHg | kPa | 0.133 |
| Amylase | U/L | nkat/L | 0.0167 | **Toxicology & Drug Monitoring** | | | |
| Bilirubin | mg/dl | μmol/L | 17.1 | Acetaminophen | mcg/ml | μmol/L | 6.62 |
| BUN | mg/dl | mmol/L | 0.357 | Amikacin | mcg/ml | μmol/L | 1.71 |
| Calcium | mg/dl | mmol/L | 0.25 | Carbamazepine | mcg/ml | μmol/L | 4.23 |
| Cholesterol | mg/dl | mmol/L | 0.0259 | Digoxin | ng/ml | nmol/L | 1.28 |
| Cortisol | mcg/dl | nmol/L | 27.6 | Gentamicin | mcg/ml | μmol/L | 2.09 |
| Cr Kinase | U/L | μkat/L | 0.0167 | Phenytoin | mcg/ml | μmol/L | 3.96 |
| Creatinine | mg/dl | μmol/L | 88.4 | Salicylate | mg/L | mmol/L | .00724 |
| Glucose | mg/dl | mmol/L | 0.0555 | Theophylline | mcg/ml | μmol/L | 5.55 |
| LDH | U/L | μkat/L | 0.0167 | Tobramycin | mcg/ml | μmol/L | 2.14 |
| Lipase | U/dl | μkat/L | 0.167 | Valproate | mcg/ml | μmol/L | 6.93 |
| Mg$^{++}$ | mEq/L | mmol/L | 0.5 | Vancomycin | mcg/ml | μmol/L | 0.690 |
| 5'-NT | U/L | μkat/L | 0.0167 | **Hematology** | | | |
| Phos | mg/dl | mmol/L | 0.322 | Folate | ng/ml | nmol/L | 2.27 |
| T$_4$ | mcg/dl | nmol/L | 12.9 | Hemoglobin | g/dl | mmol/L | 0.621 |
| T$_3$ | mcg/dl | nmol/L | 0.0154 | Iron, TIBC | mcg/dl | μmol/L | 0.179 |
| Uric acid | mg/dl | μmol/L | 59.5 | Vit B12 | pg/ml | pmol/L | 0.738 |

\* Factor to convert from standard to SI units

3  Lambert CR *et al.* Pressure measurement and determination of vascular resistance. In: *Diagnostic and Therapeutic Cardiac Catheterization*, 3$^{rd}$ ed. Pepine CJ (ed). Williams & Wilkins 1998, Baltimore.

4  *NEJM* 1998; 339(15):1063-1072

# Medical Statistics

|              | Disease Present | Disease Absent |
|--------------|-----------------|----------------|
| Test Positive | TP              | FP             |
| Test Negative | FN              | TN             |

**Prevalence** (prior probability) = (TP+FN)/(ALL) = All patients with dz / all pts
**Sensitivity** = TP / (TP + FN) = True positive / all diseased
**Specificity** = TN / (FP + TN) = True negative / all healthy
**False positive rate** = 1 - Specificity
**False negative rate** = 1 - Sensitivity
**Positive predictive value** = TP / (TP + FP) = True-positive / all positives
**Negative predictive value** = TN / (FN + TN) = True-negative / all negatives
**Accuracy** = (TP + TN) / (ALL) = True results / all patients
**Likelihood ratio** (pos. results) = Sensitivity ÷ (1 - Specificity)
**Likelihood ratio** (neg. results) = (1 - Sensitivity) ÷ Specificity
**Pre-test odds ratio** = Pre-test probability ÷ (1 - Pre-test probability)
**Post-test odds ratio** = Pre-test odds ratio x Likelihood ratio
**Post-test probability** = Post-test odds ratio ÷ (Post-test odds ratio + 1)

| Likelihood ratio | Change from Pre-test to Post-test Probability [5] |
|------------------|---------------------------------------------------|
| > 10 or < 0.1    | Large, often conclusive                           |
| 5-10 or 0.1-0.2  | Moderate                                          |
| 2-5 or 0.2-0.5   | Small; sometimes important                        |
| 0.5-2            | Rarely important                                  |

# Pediatric Vital Signs [6]

| Age | Awake HR | Asleep HR | Respiratory Rate | Systolic BP | Diastolic BP |
|-----|----------|-----------|------------------|-------------|--------------|
| Birth (12h,<1kg) |         |       |       | 39-59   | 16-36 |
| Birth (12h, 3kg) |         |       |       | 50-70   | 25-45 |
| Neonate (96hr)   | 100-180 | 80-60 |       | 60-90   | 20-60 |
| Infant 6mo       | 100-160 | 75-160 | 30-60 | 87-105 | 53-66 |
| Toddler 2yr      | 80-110  | 60-90 | 24-40 | 95-108 | 53-66 |
| Preschooler      | 70-110  | 60-90 | 22-34 | 96-110 | 55-69 |
| School-age child 7yr | 65-110 | 60-90 | 18-30 | 97-112 | 57-71 |
| Adolescent 15 yr | 60-90   | 50-90 | 12-16 | 112-128 | 66-80 |

---

5  Jaeschke R *et al*. User's guide to the medical literature III. How to use an article about a diagnostic test. B. What are the results and will they help me in caring for my patients? *JAMA* 1994; 271: 703-7.
6  ˚Cummins RO (ed). *Textbook of Advanced Cardiac Life Support*. Dallas: American Heart Association, 1994, page 1:65.

# Code Algorithms

## *Cardiac Arrest* [7]

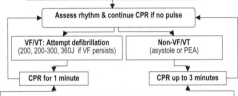

**Begin Primary ABCD Survey (BLS algorithm)**
- Check responsiveness
- Activate emergency response system
- Call for defibrillator
- Give 2 slow breaths if not breathing
- Start chest compressions if no **pulse**
- Attach monitor / defibrillator when available

**Assess rhythm & continue CPR if no pulse**

**VF/VT: Attempt defibrillation**
(200, 200-300, 360J  if VF persists)

**Non-VF/VT**
(asystole or PEA)

**CPR for 1 minute**

**CPR up to 3 minutes**

**Secondary ABCD Survey**
- **Airway**: attempt to place airway device
- **Breathing**: confirm and secure airway device, ventilation, O2
- **Circulation**: IV access; adrenergic agent; consider antiarrhythmics, bicarbonate, and pacing as appropriate

- **Vasopressin*** 40 IU IVP × 1-2 q 3 min , **followed by**
- **Epinephrine** 1 mg IV q 3-5 min. Use initially or if no response after vasopressin. May give via ETT at 2-2.5 × usual dose.

**Non-VF/VT patients:**
- **D**ifferential **D**iagnosis: search for and treat reversible causes

- **H**ypovolemia (volume infusion)
- **H**ypoxia (oxygen, ventilation)
- **H**+ - acidosis ($HCO_3$, ventilation)
- **H**yperkalemia (CaCl, *etc*)
- **H**ypothermia
- "**T**ablets" (drug OD, accidents)
- **T**amponade
- **T**ension pneumothorax
- **T**hrombosis, coronary
- **T**hrombosis, pulmonary

* This differs from AHA recommendations based on new data regarding vasopressin [8]

7  Cummins RO (ed). ACLS: Principles and Practice. American Heart Association, 2003; Guidelines 2000 for cardiopulmonary resuscitation and emergency cardiovascular care. *Circulation* 2000; 102(Suppl I).

8  Wenzel V *et al*. A comparison of vasopressin and epinephrine for out-of-hospital cardiopulmonary resuscitation. *NEJM* 2004; 350:105-13; McIntyre KM. *NEJM* 2004; 350:179-181.

# *Ventricular Fibrillation & Pulseless VT* [9]

**Primary ABCD Survey:** Basic CPR and defibrillation
- Check responsiveness
- Activate emergency response system
- Call for defibrillator
Airway: open the airway
Breathing: provide positive-pressure ventilation
Circulation: chest compressions
Defibrillation: assess for and shock VF & pulseless VT, up to 3 times (200J, 200-300J, 360J, or equivalent *biphasic*) if necessary

↓

**Persistent or recurrent VF/VT**

↓

**Secondary ABCD Survey:** more advanced assessment & treatment
Airway: place airway device as soon as possible
Breathing: confirm airway device placement by exam & confirmatory test
Breathing: secure airway device; purpose-made tube holders preferred
Breathing: confirm effective oxygenation and ventilation
Circulation: IV access
Circulation: identify rhythm → monitor
Circulation: administer drugs appropriate for rhythm and condition
Differential diagnosis: search for and treat identified reversible causes

↓

- **Vasopressin** 40 IU IVP × 1-2 q 3 min , followed by     *a*
- **Epinephrine** 1mg IV push (or 2-2.5 mg via ETT), q 3-5 minutes

↓

**Resume attempts to defibrillate**
1 × 360 J (or equivalent *biphasic*) within 30-60 seconds

↓

**Consider antiarrhythmics:**     *b*
- *Amiodarone* (IIb) 300mg IVP (may give repeat doses of 150 mg IVP)
- *Lidocaine* (recommendation indeterminate) 1-1.5 mg/kg IVP or 2-4 mg/kg via ETT (may repeat 0.5-0.75 mg/kg bolus q 3-5 min to max 3 mg/kg)
- *Magnesium* (IIb if hypomagnesemic & polymorphic VT) 1-2g IV
- *Procainamide* (IIb) for intermittent/recurrent VF) 20-50 mg/min to total 17 mg/kg
- Consider *bicarbonate*

↓

**Resume attempts to defibrillate**
360J after each med or each minute of CPR

*a:* Vasopressin before epinephrine is not yet an AHA recommendation.[10]
*b:* Levels of evidence: Class I – Interventions always acceptable, proven safe, and definitely useful. Class IIa – acceptable, safe and useful; standard of care or intervention of choice; IIb – acceptable, safe and useful; within standard of care, but considered optional or alternative intervention; Class III – not useful, potentially harmful.

---

9   Cummins RO (ed.), ACLS: Principles and Practice, American Heart Association, 2003; Guidelines 2000 for cardiopulmonary resuscitation and emergency cardiovascular care. *Circulation* 2000; 102(Suppl I)

10   Wenzel V *et al*. A comparison of vasopressin and epinephrine for out-of-hospital cardiopulmonary resuscitation. *NEJM* 2004; 350:105-13; McIntyre KM. *NEJM* 2004; 350:179-181.

# Pulseless Electrical Activity [11]
### (Rhythm on ECG monitor without detectable pulse)

---

**Primary ABCD Survey:** basic CPR and defibrillation
- Check responsiveness
- Activate emergency response system
- Call for defibrillator

Airway: open the airway
Breathing: provide positive-pressure ventilation
Circulation: give chest compression
Defibrillation: assess for VF & pulseless VT; shock if indicated

---

**Secondary ABCD Survey:** more advanced assessment and treatment
Airway: place airway device as soon as possible
Breathing: confirm airway device placement by exam & confirmatory test
Breathing: secure airway device; purpose-made tube holders preferred
Breathing: confirm effective oxygenation and ventilation
Circulation: establish IV access
Circulation: identify rhythm → monitor
Circulation: administer drugs appropriate for rhythm and condition
Circulation: assess for occult blood flow ("pseudo-PEA")
Differential diagnosis: search for and treat identified reversible causes

---

### Review for most frequent causes     *a*

- Hypovolemia (volume infusion)
- Hypoxia (oxygen, ventilation)
- $H^+$ - acidosis ($HCO_3$, ventilation)
- Hyperkalemia ($CaCl$, *etc*)
- Hypothermia
- "Tablets" (drug OD, accidents)
- Tamponade
- Tension pneumothorax
- Thrombosis, coronary
- Thromboembolism, pulmonary

---

**Vasopressin** 40 IU IVP × 1-2 q 3 min, **followed by**
**Epinephrine** 1mg IVP, repeat every 3 to 5 minutes    *b,c*

---

**Atropine** 1mg IV push (if PEA rate is **slow**), repeat every 3 to 5
minutes as needed, to a total dose of 0.04 mg/kg

---

*a:* **Sodium bicarbonate** 1 mEq/kg indications: Class I: preexisting hyperkalemia; Class
IIa: known preexisting bicarbonate-responsive acidosis; tricyclic antidepressant
overdose; to alkalinize urine in salicylate or other drug overdose. Class IIb: in
intubated and ventilated patients with long arrest interval; on return of circulation after
long arrest interval. Class III (may be harmful) in hypercarbic acidosis.

*b:* **Vasopressin** before epinephrine is not yet an AHA recommendation [12]

*c:* **Epinephrine** 1mg IVP q 3-5 minutes (recommendation indeterminate). If this
approach fails, higher doses up to 0.2 mg/kg may be used but are not recommended.
Evidence does not yet support routine use of vasopressin in PEA or asystole.

---

11 Cummins RO (ed.), ACLS: Principles and Practice, American Heart Association, 2003; Guidelines 2000
for cardiopulmonary resuscitation and emergency cardiovascular care. *Circulation*, 2000; 102(Suppl I).

12 Wenzel V *et al*. *NEJM* 2004; 350:105-13; McIntyre KM. *NEJM* 2004; 350:179-181.

# Asystole [13]

---

**Primary ABCD Survey:** basic CPR and defibrillation   **a**
- Check responsiveness  • Activate emergency response system
- Call for defibrillator

Airway: open the airway
Breathing: provide positive-pressure ventilation
Circulation: give chest compression  **Confirm:** true asystole
Defibrillation: assess for VF & pulseless VT; shock if indicated
**Rapid scene survey:** any evidence team should **not** attempt resuscitation?

---

**Secondary ABCD Survey:** more advanced assessment and rx
**Airway:** place airway device as soon as possible
**Breathing:** confirm airway device placement by exam & confirmatory test
**Breathing:** secure airway device; purpose-made tube holders preferred
**Breathing:** confirm effective oxygenation and ventilation
**Confirm asystole:** check lead & cable connections; monitor power on?
  monitor gain up? Verify asystole in another ECG lead.
**Circulation:** establish IV access
**Circulation:** identify rhythm → monitor
**Circulation:** administer drugs appropriate for rhythm and condition   **b**
**Differential diagnosis:** search for and treat identified reversible causes

---

| **Transcutaneous pacing** | **c** | **Vasopressin** 40 IU IVP × 1-2 q 3 min |
| Immediately if considered | | **Epinephrine** 1 mg IVP (2-2.5 mg via |
| | | ETT), q 3-5 minutes   **d, e** |

---

**Atropine** 1 mg IV (or 2-2.5 mg via ETT)
Repeat every 3 to 5 minutes up to 0.04 mg/kg total

---

**If asystole persists consider terminating resuscitation effort**
- Consider quality of resuscitation effort.  • Atypical clinical features absent?
  Not a victim of **drowning** or **hypothermia**?  No reversible therapeutic or
  illicit **drug OD**?  • Support for cease-efforts protocols in place?

---

**a:**  Assess clinical indicators that resuscitation not indicated, i.e. signs of death.
**b:**  **Sodium bicarbonate** 1mEq/kg indicated for tricyclic overdose, urine alkalinization in
  overdose, tracheal intubation plus long arrest intervals, or upon return of circulation if
  there is a long arrest interval. Ineffective or harmful in hypercarbic acidosis.
**c:**  **Pacing** must be early, combined with drug treatment. Not routinely indicated for
  asystole.
**d:**  **Vasopressin** initial therapy based on post-hoc evidence of improved survival to
  admission, both as primary therapy and when used before epinephrine. [14]
**e:**  **Epinephrine** 1mg IVP q 3-5 min. If this fails, higher doses (up to 0.2 mg/kg) may be
  used but not recommended.  Possibly better outcomes when used after vasopressin.[14]

---

13 Cummins RO (ed.), ACLS: Principles and Practice, American Heart Association, 2003; Guidelines 2000
  for cardiopulmonary resuscitation and emergency cardiovascular care. *Circulation*, 2000; 102(Suppl I).
14 Wenzel V *et al*. A comparison of vasopressin and epinephrine for out-of-hospital cardiopulmonary
  resuscitation. *NEJM* 2004; 350:105-13; McIntyre KM. *NEJM* 2004; 350:179-181.

# *Bradycardia* [15]

- **Absolute bradycardia** (heart rate < 60 bpm)
- **Relative bradycardia** (rate inappropriate to underlying condition, e.g. hypotension)

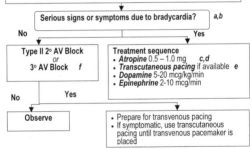

**Primary ABCD Survey**
- Assess ABCs
- Secure airway noninvasively
- Ensure monitor / defibrillator is available

**Secondary ABCD Survey**
- Assess secondary ABCs (invasive airway management if needed?)
- Oxygen — IV access — monitor — fluids
- Vital signs, pulse oximeter, monitor BP
- Obtain and review 12-lead ECG
- Obtain and review portable chest x-ray
- Problem-focused history & physical examination
- Consider differential diagnosis

**Serious signs or symptoms due to bradycardia?**   *a,b*

**No**                           **Yes**

**Type II 2° AV Block** *or* **3° AV Block**   *f*

**Treatment sequence**
- *Atropine* 0.5 – 1.0 mg   *c,d*
- *Transcutaneous pacing* if available   *e*
- *Dopamine* 5-20 mcg/kg/min
- *Epinephrine* 2-10 mcg/min

**No**       **Yes**

**Observe**

- Prepare for transvenous pacing
- If symptomatic, use transcutaneous pacing until transvenous pacemaker is placed

*a:* If the patient has serious signs or symptoms make sure they are attributable to bradycardia.

*b:* **Symptoms:** chest pain, shortness of breath, decreased level of consciousness
**Signs:** low blood pressure, shock, pulmonary congestion, congestive heart failure

*c:* Denervated **transplanted hearts** will not respond to atropine.

*d:* **Atropine** should be given in repeat doses every 3 to 5 minutes up to a total of 0.03 to 0.04 mg/kg. Use a shorter dosing interval (q 3 min) in severe clinical situations.

*e:* If the patient is symptomatic, do not delay **transcutaneous pacing** while awaiting IV access or for atropine to take effect.

*f:* Never treat the combination of **3° heart block** and ventricular escape beats with lidocaine (or any agent that suppresses ventricular escape rhythms).

*g:* Verify **mechanical capture** and patient tolerance. Use analgesia and sedation prn.

15   Cummins RO (ed.), ACLS: Principles and Practice, American Heart Association, 2003; Guidelines 2000 for cardiopulmonary resuscitation and emergency cardiovascular care. *Circulation*, 2000; 102(Suppl I).

# Tachycardia [16]

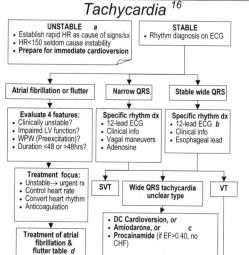

a: **Cardioversion**:
- O2 sat monitor, suction, IV access, intubation equipment
- Pre-medicate when possible (with benzodiazepine or barbiturate ± narcotic)
- Synchronized shocks in following sequence: 100, 200-300, 360J or equivalent biphasic

b: See section on Wide-complex Tachycardia, page 28.

c: Give **amiodarone** (150 mg IV over 10 minutes, then 1 mg/min x 6 hr, then 0.5 mg/min) or **procainamide** (20 mg/min to total 17 mg/kg, or development of hypotension or QRS widening).

d: See table, page 20

16  Cummins RO (ed.), ACLS: Principles and Practice, American Heart Association, 2003; Guidelines 2000 for cardiopulmonary resuscitation and emergency cardiovascular care. *Circulation* 2000; 102(Suppl I).

# Stable Ventricular Tachycardia [17]

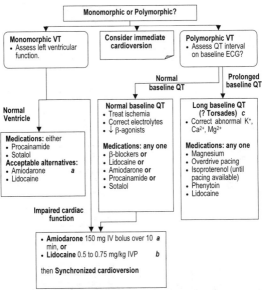

a: **Amiodarone** dosing: 150 mg IV bolus over 10 minutes. Repeat 150 mg IV every 10-15 minutes prn. Alternative infusion 360 mg over 6 hours (1 mg/min) then 540 mg over 18 hours (0.5 mg/min). Maximum total dose 2.2g in 24 hours including all resuscitation doses.

b: **Lidocaine** dosing in impaired cardiac function: 0.5-0.75mg/kg IV push. Repeat q 5-10 min then infuse 1-4 mg/min. Maximum total dose 3mg/kg over one hour.

c: If rhythm suggests *torsades de pointes*: stop/avoid all treatments that prolong QT. Identify and treat abnormal electrolytes.

17 Cummins RO (ed.), ACLS: Principles and Practice, American Heart Association, 2003; Guidelines 2000 for cardiopulmonary resuscitation and emergency cardiovascular care. *Circulation* 2000; 102(Suppl I).

# Atrial Fibrillation/Flutter [18]

| Scenario | Rate Control | Conversion to Sinus Rhythm |
|---|---|---|
| **Normal cardiac function** | *Use one of the following:* <br> • Ca-channel blockers (diltiazem or verapamil) <br> • β-blockers | **If duration < 48 hr, consider:** <br> • DC cardioversion <br> • Use only one of the following: <br>   • Amiodarone <br>   • Ibutilide <br>   • Others [19] |
| **Impaired heart (EF<40% or CHF)** | *Use one of the following:* <br> • Digoxin <br> • Diltiazem <br> • Amiodarone | **If duration > 48 hr or unknown:** <br> • **No DC cardioversion** <br> (conversion of AF to NSR may cause systemic embolism; risk reduced by ≥ 3 wks anticoagulation). <br><br> **Treatment options:** <br> • Use antiarrhythmic agent with extreme caution *or* <br> • **Delayed cardioversion:** therapeutic anticoagulation ≥ 3 weeks, then cardioversion, then additional 4 weeks anti-coagulation *or* <br> • **Early cardioversion:** IV heparin at once, TEE to exclude thrombi, then cardioversion within 24 hr; follow with 4 weeks additional anticoagulation |
| **Wolff-Parkinson-White Syndrome (Pre-excitation)** | **Do not attempt rate control** – following agents harmful (Class III): <br> • Adenosine <br> • β-blockers <br> • Ca-channel blockers <br> • Digoxin <br><br> If unstable hemodynamics or duration < 48 hr move directly to cardioversion | **If duration < 48 hr, consider:** <br> • DC cardioversion *or* <br> • Primary anti-arrhythmic treatment with only one of the following: <br>   • Amiodarone <br>   • Others (see footnote below) <br><br> **If duration > 48 hr or unknown:** <br> • Anticoagulate, then follow delayed or early cardioversion protocol as per above |

---

[18] Cummins RO (ed.), ACLS: Principles and Practice, American Heart Association, 2003; Guidelines 2000 for cardiopulmonary resuscitation and emergency cardiovascular care. Circulation 2000; 102(Supl 1).

[19] AHA guidelines include flecainide, propafenone, and procainamide. The authors recommend these agents be used with caution (if at all), and only by experienced practitioners.

# Cardiology

## *Hemodynamics — Cardiac Cycle* [20]

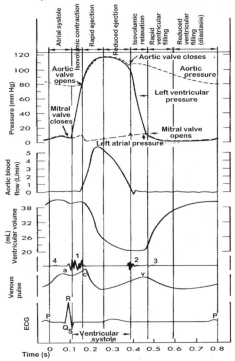

# *Coronary Artery Anatomy* [21]

### LEFT CORONARY ARTERY

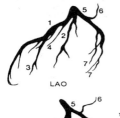

LAO

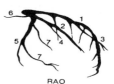

RAO

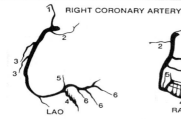

LAO-CRANIAL ANGULATION

1. LEFT ANTERIOR DESCENDING ARTERY
   WITH SEPTAL BRANCHES
2. RAMUS MEDIANUS
3. DIAGONAL ARTERY
4. FIRST SEPTAL BRANCH
5. LEFT CIRCUMFLEX ARTERY
6. LEFT ATRIAL CIRCUMFLEX ARTERY
7. OBTUSE MARGINAL ARTERY

### RIGHT CORONARY ARTERY

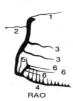

LAO                          RAO

1. CONUS ARTERY
2. S-A NODE ARTERY
3. ACUTE MARGINAL ARTERY
4. POSTERIOR DESCENDING ARTERY WITH SEPTAL BRANCHES
5. A-V NODE ARTERY
6. POSTERIOR LEFT VENTRICULAR ARTERY

[21] Reproduced with permission from Grossman WG. *Cardiac Cathoterization and Angiography*, 4th ed. Philadelphia: Lea and Febiger, 1991.

# *Echo/MRI/Nuclear Anatomy* [22]

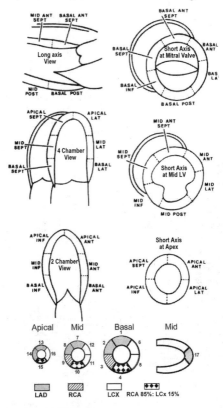

[22] Adapted with permission from Cerqueira MD et al. Standardized myocardial segmentation and nomenclature for tomographic imaging of the heart. *Circulation* 2002; 105:539-42.

# Jugular Venous Pulsations [23]

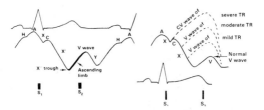

# Systolic Murmurs [24]

| Maneuver | Response | Sensitivity (%) | Specificity (%) | Positive Predictive Value (%) | Negative Predictive Value (%) |
|---|---|---|---|---|---|
| **Right-sided murmurs** | | | | | |
| Inspiration | Increase | 100 | 88 | 67 | 100 |
| Expiration | Decrease | 100 | 88 | 67 | 100 |
| Müller maneuver | Increase | 15 | 92 | 33 | 81 |
| **Hypertrophic cardiomyopathy** | | | | | |
| Valsalva | Increase | 65 | 96 | 81 | 92 |
| Squatting to Standing | Increase | 95 | 84 | 59 | 98 |
| Standing to Squatting | Decrease | 95 | 85 | 61 | 99 |
| Leg elevation | Decrease | 85 | 91 | 71 | 96 |
| Handgrip | Decrease | 85 | 75 | 46 | 95 |
| **Mitral regurgitation & ventricular septal defect** | | | | | |
| Handgrip | Increase | 68 | 92 | 84 | 81 |
| Transient arterial occlusion | Increase | 78 | 100 | 100 | 87 |
| Amyl nitrite inhalation | Decrease | 80 | 90 | 84 | 87 |

- Aortic stenosis diagnosed by exclusion
- Inspiration and Expiration: Patient breathes following listener's arm signal
- Müller maneuver: Occlude nares; Suck manometer (-)40-50 mmHg × 10 sec
- Valsalva: Exhale into manometer +40 mmHg × 20 sec. Listen at end of strain phase.
- Squatting to standing: Squat 30 sec then rapidly stand. Listen first 15-20 sec standing.
- Standing to squatting: Avoid Valsalva. Listen immediately after squatting.
- Passive leg elevation: Patient supine, elevate 45 degrees. Listen 15-20 sec later.
- Isometric handgrip: Hand dynamometer, listen after one minute max contraction.
- Transient arterial occlusion: Sphygmomanometer cuffs on both arms inflated 20-40 mm above systolic. Listen 20 sec later.
- Amyl nitrite: 0.3ml ampule broken, 3 rapid deep breaths. Listen 15-30 sec later.

23   Reproduced with permission from Constant J. Bedside Cardiology, 3rd ed. Boston: Little, Brown, 1985; pp. 95, 105.

24   Lembo N et al. Bedside diagnosis of systolic murmurs. NEJM 1988; 318:1572-8. Adapted with permission of The New England Journal of Medicine, copyright 1988, Massachusetts Medical Society.

## Selected characteristics of common systolic heart murmurs[25]

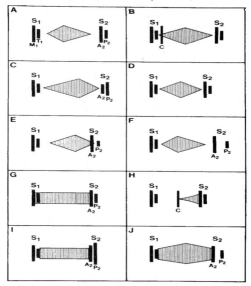

A: **Systolic ejection murmur**. Note early peaking.

B: **Mild aortic stenosis**. Note relatively early peaking and systolic ejection click.

C: **Severe aortic stenosis**. Note late peaking and decreased intensity of $A_2$.

D: **Hypertrophic cardiomyopathy**

E: **Severe pulmonary valvular stenosis**. Note late peaking with murmur extending through $A_2$ and delayed appearance of $P_2$.

F: **Atrial septal defect**. Note wide splitting of $S_2$.

G: **Uncomplicated mitral regurgitation**. Note holosystolic murmur through $A_2$.

H: **Mitral valve prolapse**. Note late systolic murmur ushered in by midsystolic click.

I: **Tricuspid regurgitation** due to pulmonary hypertension. Note holosystolic murmur beginning with $S_1$ and early, loud $P_2$.

J: **Uncomplicated ventricular septal defect**. Note loud, holosystolic murmur with midsystolic accentuation and slightly delayed $P_2$.

25 Alpert MA. Systolic murmurs. In: *Clinical Methods*. HK Walker(ed). Boston: Butterworth-Heineman, 1991. Adapted with permission.

# ECG: Hypertrophy [26]

## Left Ventricular Hypertrophy
- **Romhilt-Estes criteria:**

| | | |
|---|---|---|
| Limb lead R or S amplitude > 2.0mV or S in $V_1$ or $V_2$ > 3.0mV or R in $V_5$ or $V_6$ > 3.0mV | 3 points | **Total Points:** |
| ST segment abnormality: Without digitalis | 2 points | 4 : LVH likely |
| With digitalis | 1 point | 5 : LVH present |
| Left atrial enlargement | 3 points | |
| Left axis deviation > -30° | 2 points | Sensitivity 40-50% |
| QRS duration > 0.09s | 1 point | Specificity 80-90% |
| Intrinsicoid deflection $V_5$ and $V_6$ > 0.05s | 1 point | |

- **Cornell criteria:** [27] R ($aV_L$) + S ($V_3$) ≥ 2.8 mV (men), ≥ 2.0 mV (women)
  Sensitivity 42%, specificity 96%
- **Other:** R in $aV_L$ > 1.1 mV (97% specific)

## Right ventricular hypertrophy (any of the following)
- Right axis deviation > 90° without anterior/inferior MI, left posterior fascicle block, or RBBB (99% specific)
- R > S in $V_1$ **and** R in $V_1$ > 0.5 mV (90% specific; highest sensitivity at 44%)
- S in $V_5$ or $V_6$ ≥ 0.7 mV (95% spec)
- S1Q3 pattern (93% specific)
- P-pulmonale (97% specific)

**Note:** Sensitivity and specificity generally higher in absence of LVH

## Causes of dominant R in V1 and V2 [28]
- Normal variant • RVH • Posterior or lateral infarction • WPW • LV diastolic overload
- Hypertrophic cardiomyopathy • Duchenne's muscular dystrophy

# ECG: BBB, Fascicle Block & IWMI [29]

## Left bundle branch block
- QRS > 120 msec
- Absent septal Q (abnormal septal activation R → L)
- Slurred R wave leads I & $V_6$ (slow R → L activation)
- Notched R in I and $V_6$ (prominent delay late in QRS)
- Unpredictable A-P, inferosuperior activation patterns:
  - frontal axis may be normal or leftward
  - right-precordial R waves may be present or absent
- Absent Q waves in LBBB obscure myocardial scar
- ST- and T-wave vector opposite to QRS vector
- **Incomplete LBBB** • QRS 100-120 msec • loss of septal Q wave • slurred/notched QRS in I and $V_6$

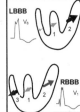

26  Romhilt *et al.* A critical appraisal of the ECG criteria for the diagnosis of left ventricular hypertrophy. *Circulation* 1969;40:185.

27  Casale PN *et al.* Improved sex-specific criteria of left ventricular hypertrophy for clinical and computer interpretation of electrocardiograms: Validation with autopsy findings. *Circulation* 1987; 75:565-72.

28  Marriot HJL. *Practical Electrocardiography*, 8th ed. Baltimore: Williams & Wilkins; 1988.

29  Warner RA. Recent advances in the diagnosis of myocardial infarction. *Cardiology Clinics* 1987;5:381; Warner RA *et al.* Improved ECG criteria for the diagnosis of left anterior hemiblock. *Am J Cardiol* 1983; 51:723.

## LBBB and acute MI [30]

- ST-segment elevation ≥ 1 mm **concordant** with QRS complex – highly sensitive and specific for acute MI under appropriate clinical circumstances (e.g. chest pain)
- ST-segment depression ≥ 1 mm in lead $V_1$, $V_2$ or $V_3$ – highly specific but less sensitive (36-78%) for MI
- ST-segment elevation ≥ 5 mm **discordant** with QRS complex – suggestive of MI but confirmatory data needed

## Right bundle branch block

- QRS > 120 msec
- Normal septal activation
- Terminal portion of QRS vector rightward and anterior
  - $V_1$: initial R from normal septal activation; subsequent S from LV activation; terminal R' from delayed RV activation
  - I, $V_5$, $V_6$: initial Q from normal septal activation, R from normal LV activation, prolonged shallow S wave from delayed RV activation
- T wave vector opposite the **terminal** portion of QRS
- Early activation intact (including Q wave of myocardial scar)
- **Incomplete RBBB**: • QRS 100-120 msec • morphology criteria of RBBB (RsR' pattern) in $V_1$, prolonged shallow S wave in lateral leads)

## Left anterior fascicular block (LAFB)

- Vectorcardiogram: frontal plane forces counterclockwise, initially inferior and terminally superior; therefore $_aV_L$ peaks before $_aV_R$
- ECG: **(1)** QRS complexes in $_aV_R$ and $_aV_L$ each end in an R wave **and (2)** peak of the terminal R wave in $_aV_R$ occurs later than the peak of terminal R wave in $_aV_L$
- Scalar criteria: • QRS axis -45⁰ to -90⁰ • QRS<120 msec • small Q in lead I • small R in II, III, $_aV_F$ • late intrinsicoid deflection in $_aV_L$ (>45 msec)

## Left posterior fascicular block (LPFB)

- Vectorcardiogram: QR complex in II, III, $_aV_F$ from initial superior and final inferior force
- Scalar criteria: • QRS axis > +90⁰ • initial R in I, $_aV_L$+ small Q in II, III, $_aV_F$ • QRS < 120 msec • late intrinsicoid deflection in $_aV_F$ (>45 msec) • Absence of pulmonary disease, vertical heart position, RVH, W-P-W

## Inferior wall MI (sensitivity & specificity > 90%)

- Vectorcardiogram: initial frontal forces clockwise and superior
- Clockwise rotation of frontal plane (lead II peaks before lead III) **and**
- Q waves > 30 msec in lead II **or** regression of initial inferior forces from lead III to lead II (initial portion of QRS is more negative in lead II than in lead III)
- Right coronary culprit: ST elevation lead III > lead II & ST depression in lead I and lead $_aV_L$
- Left circumflex culprit: ST elevation lead II > lead III & isoelectric or elevated ST in lead $_aV_L$

## Inferior wall MI + left anterior fascicular block (requires both)

- $_aV_R$ and $_aV_L$ both end in R waves; terminal R of $_aV_L$ before $_aV_R$; **and**
- Q of any magnitude in lead II
- VCG: initial superior and clockwise; terminal superior and counterclockwise

---

30 Sgarbossa E *et al.* Electrocardiographic diagnosis of evolving acute myocardial infarction in the presence of left bundle branch block. *NEJM* 1996; 334: 481-7; Zimetbaum P, Josephson M. Use of the electrocardiogram in acute myocardial infarction. *NEJM* 2003;348:933-40.

# ECG: Wide-Complex Tachycardia

**Inexact features suggestive of ventricular tachycardia (VT)**
- Extreme left axis deviation
- QRS duration > 140 msec (RBBB morphology) or >160 msec (LBBB morph)
- "Capture" (narrow complex) and "fusion" (hybrid narrow-wide complex) beats
- Net area under QRS negative both in leads I and II

**Brugada criteria** (99% sensitive, 97% specific) [31]
- Rhythm is **ventricular tachycardia** if **any** of the following is present (in stepwise fashion):
  1) RS absent in **all** precordial leads (may include QS, QR, monophasic R)
  2) R-S interval > 100 msec (onset of R to nadir of S)
     in **any** precordial leads
  3) Evidence of atrioventricular (A-V) dissociation
  4) Morphology criteria for VT in **both** leads V1-2 and V6:
     - RBBB - like QRS (predominantly positive in V1)

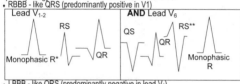

Other classic morphologies typical of VT not listed by Brugada are:
  \*    RBBB: RSR' with R>R'   \*\* RBBB: R/S<1 more suggestive of VT than R/S>1
  \*\*\* LBBB: QS in V1-2
- If **all** of above criteria are absent, 99% likelihood that rhythm is **supraventricular**

## Pearls and Nonsense
- In patients with **structural heart disease** and reduced LV systolic function, a wide complex tachycardia is VT in 95% of cases
- Clinical appearance (i.e. whether patient is symptomatic or hemodynamically stable) is poor predictor of ventricular vs. supraventricular tachycardia
- If there is uncertainty about whether an arrhythmia is VT or SVT and patient does not require immediate electrical cardioversion, IV amiodarone or procainamide are the drugs of choice to terminate arrhythmia. **Avoid verapamil and diltiazem.** Adenosine may be tried, but **(1)** response may not reliably determine VT vs. SVT and **(2)** there is a small (1%) but definite risk of ventricular fibrillation (VF).

---

[31] Brugada et al. A new approach to the differential diagnosis of a regular tachycardia with a wide QRS complex. *Circulation* 1991;83:1649-1659. **Note:** these patients were not taking antiarrhythmic drugs. Diagrams adapted with permission from Tom Evans, MD.

# Torsades & Long QT syndromes[32]

## Acquired
**Pathophysiology**: Usually "pause-dependent," i.e. triggered by long→ short R-R intervals, e.g. PVC followed by compensatory pause, or frequent sinus pauses

**Etiology**:
- **Bradyarrhythmias**: Severe bradycardia . Sinus node dysfunction . A-V block
- **Metabolic**: Hypokalemia . Hypomagnesemia . Hypocalcemia
- **Nutrition**: Starvation . Anorexia nervosa . Liquid protein diet
- **Drugs**: [33]  Effect often dose dependent . Toxicity may be triggered by drug interactions, e.g. erythromycin

| Drugs associated with Torsades de Pointes | |
|---|---|
| Antiarrhythmics (not Ic) | Class IA: disopyramide, procainamide, quinidine<br>Class III: amiodarone, bretylium, dofetilide, ibutilide, sotalol |
| Anti-infectives | amantadine, chloroquine, fluoroquinolones (gati/levo/moxifloxacin), foscarnet, macrolides (erythro/clarithro/azithromycin), pentamidine, voriconazole |
| GI/Antiemetics | cisapride, dolasetron, droperidol, granisetron, octreotide, ondansetron |
| Psychiatric | chloral hydrate, chlorpromazine, haloperidol, lithium, mesoridazine, quetiapine, risperidone, thioridazine, venlafaxine, ziprasidone |
| Other | alfuzosin, arsenic trioxide, cocaine, indapamide, felbamate, fosphenytoin, methadone (high dose), nicardipine, organophosphates, salmeterol, tacrolimus, tamoxifen, tizanidine, vardenafil |

- **Other**: . subarachnoid hemorrhage, stroke or head trauma . autonomic manipulation from surgery (vagotomy, carotid endarterectomy)

**Treatment**:
- Discontinue offending drug
- Magnesium sulfate 1-2 gm IV push
- Correct electrolyte disorder; consider empiric K+ supplementation
- Cardiac pacing or isoproterenol infusion to maintain HR > 80 bpm
- Class IB antiarrhythmics (lidocaine or phenytoin)

## Inherited/Congenital [34]
**Pathophysiology**: Defective repolarization currents, often silent until trigger (above). Usually "catecholamine-dependent," i.e. episodes follow adrenergic surge; may also be "pause-dependent"

**Etiology**: May be sporadic or inherited syndrome e.g. Jervell-Lange-Nielsen (autosomal-recessive with congenital deafness) or Romano-Ward (autosomal-dominant without deafness).

**Treatment (chronic)**: . β-adrenergic blockade . ICD . pacing . sympathectomy

---

[32] el-Sherif N et al. Torsade de pointes. Curr Opin Cardiol 2003; 18(1):6-13 ; Al-Khatib S et al. What clinicians should know about the QT interval. JAMA 2003; 289:2120-2127.

[33] Roden DM. Drug-induced prolongation of the QT interval. NEJM 2004; 350:1013-1022. See database at www.torsades.org.

[34] Moss A. Long QT Syndrome. JAMA 2003;289:2041-2044.

# Brugada Syndrome[35]

## Description and epidemiology

- Syndrome of sudden death or ventricular tachycardia or fibrillation with abnormal EKG (RBBB pattern with ST- elevation in $V_1$-$V_3$), normal $QT_c$ and no evidence of structural heart disease
- May account for 40-60% of "idiopathic" VT/VF (although < 5% of total sudden deaths in U.S.)
- High incidence in S.E. Asia (leading cause of death in young men in Thailand)
- Pathophysiology: Abnormal repolarization via mutations in $Na^+$ channel

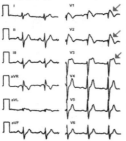

### ECG features

- RBBB pattern, although widened S-wave in left lateral leads often absent
- Left axis deviation often present
- ST segment characteristically elevated ≥ 0.1 mV in $V_1$-$V_3$, although ST elevation variable in individuals patients and transient normalization common
- ST segment elevation provoked by procainamide or flecainide
- ECG mimicked by tricyclic overdose [36]

## Clinical features

- 10:1 male-female ratio
- Most patients Asian
- Age at first arrhythmic event 22-65, peak in 4th decade
- Family history of sudden death, syncope or documented VT/VF in only 20%
- Events often occur in sleep; may be provoked by alcohol

## Additional testing

- Echo, ETT, MRI and endomyocardial biopsies typically normal
- EP study: prolonged His-ventricular (H-V) interval (95%), inducible VF (66%) or VT (11%)

## Treatment

- ICD only documented effective therapy
- Antiarrhythmics including β-blockers and amiodarone do **not** prevent sudden death

---

35  Brugada J, Brugada R, Brugada P.  Right bundle-branch block and ST-segment elevation in leads V1-V3: A marker for sudden death in patients without demonstrable structural heart disease. *Circulation* 1998; 97:457-60. Alings M, Wilde A.  "Brugada" syndrome. *Circulation* 1999;99:666-73. Website: http://www.brugada.org.

36  Goldgran-Toledano D. Overdose of cyclic antidepressants & Brugada syndrome. *NEJM* 2002;346:1591.

# Syncope[37]

## Risk of Death
Increases with number of risk factors: • Heart disease • Abnormal ECG • Ventricular arrhythmia • Age > 45

## Etiology [38]

| Cause | Frequency |
|---|---|
| Cardiovascular | 18% (5–46) |
| Structural heart disease (MI, valve disease, pulmonary embolism) | 4% (1–8) |
| Arrhythmia: brady or tachycardia | 14% (4–38) |
| **Neurally-mediated** | 24% (10–56) |
| Neurocardiogenic (vasovagal) | 18% (8–37) |
| Situational | 5% (1–8) |
| Carotid sinus | 1% (0–4) |
| **Psychiatric disorders** | 2% (1–7) |
| **Postural hypotension:** includes drugs & autonomic failure | 11% (1–17) |
| **Neurologic disease** | 10% (3–32) |
| **No diagnosis** | 24% (13–41) |

### Pearls & Nonsense
- In syncope with underlying structural heart disease, VT or myocardial ischemia should be excluded before attributing symptoms to bradycardia
- Convulsions, loss of consciousness, trauma do not help identify etiology
- Carotid TIAs rarely

## Syncope vs. Seizure

| Feature | Favors Syncope | Favors Seizure |
|---|---|---|
| Precipitant or prodrome | Pain, emotional stress, micturition, defecation; diaphoresis, nausea | Aura |
| Duration of unconsciousness | Brief | Long (> 5 minutes) |
| Seizure activity | Noncontributory: seizure-like activity often observed, onset after loss of consciousness | Organized, repetitive, localized; onset w/ loss of consciousness; Todd's paralysis, postictal confusion |

## Goal of diagnostic evaluation: Identify structural heart disease
- History, physical exam, resting ECG, postural blood pressures
- If above unrevealing, test for structural heart disease: echo, MRI, etc.
- If evidence of ischemia or effort symptoms: ETT, stress-imaging, cardiac cath
- If abnormal heart or ECG & no ischemia: Holter, loop records, EP study
- Older patients: carotid sinus massage
- If normal heart and ECG: probably neurally-mediated
- Consider multifactorial etiology in elderly

## Indications for hospital admission
- Known heart disease: CAD, CHF, valvular stenosis, prior ventricular arrhythmia
- Symptoms of ischemia, e.g. dyspnea, angina, exertional syncope
- Abnormal ECG: ischemia, conduction abnormality, non-sustained tachycardia, QT prolongation, Brugada morphology (RBBB + ST elevation $V_1$-$V_3$)
- Pacemaker malfunction

---

37 Brignole M et al. Guidelines on management (diagnosis and treatment) of syncope. Eur Heart J. 2001;22:1256-306; Kapoor WN. Syncope. NEJM 2000;343:1856-62; Kapoor WN. Current evaluation and management of syncope. Circulation 2002;106:1606-9.

38 Linzer M et al. Diagnosing syncope. Value of history, physical examination, and electrocardiography. Clinical Efficacy Assessment Project of the American College of Physicians. Ann Intern Med. 1997;126:989-96.

# Probability of Coronary Disease [39]

## Likelihood of significant coronary disease based on history

| Age | Asymptomatic | Non-Anginal | Atypical Angina | Typical Angina |
|---|---|---|---|---|
| **Men** | | | | |
| 60-69 | .12 | .28 | .67 | .94 |
| 50-59 | .10 | .22 | .59 | .92 |
| 40-49 | .06 | .14 | .46 | .87 |
| 30-39 | .02 | .05 | .22 | .70 |
| **Women** | | | | |
| 60-69 | .08 | .19 | .54 | .91 |
| 50-59 | .03 | .08 | .32 | .79 |
| 40-49 | .01 | .03 | .13 | .55 |
| 30-39 | .00 | .01 | .04 | .26 |

## Post-exercise test probability (%) of significant CAD

| Age Sex | Asymptomatic M | F | Non-Anginal M | F | Atypical Angina M | F | Typical Angina M | F |
|---|---|---|---|---|---|---|---|---|
| **ST depression > 2.5 mm** | | | | | | | | |
| 30-39 | 43±25 | 11±9 | 68±22 | 24±20 | 92±8 | 63±25 | 99±1 | 93±7 |
| 40-49 | 69±21 | 28±21 | 87±12 | 53±26 | 97±3 | 86±13 | 100±.4 | 98±2 |
| 50-59 | 81±16 | 56±25 | 91±8 | 78±17 | 98±2 | 95±5 | 100±.2 | 99±.7 |
| 60-69 | 85±13 | 76±18 | 94±6 | 90±9 | 99±1 | 98±2 | 100±.2 | 100±.3 |
| **ST depression 2-2.5 mm** | | | | | | | | |
| 30-39 | 18±10 | 3±2 | 38±17 | 8±6 | 76±13 | 33±17 | 96±3 | 79±13 |
| 40-49 | 39±17 | 10±7 | 65±16 | 24±14 | 91±6 | 63±17 | 98±1 | 93±5 |
| 50-59 | 54±17 | 27±14 | 75±13 | 50±18 | 94±4 | 84±9 | 99±.5 | 98±2 |
| 60-69 | 61±16 | 47±17 | 81±11 | 72±14 | 96±3 | 93±5 | 100±.4 | 99±.6 |
| **ST depression 1.5-2.0 mm** | | | | | | | | |
| 30-39 | 8±5 | 1±1 | 19±11 | 3±2.5 | 55±18 | 16±10 | 91±6 | 59±19 |
| 40-49 | 20±11 | 4±3 | 41±17 | 11±7.2 | 78±12 | 39±18 | 97±2 | 84±10 |
| 50-59 | 31±15 | 12±8 | 53±18 | 28±14 | 86±9 | 67±16 | 98±1 | 94±4 |
| 60-69 | 37±16 | 25±13 | 62±17 | 49±18 | 90±7 | 83±10 | 99±1 | 98±2 |
| **ST depression 1.0-1.5** | | | | | | | | |
| 30-39 | 4±1 | 0.6±.2 | 10±2 | 2±.7 | 38±5 | 9±3 | 83±3 | 42±9 |
| 40-49 | 11±2 | 2±.5 | 26±4 | 6±2 | 64±4 | 25±6 | 94±1 | 72±6 |
| 50-59 | 19±2.6 | 7±1 | 37±5 | 16±3 | 75±3 | 50±5 | 96±.7 | 89±2 |
| 60-69 | 23±3 | 15±2 | 45±5 | 33±5 | 81±3 | 72±4 | 97±.5 | 95±1 |
| **ST depression 0.5-1.0** | | | | | | | | |
| 30-39 | 2±.6 | 0.3±.1 | 5±2 | 0.7±.4 | 21±6 | 4±2 | 68±7 | 24±8 |
| 40-49 | 5±2 | 1±.3 | 13±4 | 3±1 | 44±8 | 12±4 | 86±4 | 53±10 |
| 50-59 | 9±3 | 3±1 | 20±5 | 8±2 | 57±8 | 31±7 | 91±3 | 78±6 |
| 60-69 | 11±3 | 7±2 | 26±6 | 17±5 | 65±7 | 52±8 | 94±2 | 90±3 |

39  Diamond GA, Forrester JS. Analysis of probability as an aid in the clinical diagnosis of coronary artery disease. N Engl J Med 1979;300:1350. Adapted with permission of The New England Journal of Medicine, copyright 1979, Massachusetts Medical Society.

# *Exercise Stress Testing*

**Objectives:**
**(1)** Diagnose functionally significant coronary artery disease
**(2)** Assess functional capacity, need for medical therapy or revascularization, safety of work/recreation, or adequacy of treatment
**(3)** Determine prognosis

## Limitations of exercise tests in detecting coronary disease

• Limited value in certain common situations: **. Women:** high false-positive rate (ST segment response; positive tests add little to predictive value of history alone **. Beta-blockers:** limit max work (heart rate × blood pressure) → sensitivity decreased **. Digitalis:** depresses ST segments, usually ≤ 0.1 mV. Further exertional ST-depression usually reflects ischemia. Consider stopping digoxin > one week before test **. Conduction abnormalities (BBB, pre-excitation):** ST segments uninterpretable (except lateral precordial leads in RBBB) **. Pressure overload (LVH, aortic stenosis):** subendocardial ischemia and ST depression even in absence of CAD (true-positive test for ischemia; false-positive for epicardial coronary obstruction) **. Metabolic abnormalities:** anemia, hypoxia, hypokalemia and hyperventilation
• The patient has to be **able to exercise**
• **Uncertainty** about whether a positive test reflects an anatomic abnormality
• ST-segment depression suggests presence of but **does not localize** ischemia

## Modifications to exercise testing

• **Myocardial imaging** with radioisotopes (thallium/sestamibi) or echocardiography
  . Modest ↑ in sensitivity and specificity for CAD compared to ECG alone
  . Helpful when expected likelihood of CAD is intermediate; conversely **unlikely to help** when suspicion of CAD is low or high
  . Preferable to standard exercise test in patients with abnormal resting ECG, e.g. BBB, LVH, pacemaker (generally similar specificity but lower sensitivity)
  . Localizes ischemia (may help to direct percutaneous intervention)
• **Pharmacologic stimulation** with dobutamine, adenosine or dipyridamole
  . Increases myocardial workload in patients unable to exercise (arthritis, PAD, deconditioning). Increases sensitivity for detecting significant CAD but functional implications less clear; most useful for pre-op risk stratification.
  . Dobutamine less effective if on beta blockers
  . Adenosine and dipyridamole contraindicated in patients with bronchospasm or high-grade A-V block; theophylline & caffeine decrease effectiveness

## The Duke Prognostic Score[40]

> *Score =   (Exercise duration in min) — (5 × max ST-deviation in mm)*
> *— (4 × treadmill angina index)*

Treadmill angina index: 0 = none;  1 = non-limiting angina;  2 = angina stops test

| Risk of death | Inpatients | | Outpatients | |
|---|---|---|---|---|
| (score) | *Patients* | *4-yr Survival* | *Patients* | *4-yr survival* |
| Low (≥ +5) | 470 (34%) | 98 % | 379 (62%) | 99 % |
| Mod (-10 to +4) | 795 (57%) | 92 % | 211 (34%) | 95 % |
| High (< -10) | 129 (9%) | 71 ± 6 % | 23 (4%) | 79 ± 11 % |

40  Mark DB *et al.* Prognostic value of exercise score in outpatients with suspected coronary artery disease. *NEJM* 1991;325(12): 849.

# Emergency Cardiac Pacing Technique

## Transcutaneous pacing method

1) Attach anterior electrode over cardiac apex, second directly posterior to first
2) Turn on pacemaker at desired rate (typically 70-100 bpm)
3) Assess capture by presence of consistent ST-segment and T-wave following each pacer spike on ECG tracing. Do not confuse with stimulation of skeletal muscles!
4) Confirm adequate BP and pulse
5) **Brady-asystolic arrest**: Set initial output to maximum; confirm capture, then decrease output slowly until threshold determined. **Conscious patient**: Set output to minimum and increase until capture.
6) Set output at 20% above capture threshold
7) Give sedatives and analgesia as needed for patient comfort
8) If immediate reversible causes of bradycardia are not identified, arrange for prompt placement of transvenous pacing lead

## Insertion of transvenous pacing wires

• If fluoroscope unavailable, use balloon flotation for ventricle and J-wire for atrium.
• **"Pace-capture" technique**:
1) Attach leads to pacemaker generator. Monitor ECG. Turn generator on at rate 70-100 bpm, maximum output, minimum sensitivity (demand pacing).
2) Advance pacing catheter until ventricle is successfully captured.
3) After placement, leave balloon deflated and test thresholds (see below).
• **"Injury current" technique**:
1) Attach distal (negative/black) lead to V (chest) input of ECG. This will show a unipolar electrogram on the corresponding V lead. **Or** attach distal (negative/black) electrode to R arm input and proximal (positive/red) electrode to L arm input, yielding lead 1 bipolar, and leads II & III unipolar electrograms.
2) Advance catheter with ECG running. QRS voltage should increase as catheter enters the right ventricle. Voltage decreases if catheter enters the IVC or pulmonary artery. Suspect incorrect positioning if catheter depth exceeds 35 cm from the right internal jugular approach. *Note: Catheter trauma may precipitate VT; withdrawal usually stops it.*
3) Deflate balloon and advance catheter. Injury current (ST segment elevation resembling MI) reflects endocardial contact. Advance ~1cm further for good contact.

## Threshold testing

**Pacing (stimulation) threshold**: minimum energy for successful capture. *Note: temporary pacing thresholds increase with time and should be checked daily.*
1) Set pacing rate 10-20 bpm higher than intrinsic heart rate.
2) Set generator at maximum until successful capture. If capture is unsuccessful, check for: stimulus artifact on ECG, battery, connections, placement; consider myocardial unresponsiveness (e.g., acidosis).
3) While monitoring ECG gradually decrease pacemaker output (mA) until capture fails – this is the *stimulation threshold*.
4) Set output to 2-3 times stimulation threshold. Maximum output setting is more reliable but may also increase risk of VF.

**Sensing (inhibition) threshold**: detected voltage at which pacing is inhibited (when intrinsic heart rate is adequate).
- Proper sensing permits pacer inhibition by normal QRS complexes but not T waves and other noise. Also avoids pacing during repolarization (R-on-T phenomenon) which can induce VF.
- **Terminology:**
   "Demand mode" = highest sensitivity: minimal energy will inhibit pacer, e.g. unwanted stimuli such as muscle movement or T waves.
   "Asynchronous mode" = lowest sensitivity: pacemaker will fire even though it detects considerable energy, e.g. from the QRS complex.
- **Technique:**
   1) Set pacemaker rate to 10-20 bpm below the patient's intrinsic heart rate (abort test if that rate is hemodynamically unacceptable). Decrease the pacemaker rate gradually to allow the patient's intrinsic rate to increase appropriately.
   2) Begin with highest sensitivity (lowest mV setting or "demand"); this should inhibit pacing. With real-time ECG monitoring, gradually increase sensing millivoltage until inappropriate pacing occurs. This is the *sensing threshold*, usually 0.5-2mV.
   3) Set sensitivity to approximately half of the sensing threshold. For example, if sensing is appropriate at 6 mV and inappropriate at 7 mV, half the sensing threshold (= twice the safety margin) is 3 mV. Check to make sure the device is not inhibited by artifacts like T waves.

# *Intra-Aortic Balloon Pump*

### Indications
- **Myocardial ischemia**: refractory unstable angina or postinfarction angina; refractory polymorphic VT; support for PTCA
- **Cardiogenic shock**: pump failure; acute mitral regurgitation or acute ventricular septal rupture (as a bridge to definitive treatment)
- **Postoperative**: myocardial depression and weaning from bypass

### Contraindications
- No definitive treatment available for underlying pathology
- Moderate-severe aortic insufficiency
- Severe aortic or ilio-femoral vascular disease

### Operating the intra-aortic balloon pump (IABP)
- **Balloon deflation**: nadir of end-diastolic pressure should occur just before arterial upstroke (aortic valve opening) begins • Late deflation: ventricle contracts against inflated balloon • Premature deflation: suboptimal afterload reduction
- **Balloon inflation**: should occur just after dicrotic notch • Early inflation: ventricle contracts against inflated balloon • Late inflation: excessive diastolic hypotension and suboptimal augmentation of coronary flow
- Full anticoagulation should be used
- During CPR the IABP should be turned off or set in "standby" mode

### Complications
- Leg ischemia • Aortic dissection • Femoral or retroperitoneal hemorrhage
- Infection • Pseudoaneurysm • Thromboembolism • ↓ Platelets • Lymphedema

**Timing examples:** [41] Arterial pressure waveforms with 1:2 counterpulsation

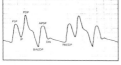

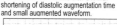

**Correct timing.** Balloon aortic end-diastolic pressure (BAEDP) is lower than aortic end-diastolic pressure (PAEDP). Assisted peak systolic pressure (APSP) is lower than native peak systolic pressure (PSP). IP = inflation point.

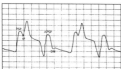

**Early inflation.** Inflation point (IP) occurs before aortic valve closure, before dicrotic notch (DN).

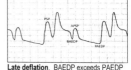

**Late inflation.** IP occurs after DN with shortening of diastolic augmentation time and small augmented waveform.

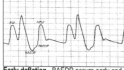

**Early deflation.** BAEDP occurs early and equilibrates rapidly with nonaugmented PAEDP; augmented peak systolic pressure (APSP) is improperly higher than nonaugmented PSP.

**Late deflation.** BAEDP exceeds PAEDP (should be lower).

# Hypertensive Emergencies [42]

## Diagnosis

- Defined end-organ damage, e.g. encephalopathy, renal dysfunction, CHF, cardiac ischemia, decreased placental perfusion
- DBP usually > 120 mmHg but BP can be as low as 160/100 in previously normotensive patient (e.g. pregnant woman, drug reaction in young adult)
- "Hypertensive urgency": elevated BP without end-organ damage; usually appropriate to treat with oral medications

---

41 Sorrentino M, Feldman T. Techniques for IABP timing, use, and discontinuance. *J Critical Illness* 1992; 7(4): 597-604; with permission of Cligott Publishing.

42 Alper AB, Calhoun DA. Hypertensive Emergencies. In: Antman EM, ed. *Cardiovascular Therapeutics : A Companion to Braunwald's Heart Disease.* Philadelphia: W.B. Saunders Co., 2002. Gifford RW. Management of hypertensive crises. *JAMA* 1991; 266:829-835. Adams HP, Jr. *et al.* Guidelines for the early management of patients with ischemic stroke. *Stroke* 2003; 34:1056-83.

**Etiology:** • Chronic HTN • Renal or renovascular disease • Drug ingestion (cocaine, amphetamines) • Non-compliance or withdrawal (esp. clonidine, β-blocker) • Pheochromocytoma • Scleroderma or other collagen-vascular disease • S/p carotid artery or neurosurgery • Head or spinal cord injury • Guillain-Barré

| Clinical Scenario | Goal of Treatment | 1st Line Rx [43] | Comments |
|---|---|---|---|
| Hypertensive encephalopathy | 20-25% reduction in MAP over 2-3 hr (but keep DBP > 100 mmHg) | SNP, FD, labetalol, nicardipine | Treatment may worsen neuro fxn. Avoid clonidine, βB (CNS effects). |
| Ischemic stroke | BP no lower than 220/120 mmHg, achieved slowly over 24 hr | Labetalol, nicardipine. | SNP, FD and NTG may increase ICP. Goal BP 185/110 if thrombolytic given. |
| Intracerebral hemorrhage | SBP 140-160 mmHg (or pre-stroke level) | Labetalol, SNP, nicardipine | Monitor for worsening neuro function after lowering BP |
| Subarachnoid hemorrhage | Generally withheld; if patient alert, consider rx to ↓ re-bleeding risk[44] | Nimodipine 60 mg PO/PNGT q 4 hr (to prevent spasm) ± labetalol | Avoid SNP, FD and NTG (increase ICP) |
| Pulmonary edema | DBP ≤100 mmHg or resolution of symptoms | SNP **plus** NTG **plus** diuretic | Avoid (-) inotropes in LV dysfunction. Search for myocardial ischemia. In CAD or PAD, search for RAS. |
| Myocardial infarction or unstable angina | DBP ≤100 mmHg or resolution of symptoms | NTG, β-B. Add SNP if DBP remains elevated | |
| Aortic dissection | SBP 100-120 or MAP 80 mmHg (watch urine output) | SNP or FD **plus** βB or labetalol | Decrease dP/dT. Avoid vasodilator monotherapy. |
| Sympathomimetic crisis (cocaine, amphet., pheochromocytoma, MAOI reaction, βB or clonidine withdrawal) | DBP ~100-105 (but ≤ 25% reduction in presenting BP) over 2-6 hr | Phentolamine (first) then βB **or** labetalol. Add benzodiazepine for drug overdose/withdrawal. | Avoid βB or labetalol alone [45] (unopposed α stimulation). Restart βB or clonidine if withdrawing. |
| Pregnancy (eclampsia) | DBP 90-105 or MAP ≤ 126 mmHg | Hydralazine [46], labetalol, nifedipine | **PO:** methyldopa. Avoid SNP, ACE-I. |
| Post-operative | Pre-op BP | SNP, labetalol | Treat pain, ↑ volume, & ↓O₂ |
| Acute renal insufficiency | DBP ~100-105 (but ≤ 25% reduction in presenting BP) | FD, Ca⁺⁺ channel blockers, SNP | Avoid diuretics. Maintain renal blood flow. |

SNP= sodium nitroprusside  FD= fenoldopam  βB=β-blocker
NTG= nitroglycerin  ICP=intracranial pressure

43  For specific drug dosages and administration guidelines see Groovy Drugs
44  Van Gijn. Sub-arachnoid hemorrhage. Lancet 1992; 339:653.
45  Hollander JE. Management of cocaine-associated myocardial ischemia. NEJM 1995; 333: 1270-6
46  Magee LA et al. Hydralazine for severe hypertension in pregnancy: meta-analysis. BMJ 2003;327:955-0.

# Perioperative Cardiovascular Risk [47]

## Goals
- Identify high risk patients → modify risk, provide special peri-operative care, postpone elective surgery, or consider revascularization
- Identify low risk patients → proceed with surgery
- Intermediate risk patients → empiric beta-blockade versus further risk stratification via non-invasive testing
- Coronary catheterization and revascularization (PTCA, CABG) should be considered only if indicated apart from surgery

## Interventions to reduce perioperative cardiac complications
- Mechanical revascularization (e.g. coronary bypass surgery, coronary stent). Delay surgery 4-6 wks after stent, if possible, due to risk of acute thrombosis.
- In high risk patients, perioperative β-**blockers** reduce perioperative death and myocardial infarctions as well as long-term morbidity & mortality.[48] Tested regimens: (1) atenolol 5-10 mg IV over 5-10 min as long as HR > 55 and SBP > 100, given 30 minutes pre-op and immediately post-op, followed by 50-100mg po qd; or (2) bisoprolol 5-10 mg po qd, titrated to HR < 60, started 1 week pre-op and continued 4 weeks post-op.
- Nitrates and Ca-blockers probably have limited benefit
- Aspirin if acceptable to surgeons
- Avoid negative inotropes in severe LV dysfunction (e.g. consider spinal or opiate-based anesthesia)
- Consider hemodynamic monitoring (PA catheter, continuous 12-lead ECG, intraoperative trans-esophageal echocardiography) in (1) recent MI without revascularization (2) large unrevascularized myocardial territory (3) severe LV dysfunction (4) severe aortic or mitral valve disease (5) aortic cross-clamping (f) emergency surgery without optimized hemodynamics. However **no benefit** of PA catheters in randomized trial. [49]
- Scrupulous postoperative BP, pain, volume management

47  Graybum PA, Hillis LD.  Cardiac event sin patients undergoing noncardiac surgery:  Shifting the paradigm the paradigm from noninvasive risk stratification to therapy.  Ann Int Med 2003; 138:506-11.

48  Mangano DT et al. Effect of atenolol on mortality after cardiovascular morbidity after noncardiac surgery. NEJM 1996; 335(23):1713-20.  Poldermans D et al.  The effect of bisoprolol on perioperative cardiac death and myocardial infarction in high-risk patients undergoing vascular surgery. NEJM 1999; 341(24): 1789-94.

49  Sandham JD et al. A randomized, controlled trial of the use of pulmonary-artery catheters in high-risk surgical patients. NEJM 2003; 348:5-14.

## ACC-AHA guidelines for perioperative cardiac evaluation [50]

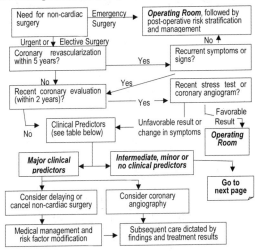

### Clinical predictors (increased risk of MI, CHF or death)

| Major | Intermediate | Minor |
|---|---|---|
| • Unstable coronary syndrome * | • Mild angina † | • Advanced age |
| • Decompensated CHF | • Prior MI (by history or EKG) | • Abnormal ECG ‡ |
| • Significant arrhythmias # | • Compensated or prior CHF | • Rhythm other than sinus |
| • Severe valvular disease | • Diabetes mellitus | • Low functional capacity |
| | • Renal insufficiency | • History of stroke |
| | | • Uncontrolled hypertension |

\* Recent MI w/ important ischemic risk; unstable or severe (class III/IV) angina
\# High-grade A-V block, symptomatic ventricular arrhythmias w/ underlying heart disease, or SVT with uncontrolled ventricular rate
† Canadian class I/II angina
‡ LVH, LBBB, ST-T abnormalities

50  Adapted from Eagle KA *et al*. Guidelines for perioperative cardiovascular evaluation for noncardiac surgery -- Executive summary. A report of the ACC/AHA Task Force on Practice Guidelines. *Circulation* 2002; 105:1757-67.

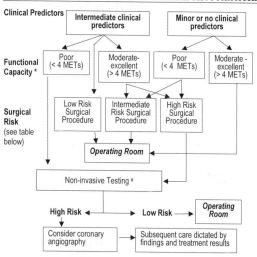

\* MET= metabolic equivalents. 1-4 METs: daily activities, walking 1-2 blocks on level ground at 2-3 mph, light house work.  4-10 METs: climbing stairs or hill, running short distance, heavy house work, bowling, dancing, golf, tennis, swimming, skiing
\# Assessment of LV function, exercise or pharmacologic stress testing, or ambulatory ECG monitoring

### Surgical risk for non-cardiac procedures

| High Risk (> 5%) | Intermediate Risk (<5%) | Low Risk (< 1%) |
|---|---|---|
| • Emergent major operations, especially in elderly patients<br>• Major vascular or peripheral vascular surgery<br>• Prolonged surgical procedures with large fluid shifts or blood loss | • Carotid endarterectomy<br>• Head and neck operations<br>• Intraperitoneal and intrathoracic operation<br>• Orthopedic operation<br>• Prostate operation | • Endoscopic procedures<br>• Superficial procedures<br>• Cataract operation<br>• Breast operation |

# Acute MI & Unstable Angina [51]

## Principal presentations of UA/NSTEMI
• Rest angina • New onset angina (to CCS 3) • Increasing angina (to CCS 3)

## Likelihood that signs & symptoms represent CAD

| Features | High Likelihood | Intermediate Absence of high-likelihood features *and* any of following | Low likelihood Absence of high intermediate features *and* any of following: |
|---|---|---|---|
| History | • Chest or left arm discomfort as chief symptom reproducing past angina<br>• Known history of CAD, including MI | • Chest or left arm discomfort as chief symptom<br>• Age > 70<br>• Male gender<br>• Diabetes | • Probable ischemic symptoms in absence of any intermediate likelihood characteristics<br>• Recent cocaine use |
| Examination | • Transient mitral regurgitation, hypotension, diaphoresis, pulmonary edema, or rales | • Extracardiac vascular disease | • Chest discomfort reproduced by palpation |
| ECG | Presumably new:<br>• Transient ST-segment deviation ($\geq 0.05$ mV), or<br>• T-wave ($\geq 0.2$ mV) w/symptoms | • Fixed Q waves<br>• Abnormal ST segments<br>• T wave abnormality not known to be new | • T-wave flattening or inversion in leads with dominant R waves<br>• Normal ECG |
| Cardiac markers | • Elevated cardiac troponins or CK-MB | • Normal | • Normal |

## Prognostication
***TIMI-Risk Score*** [52] (markers of 14 day risk of death, MI or urgent revascularization): • Age$\geq$65 • 3 coronary risk factors • Coronary disease with > 50% stenosis • ST elevation on initial ECG • Two angina episodes in preceding 24 hr • Aspirin in past 7 d • Elevated serum cardiac markers

| # of Markers | 0/1 | 2 | 3 | 4 | 5 | 6/7 |
|---|---|---|---|---|---|---|
| 14 d risk | 4.7% | 8.3% | 13.2% | 19.9% | 26.2% | 40.9% |

### Adverse Prognostications From PURSUIT: [53]
• Age > 60 • Male • Prior CCS 3 angina • HR > 100-120 • SBP < 80-100 • CHF signs • ST depression

---

51  Braunwald E *et al.* ACC/AHA 2002 guideline update for the management of patients with unstable angina and non–ST-segment elevation myocardial infarction: A report of the American College of Cardiology/American Heart Association Task Force on Practice Guidelines. Available at: http://www.acc.org/clinical/guidelines/unstable/unstable.pdf.

52  Antman EM *et al.* The TIMI risk score for unstable angina/non-ST elevation MI. *JAMA* 2000; 284:835-842.

53  The PURSUIT Trial Investigators. Inhibition of platelet glycoprotein IIb/IIIa with eptifibatide in patients with acute coronary syndromes. *NEJM* 1998; 339:436-443.

*Short-Term Risk of Death or MI*

- Traditional risk factors (e.g. HTN, lipids, tobacco) are weakly predictive of acute coronary sundromes and are far less important than symptoms, ECG findings, and cardiac markers.

| Feature | High Risk (any) | Intermediate Risk | Low Risk |
|---|---|---|---|
| History | Accelerating tempo of ischemic Symptoms in past 48h | Prior MI, CABG, PAD or cerebro-vascular disease, or prior ASA use | |
| Character of Pain | Ongoing rest angina > 20 min | Rest angina > 20 minute now resolved | New or pro-gressive angina ≥ CCS 3 without prolonged rest angina |
| Findings | • Ischemic pulmonary edema<br>• New mitral regurgitation murmur<br>• S3 or new/worsening rales<br>• ↓ BP, or ↑/↓ HR<br>• Age > 75 years | • Age > 70 years | |
| ECG | • Transient ST changes > 0.05 mV<br>• Presumed new BBB<br>• Sustained ventricular tachycardia | • T wave inversions > 0.2 mV<br>• Pathological Q waves | • Normal or unchanged ECG during chest discomfort |
| Cardiac Markers | • Troponin > 0.1 ng/mL | • Troponin > 0.01 but < 0.1 ng/mL | • Normal |

## Syndrome-specific emergency treatment
### All patients
- 12-lead ECG; leads $V_3R$, $V_4R$, $V_5R$ in inferior wall MI; leads $V_7$-$V_9$ in suspected circumflex territory MI
- Oxygen 2-4 L nasal cannula
- Nitroglycerin SL/IV, if not hypotensive and has not taken sildenafil or related drugs within 24 hr. Avoid in inferior wall MI with right ventricular involvement
- Morphine IV if pain not relieved with NTG

### ST-Elevation Acute Myocardial Infarction (STEMI)
Indications: Acute coronary syndrome with ST elevation or presumably-new LBBB
**(1)** Adjunctive treatments:
- Aspirin 160-325 mg po/pr, not enteric-coated. Large mortality benefit.
- β-adrenergic blocker IV targeted to heart rate 50-60
- ACE inhibitors after stabilized or revascularized for 6 hours
- Glycoprotein IIb/IIIa inhibitors: Only if percutaneous coronary intervention (PCI) planned. May interfere with emergency surgery. Safety and utility in combination with thrombolytics unproven.
- Clopidogrel in ASA-intolerant patients and probably in all patients. **Note:** Clopidogrel may interfere with emergency CABG and may be deferred until after angiography.

(2) *Emergency revascularization if onset of symptoms < 12 hours:*
- Transfer for emergency PCI within 2 hours [54]
- Thrombolytics (page 209) if no contraindications and emergency PCI unavailable

(3) *Cardiogenic Shock:*
- Intra-aortic balloon pump (See page 35)
- Emergency revascularization (especially if age < 75) [55]

### Non-ST-Elevation Acute Myocardial Infarction (NSTEMI)

*Indications:* ST-depression or dynamic T-wave inversion or Troponin elevation

*(1) Adjunctive anti-ischemic treatments:*
- β-adrenergic blocker PO or IV targeted to heart rate 50-60
- Non-dihydropyridine calcium-channel blocker (diltiazem or verapamil) if β-blocker contraindicated.
- Intravenous nitrates for ongoing pain
- ACE inhibitors in levt ventricular dysfunction, CHF, diabetes, or hypertension after other anti-ischemic agents

*(2) Adjunctive anti-thrombotic treatments:*
- Aspirin 160-325 mg po/pr, not enteric-coated
- Clopidogrel 300mg in ASA-intolerant patients and probably in all patients. **Note:** Clopidogrel may interfere with CABG; often deferred until after angiography.
- Heparin: unfractionated (UFH) or low-molecular weight (LMWH). LMWH has marginal incremental benefit and may interfere with PCI or emergency CABG at some institutions.
- Glycoprotein IIb/IIIa inhibitors: Utility controversial unless PCI is planned or high-risk. Abciximab not indicated without PCI.
- **Note:** Thrombolytic therapy is contraindicated

*(3) CCU observation if not revascularized*

*(4) Early-invasive strategy:* Urgent catheterization ± revascularization before discharge irrespective of non-invasive testing
- Recommended in high-risk patients (recurrent or persistent angina, recurrent ischemia, LV dysfunction, multi-lead ECG repolarization abnormalities, prior MI, PCI, CABG)
- Controversial in intermediate and low-risk patients.
- Distinguished from "early-conservative" strategy of pharmacologic stabilization and angiography ± revascularization only if recurrent symptoms or abnormal stress test

### Unstable Angina (USA)

*Indications:* Suspected angina syndrome without abnormal troponins.
**Note:** Clinical judgment alone does not exclude UA/NSTEMI.
- All patients with suspected acute coronary syndromes must undergo observation with 6-12 hour follow-up ECG and cardiac enzyme measurement before discharge
- Cardiac MRI in experienced centers is more sensitive than troponins[56]
- Select treatment strategy (from NSTEMI) based on risk criteria above

---

54 Andersen HR *et al.* A comparison of coronary angioplasty with fibrinolytic therapy in acute myocardial infarction. *NEJM* 2003;349:733-742.

55 Hochman JS et al. Early revascularization in acute myocardial infarction complicated by cardiogenic shock. *NEJM* 1999;341:625-634; Ryan TJ. Early revascularization in cardiogenic shock -- A positive view of a negative trial. *NEJM* 1999;341:687-688.

56 Kwong RY *et al.* Detecting acute coronary syndrome in the emergency department with cardiac magnetic resonance imaging. *Circulation* 2003;107:531-537.

# Critical Care

## *Checklists for Critical Care*

### General Care
- DVT prophylaxis with heparin and/or compression boots
- GI bleeding prophylaxis with $H_2$ blocker, proton pump inhibitor or sucralfate
- Intensive insulin therapy for hyperglycemia – *see page 192*
- Early attention to nutrition
- Elevate head of bed 30° to prevent aspiration
- Daily reversal of sedation in intubated patients [57]

### Occult causes of fever in the ICU patient [58]
- Infected intravascular catheters
- Drug reaction
- Sinusitis or otitis media, especially if nasogastric tube present
- Pulmonary embolism and deep venous thrombosis
- Acalculous cholecystitis or pancreatitis
- *Clostridium difficile* colitis
- Fungal infection or secondary infection by resistant organisms
- Postcardiotomy syndrome
- Central fever (in patients with head trauma)

## *Shock*

### Classification of Shock

| Cause | PCWP | CO | SVR | Comments |
|---|---|---|---|---|
| **Cardiogenic** | | | | |
| Myocardial dysfunction | ↑ | ↓ | ↑ | Hemodynamic goals: • PCWP 15-18 • MAP ≥ 70 mm Hg • CI ≥ 2.2 • SVR 1000-1200 |
| Acute MR | ↑ | ↓(forward) | ↑ | |
| Acute VSD | ↑ | ↓ | ↑ | $CO_{RV} > CO_{LV}$. $O_2$ "step-up" at RV. |
| RV infarction | ↔/↓ | ↓ | ↑ | RA pressure >> PCWP |
| Tamponade | ↑ | ↓ | ↑ | RAP=RVEDP=PAD=PCWP Pulsus paradoxicus increased |
| **Distributive** | | | | |
| Sepsis (early) | ↔/↓ | Usually ↑ | ↓ | CO may ↓ due to sepsis-mediated LV dysfunction, esp. in later phases (mixed cardiogenic-septic physiol.) |
| Anaphylaxis, liver disease, spinal shock, adrenal insuff. | ↔/↓ | ↑ | ↓ | Epinephrine for anaphylaxis after treating underlying cause; pure α agonists in spinal shock |
| **Hypovolemic** | | | | |
| Hemorrhage, dehydration | ↓ | ↓ | ↑ | Invasive monitoring needed only if co-existing LV dysfunction |

[57] Kress JP et al. Daily interruption of sedative infusions in critically ill patients undergoing mechanical ventilation. *NEJM* 2000; 342:1471-1477.

[58] Hotchkiss RS, Karl IE. The pathophysiology and treatment of sepsis. *NEJM* 2003; 348:138-150.

## Choice of drugs in shock

| Hemodynamics | Initial Treatment | Comments |
|---|---|---|
| PCWP (or CVP) ↓ | Aggressive volume expansion | Consider pressors initially, but re-eval once PCWP ≥ 18 or CVP ≥ 12 |
| CO ↓, SVR ↑ | Dobutamine | Alternatives include milrinone or dopamine plus nitroprusside |
| CO ↓, SVR ↔or ↓ | Dopamine | Norepinephrine is 2nd line agent |
| SVR ↓, CO ↑ | High dose dopamine or norepinephrine | Add epinephrine or phenylephrine for refractory hypotension |

## Relative action of catecholamine vasopressors

| Drug | Receptor | HR | Inotropy | SVR | Comments |
|---|---|---|---|---|---|
| Dopamine - Low dose | DA | 0 | 0 | ↔↓ | Renal and splanchnic vasodilatation |
| Dopamine - High dose | $\beta_1 \rightarrow \alpha_1$ | ↑ | ↑↑ | ↑↑ | First-line pressor for SBP 70-90 mmHg |
| Dobutamine | $\beta_1, \beta_2 > \alpha_1$ | ↔↑ | ↑↑ | ↓↓ | Inotrope & vasodilator; may lower BP |
| Norepi-nephrine | $\alpha_1, \alpha_2, \beta_1$ | ↔↑ | ↑↑ | ↑↑↑ | For hypotension refractory to fluids |
| Epinephrine | $\alpha_1, \alpha_2$ $\beta_1, \beta_2$ | ↑↑ | ↑↑↑ | ↑↑↑ | For refractory cardiac failure (e.g. post CABG) or anaphylaxis |
| Phenylephrine | $\alpha_1$ | 0 | 0 | ↑↑↑ | For refractory hypotension, esp. vasculogenic |
| Isoproterenol | $\beta_1, \beta_2$ | ↑↑↑ | ↑↑ | ↔↓ | Primarily increases HR. May cause reflex hypotension |

## Additional treatment considerations in severe septic shock

- Early "goal-directed" therapy based on hemodynamic parameters: [59]
  - Titration of CVP to 8-12 mmHg
  - Pressors for MAP < 65 mmHg and vasodilators for MAP > 90 mmHg
  - Transfusion to hematocrit > 30% if central venous $O_2$sat < 70%
  - Inotropic agents if central venous $O_2$sat remains < 70%
- Activated protein C (drotrecogin alpha) – see page 182
- Corticosteroids for relative adrenal insufficiency:[60] In critically-ill patients with hypotension unresponsive to fluids, consider hydrocortisone 50 mg IV q 6h ± fludrocortisone 50 mcg PNGT qd until results of ACTH stimulation test available - see Adrenal Insufficiency, page 61

59  Rivers E et al. Early goal-directed therapy in the treatment of severe sepsis and septic shock. NEJM 2001; 345:1368-77.

60  Annane D et al. Effect of treatment with low doses of hydrocortisone and fludrocortisone on mortality in patients with septic shock. JAMA 2002; 288:862-871. Cooper MS, Stewart PM. Corticosteroid insufficiency in acutely ill patients. NEJM 2003; 348:727-734.

# APACHE II Score [61]

**Acute Physiology Score (APS):** Sum variables 1-12 (use one each for 5 & 9), add to Age and Chronic Health Points below. *Use worst value from preceding 24 hr.*

| | Physiologic Variable | 0 | 1 | 2 | 3 | 4 |
|---|---|---|---|---|---|---|
| 1 | Temperature (°F) | $96^8$-$101^2$ | $101^3$-$102^1$ $93^2$-$96^7$ | $89^6$-$93^1$ | $102^2$-$105^7$ $86^0$-$89^5$ | $\geq105^8$ $\leq85^9$ |
| 2 | Heart Rate *Ventricular response* | 70-109 | n/a | 110-139 55-69 | 140-179 40-54 | $\geq180$ $\leq39$ |
| 3 | Mean Art Pressure $(2 \times DBP + SBP) \div 3$ | 70-109 | n/a | 110-139 50-69 | 130-159 | $\geq160$ $\leq49$ |
| 4 | Resp Rate *On or off ventilator* | 12-24 | 25-34 10-11 | 6-9 | 35-49 | $\geq50$ $\leq5$ |
| 5 | Oxygenation: Use 5a if $FiO_2 \geq 0.5$, **or** 5b if $FiO_2 < 0.5$ *A-a gradient = $(713 \times FiO_2) - (1.25 \times PaCO_2) - PaO_2$* | | | | | |
| | 5a: A-a gradient | < 200 | | 200-349 | 350-499 | $\geq500$ |
| | 5b: $PaO_2$ | > 70 | 61-70 | | 55-60 | $\leq 54$ |
| 6 | Serum Na+ | 130-139 | 150-154 | 155-159 120-129 | 160-179 111-119 | $\geq180$ $\leq110$ |
| 7 | Serum K+ | 3.5-5.4 | 5.5-5.9 3.0-3.4 | 2.5-2.9 | 6.0-6.9 | $\geq7.0$ $\leq2.4$ |
| 8 | Serum Creatinine *Double if Acute RF* | 0.6-1.4 | n/a | 1.5-1.9 <0.6 | 2.0-3.4 | $\geq3.5$ |
| 9 | 9a: Arterial pH *Preferred* | 7.33-7.49 | 7.50-7.59 | 7.25-7.32 | 7.60-7.69 7.15-7.24 | $\geq7.70$ $\leq7.14$ |
| | 9b: Venous $HCO_3$ *Use only if no ABG* | 22-31.9 | 32-40.9 | 18-21.9 | 41-51.9 15-17.9 | $\geq52$ $\leq14$ |
| 10 | WBC | 3.0-14.9 | 15 -19.9 | 20-39.9 1.0-2.9 | n/a | $\geq40$ <1.0 |
| 11 | Hematocrit | 30-45.9 | 46-49.9 | 50-59.9 20-29.9 | n/a | $\geq60$ <20 |
| 12 | GCS (see below) | Score = 15 – GCS Score (Eye + Motor + Verbal) | | | | |

| Glasgow Coma Scale (GCS) | | Chronic Health Points | | Age Points | |
|---|---|---|---|---|---|
| **Eye Opening** | **Verbal** | Non-operative, or emergency post-op & any conditions below* | 5 | $\leq 44$ | 0 |
| 4:Spontaneously | 5: Oriented & conversant; seems able to talk if intubated | | | 45-54 | 2 |
| 3:To command | | | | 55-64 | 3 |
| 2:To pain | | Elective operation & any conditions below* | 2 | 65-74 | 5 |
| 1:No response | | | | $\geq 75$ | 6 |
| **Motor Response** | 4: Confused | *Cirrhosis with portal hypertension or encephalopathy; class IV angina; chronic hypoxia, hypercarbia or polycythemia; chronic dialysis; immunocompromised | | | |
| 6: Obeys commands | 3: Inappropriate speech; question-able ability to speak if intubated | | | | |
| 5: Localizes to pain | | | | | |
| 4: Withdraws to pain | | **Total APACHE II Score =** | | | |
| 3: Flexion to pain | | **Acute Physiology Score + Chronic Health Points + Age Points** | | | |
| 2: Extension to pain | 2: Incomprehensible | | | | |
| 1: No response | 1: No response | | | | |

61 Knaus WA, Draper EA, Wagner DP, Zimmerman JE. APACHE II: a severity of disease classification system. *Crit Care Med* 1985; 13:818-29.

# Pulmonary Artery Catheters [62]

**Utility:** (1) Determine causes of **pulmonary edema** (cardiogenic vs. non-cardiogenic), **hypotension** (cardiac function vs. volume status vs. vascular tone) or **oliguria** (cardiac function vs. volume status vs. renal disease) (2) As an adjunct to the management of critically ill patient with **MI**, **heart failure** or **sepsis** complicated by **shock**

**Effectiveness:** RCTs in medical [63] and surgical [64] patients have shown no benefit on morbidity and mortality; one study [65] suggested **increased** mortality

**Increased complications with:** • High risk of VT with uncorrected ischemia, acidosis (pH ≤ 7.2), hypoxemia ($PaO_2$ < 60 mmHg), uncorrected $Ca^{++}$ ≤ 8.0 mg/dL or $K^+$ ≤ 3.5 mEq/L • LBBB – 5% risk of complete heart block
 • Coagulopathy • Balloon overinflation

## PCWP is accurate if
- Catheter is calibrated, level and flushes easily
- Correct position on CXR (AP: < 3-5 cm from midline; lateral: below LA)
- Characteristic waveforms with balloon deflated
- PCWP < PADP
- Mean PCWP < mean PAP

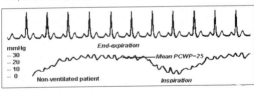

## Evaluate tracing
- Measure mean "*a*" wave pressure at end expiration (peak "*a*" wave follows ECG "*p*" wave by ~ 0.24 ms and *v*-wave follows ECG *T*-wave)
- Correct PCWP by subtracting ½ of PEEP (multiply x 0.8 to convert cm $H_2O$ to mmHg) from measured PCWP. Less PEEP is transmitted if low compliance (e.g. ARDS); more if high compliance (e.g. emphysema).
- Use caution when interpreting the wedge pressure if there is excessive catheter whip or marked respiratory variation

62 Sharkey. Beyond the wedge: clinical physiology and the Swan-Ganz catheter. *Am J Med* 1987; 83:111; Leatherman JW, Marini JJ. Clinical use of the pulmonary artery catheter. In: Hall, ed. *Principles of Critical Care*, 2nd ed. NY: McGraw-Hill; 1998. Voyce S, McCaffree DR. Pulmonary artery catheters. In: Irwin RS, Rippe JM, eds. *Irwin and Rippe's Intensive Care Medicine*. Philadelphia: Lipincott, Williams & Wilkins, 2003. Figures copyright 1987 Lawrence Martin MD, with permission.

63 Richard C *et al.* Early use of the pulmonary artery catheter and outcomes in patients with shock and acute respiratory distress syndrome: A randomized controlled trial. *JAMA* 2003; 290:2713-2720.

64 Sandham JD *et al.* A randomized, controlled trial of the use of pulmonary-artery catheters in high-risk surgical patients. *NEJM* 2003; 348:5-14.

65 Connors AF *et al.* The effectiveness of right heart catheterization in the initial care of critically ill patients. *JAMA* 1996; 276(11):889.

## Interpretation of PCWP

- **PCWP correlates with LV filling pressures (LVEDP)** – see exceptions below
- **"Physiologic" LVEDP is rate-dependent**
    - Bradycardia increases LVEDP, tachycardia decreases LVEDP
- **High LVEDP does not always correlate w/ occurrence of pulmonary edema**
    - No edema with chronically ↑ LVEDP (↑ lymph drainage, ↓ vasc. permeability)
    - Non-cardiogenic pulmonary edema (normal LVEDP) occurs with endothelial injury (e.g. ARDS) or low albumin states
- **PCWP underestimates LVEDP (pre-load) in presence of**
    - Decreased LV compliance (MI, LVH, diastolic dysfunction, pericardial disease)
    - Severe aortic insufficiency
    - High intrapericardial or intrathoracic pressure, e.g. obstructive lung disease, high levels of applied PEEP, or pericardial disease. **Note:** LVEDP is proportional to gradient between intracardiac and *intrapericardial* pressure; PCWP proportional to gradient between intracardiac and *atmospheric* pressure
- **PCWP overestimates LVEDP (pre-load) in presence of**
    - Mitral stenosis or regurgitation
    - Catheter in non-"zone III" position, "over wedged" waveform (unnaturally smooth with marked respiratory variation) or anterior balloon migration (PCWP>PAD)
    - PEEP or auto-PEEP
    - Increased PA vascular tone (hypoxia, hypovolemia, dopamine)
    - "Catheter whip" esp. in hyperdynamic states
    - Catheter tip obstruction (left atrial myxoma, thoracic tumors, mediastinal fibrosis)
    - Ruptured balloon

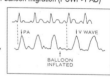

"Giant" v waves

| Specific findings on PA catheterization<br>Also see jugular vein pulsations, page 24 | Cause |
|---|---|
| Giant "v" waves with obliteration of *a* waves (balloon inflated), and bifid PA waveform (balloon deflated) *See diagram* | • Acute mitral regurgitation<br>• LA enlargement or LV failure<br>• Acute ventriculoseptal defect |
| PA diastolic pressure exceeds PCWP by > 5-7 mmHg | • Elevated pulmonary vascular resistance (pulmonary embolism, veno-occlusive disease, hypoxic vasoconstriction or 1° vs. 2° pulmonary hypertension)<br>• Pulmonary parenchymal disorders<br>• Tachycardia |
| O₂sat "step-up" (> 10%) between RA and RV | • Acute ventriculoseptal defect<br>• Primum atrial septal defect (ASD)<br>• Coronary fistula to right ventricle<br>• Patent ductus arteriosus (PDA) with pulmonic insufficiency |
| Elevated RA pressure with prominent *x* and *y* descents (*y* usually > *x*). RA pressure does not decrease with negative intrathoracic pressure (Kussmaul's sign). | • Right ventricular infarction<br>• Restrictive physiology |
| Elevated RA pressure with prominent *x* descent & diminished or absent *y* descent. RAP = RVEDP = PAD = mean PAWP. Absent Kussmaul's sign. Pulsus paradox. | • Pericardial Tamponade |

## Common PA catheter problems

| | |
|---|---|
| Catheter is persistently wedged | • Flush tip<br>• Make sure that balloon is deflated<br>• Pullback to PA tracing, then inflate and re-float |
| Catheter will not wedge | • Make sure that balloon is intact (air returns from balloon) and that tip is not over wedged<br>• Inflate balloon while in PA and advance<br>• Use fluoroscopy guidance<br>• If repeatedly unsuccessful, consider using PAD to estimate PCWP |
| Ectopy during or after placement | • Pull back catheter to SVC or advance into PA<br>• Check electrolytes<br>• Replace/remove catheter |

# Using Mechanical Ventilators[66]

## Indications

| Category | Mechanisms | Common clinical scenarios |
|---|---|---|
| Acute hypoxemic respiratory failure | • Shunt<br>• V/Q mismatch<br>• Diffusion impairment | • Pneumonia<br>• ARDS<br>• CHF<br>• Pulmonary fibrosis<br>• Hemorrhage<br>• Aspiration |
| Acute ventilatory (hypercarbic) respiratory failure | • Decreased alveolar ventilation<br>• Increased dead space ventilation | • Respiratory muscle fatigue<br>• Acute on chronic respiratory disease (e.g. COPD)<br>• Drug-induced respiratory depression<br>• Neuromuscular or chest wall disease<br>• Obesity-hypoventilation<br>• Massive thromboembolism<br>• CNS injury |
| Shock | • Cardiogenic and non-cardiogenic pulmonary edema | See page 44 |
| Airway protection | • Obstruction<br>• Aspiration | • Altered mental status<br>• Aspiration<br>• Pulmonary hemorrhage<br>• Airway mass or extrinsic compression<br>• Soft tissue infection or edema |

---

66 Hall JB, Wood LDH. Management of the patient on a ventilator. In: Hall (ed). *Principles of Critical Care*, 2nd ed. NY: McGraw-Hill, 1998. Hubmayr RD. Setting the ventilator. In: Tobin (ed). *Principles and Practice of Mechanical Ventilation*. NY: McGraw Hill, 1994; Tobin MJ. Advances in mechanical ventilation. *NEJM* 2001; 344:1986-1996.

## Modes of Mechanical Ventilation

| Mode | Advantages | Disadvantages |
|------|-----------|---------------|
| Assist-control (AC) | • Full tidal volume regardless of respiratory effort or drive<br>• Can preset minute volume | • Tachypnea may lead to respiratory alkalosis<br>• Poor synchrony between patient and vent may lead to "breath-stacking" and auto-PEEP |
| Intermittent Mandatory Ventilation (IMV) | • Patient determines tidal volume for spontaneous breath<br>• Potentially less respiratory alkalosis<br>• May facilitate weaning or respiratory conditioning | • May increase work of breathing and respiratory muscle fatigue<br>• Must overcome resistance of respiratory circuit for spontaneous breath (unless added pressure support) |
| Pressure Support Ventilation (PSV) | • Patient determines own volumes, rate and flow (more physiologic)<br>• Potentially reduces peak inspiratory pressures (PIPs) | • Needs careful monitoring to guarantee adequate tidal volumes and minute ventilation<br>• Requires consistent respiratory effort |
| Pressure Control Ventilation (PCV) | • Can more easily control inspiratory time and peak airway pressures<br>• May be used with AC or IMV modes | • Needs careful monitoring to guarantee adequate tidal volumes and minute ventilation<br>• May increase risk of auto-PEEP |
| Non-invasive Positive Pressure Ventilation (NIPPV) - see page 54 | • Allows ventilation without intubation<br>• Easily taken on/off | • Requires careful patient selection and trained respiratory therapists<br>• No airway control |

## Ventilator parameters and initial settings

| Parameter | Suggested Initial Settings or Normal Range | Comments |
|---|---|---|
| FiO$_2$ | 100% | • May taper rapidly to level adequate to maintain PaO$_2$/O$_2$sat<br>• Ideally keep < 60% to prevent oxygen toxicity and lung injury |
| Respiratory Rate (RR) | 8-12/min | • Titrate to pH<br>• Consider 18-24/min for "therapeutic" hyperventilation (will decrease respiratory effort in shock)<br>• Rate > 20/min may increase auto-PEEP |
| Mode | IMV or AC | • Consider PSV in neuromuscular disease if respiratory effort enough to trigger cycle |
| Tidal Volume (TV) | 6 ml/kg ideal body weight | • Higher volumes may increase risk of alveolar overdistention ("barotrauma") and worsen ventilator-associated lung injury |
| Inspiratory Flow Rate (IFR) | 60 L/min | • Set only on volume cycled ventilators<br>• IFR set too low may increase auto-PEEP by allowing insufficient exhalation time<br>• IFR set too high may increase PIPs |
| Inspiratory to Expiratory (I:E) Ratio | 1:3 | • Determined by IFR and respiratory rate during volume-cycled ventilation<br>• Can be specifically adjusted during PCV<br>• Increased I:E ratio (e.g. 1:4) may be useful in severe obstruction (↑expiratory phase)<br>• Inverse ratio (2:1) may be used to increase PaO$_2$ in severe hypoxemia |
| Plateau Pressure | < 35 cm H$_2$O | • A non-invasive measure of transpulmonary pressure<br>• Ideally kept low to decrease risk of barotrauma |
| Peak Inspiratory Pressure (PIP) | < 45 cm H$_2$O | • Ideally kept low, but may not be achievable (less important than plateau pressure) |
| Positive End Expiratory pressure (PEEP) | 5 cm H$_2$O (considered "physiologic") | • Improves oxygenation by preventing alveolar collapse and V/Q mismatch<br>• Titrate PEEP by 5 cm H$_2$O increments until F$_i$O$_2$ requirement ≤ 0.6 *or* plateau pressure > 35 cm H$_2$O *or* compliance decreases<br>• Increases airway pressures and risk of barotrauma<br>• Decreases venous return and cardiac output |
| Compliance | 70-100 ml/cm H$_2$O | • Δvolume/Δpressure = TV÷(plateau pressure - PEEP)<br>• Decreased in CHF, pneumothorax, ARDS, effusions, pneumonia, chest wall disorders |
| Resistance | < 5-10 cm H$_2$O/L/sec | • Δpressure/flow rate = (PIP - plateau) ÷IFR<br>• Increased in bronchoconstriction, mucous plugging |

## Acute hypoxemic respiratory failure
- **Common clinical scenarios:** . ARDS . Pneumonia . CHF . Pulmonary fibrosis . Pulmonary contusion . Aspiration
- **Things to consider:**
  - Pulmonary overdistention (**"barotrauma"**) appears to promote ventilator-associated lung injury, but can be prevented with lower tidal volumes (5-7 ml/kg) and lower plateau pressures ($\leq$ 35 cm $H_2O$). Hypercapnia and respiratory acidosis (**"permissive hypercapnia"**) may be acceptable as part of a protective ventilation strategy if $P_aCO_2$ cannot be normalized with such pressures.[67] pH as low as 7.2 is usually well tolerated but increased sedation may be needed to suppress respiratory drive.
  - High respiratory rates (>20) needed to normalize $P_aCO_2$ may also increase auto-PEEP (see page 53)
  - **PEEP** redistributes fluid from alveolar to interstitial compartments, and recruits collapsed or flooded alveoli. In ARDS, PEEP levels of 12-20 cmH$_2$O prevent recurrent collapse/reopening of alveoli, resulting in improved oxygenation and possible prevention of ventilator-associated lung injury.[68] **Caveats:**
    - PEEP may interfere with RA/LA filling, causing hypotension or tachycardia
    - In inhomogeneous lung disease (e.g. lobar pneumonia) PEEP may not improve oxygenation and may increase intrapulmonary shunt
    - Interrupting the PEEP circuit even transiently (e.g. manual bagging during transport) can cause deterioration in marginally oxygenated patients
  - To reduce pulmonary edema, titrate PCWP to minimum that achieves an adequate cardiac output
  - **Flow rate/wave-form:** Slower inspiratory flow rates (e.g. 40 L/min) and/or a decelerating wave flow pattern will increase inspiratory time and may improve oxygenation
  - If **refractory hypoxemia** consider:
    - Trial of **prone position** for 20-40 minutes (if oxygenation is improved begin regular prone positioning 2-3 hr bid-tid). Note requires team effort to avoid dislodging ETT.
    - **Pressure control ventilation** (PCV) with inverse I:E ratio (1:1 or less) - will further increase inspiratory time and possibly oxygenation)
    - Inhaled nitrous oxide
    - Recruitment maneuvers to open lung units using high pressures delivered by ventilator
    - Extracorporeal membrane oxygenation (ECMO)

## Severe airflow obstruction
- **Common clinical scenarios:** . Status asthmaticus or COPD . Thermal injury of the upper airway . Central airway obstruction by mass . Tracheal stenosis
- **Things to consider:**
  - "Permissive" hypercapnia should be tolerated to pH as low as 7.2 as part of a protective ventilation strategy. This appears preferable to gas trapping, intrinsic PEEP and high airway pressures.
  - High PIPs may be needed to allow for lower plateau pressures

---

67 ARDS Network. Ventilation with lower tidal volumes as compared to traditional tidal volumes for acute lung injury and the adult respiratory distress syndrome. NEJM 2000;342:1301-8. Steinbrook R. How best to ventilate? Trial design and patient safety in studies of the acute respiratory distress syndrome. NEJM 2003; 348:1393-1401.

68 Amato MB et al. Effect of a protective-ventilation strategy on mortality in the acute respiratory distress syndrome. NEJM 1998; 338:347-54. Amato MB et al. Beneficial effects of the "open lung approach" with low distending pressures in acute respiratory distress syndrome. A prospective randomized study on mechanical ventilation. Am J Respir Crit Care Med 1995; 152:1835-46.

. Intrinsic PEEP (**"auto-PEEP"**) reflects elevated alveolar pressure at end-expiration in severe airway obstruction. Measure at airway opening during an expiratory hold maneuver (i.e. while occluding the expiratory and inspiratory limbs of the ventilator). Intrinsic PEEP effectively raises the pressure needed to trigger ventilator, requires increased work of breathing, and potentiates muscle fatigue. Keep intrinsic PEEP < 15 cm $H_2O$ by:
- Lowering respiratory rate ($\leq$ 8/min) or lengthening expiratory time
- Increasing inspiratory flow rate (e.g. 80 L/min) to decrease inspiratory time and lengthen expiratory time
- Avoiding extrinsic PEEP and sighs, since pressures are already excessive
. Diminished venous return is common on initiation of mechanical ventilation; hypotension responds to intravascular volume expansion or temporary disconnection from ventilator
. Early sedation and muscle relaxation will decrease airway pressure, $O_2$ consumption and patient discomfort
. Refractory obstruction may respond to helium-oxygen (heliox) therapy, but this strategy is controversial in small-airways obstruction (e.g. asthma)

## Restrictive lung disease
. **Indications:** . Progressive restrictive lung (e.g. pulmonary fibrosis) or chest wall (e.g. kyphoscoliosis) disease . Rarely, massive and tense fluid collection in the abdomen or recent abdominal surgery
. **Things to consider:**
. Relieve restriction if possible (e.g. paracentesis, escharotomy)
. Upright posture may improve restriction from intra-abdominal processes
. Restriction increases risk of **(1)** reduced venous return impairing cardiac output and **(2)** increased physiologic dead space from high minute ventilation and PEEP, especially with concurrent hypovolemia

## Indications for sedation and muscle relaxation
. Patients at high-risk for ventilator-associated lung injury
. Airway disease with increased airway pressure and intrinsic PEEP (e.g. status asthmaticus)
. Hypoxemic respiratory failure and clinical instability
. Toxic $F_iO_2$ (> 0.6) despite PEEP
. Hypoxemic respiratory failure with high intrinsic PEEP and increased work of breathing
. Bronchopleural fistula in patients with chest tubes
. Control of central neurogenic hyperventilation
. Ventilatory mode that heightens patient discomfort, e.g. pressure control with inverse ratio, permissive hypercapnia

## Non-invasive ventilation [69]

- **Indications:** . Effective in acute respiratory failure due to COPD, ARDS, CHF, complications of BMT, asthma . May decrease need for endotracheal intubation, decrease mortality, and shorten ICU/hospital length of stay
- **Contraindications:** . Uncooperative patient . Impaired mental status . Hemodynamic instability . Inability to protect airway . Upper airway obstruction . Excessive secretions . Facial deformity . Absence of skilled respiratory therapist or appropriate monitoring
- **Administration:** . Usually delivered as bi-level positive airway pressure (BiPAP®) via nasal mask/pillows or full face mask . Critical care ventilator (rather than portable unit) allows higher and more precise $O_2$ delivery, higher inspiratory flow rate (improved patient comfort), and monitoring and alarms
- **Settings:** . Start with rate 10 bpm, rise time 0.4 sec, inspiratory pressure (IPAP) 8-10 cmH2O and expiratory pressure (EPAP=CPAP) 2-4 cm $H_2O$ . Titrate rate and IPAP to provide ventilation and EPAP to maintain $O_2$ sat and airway patency
- **Complications:** . Local irritation from mask . Gastric distention (rare if peak pressure < 20 cm $H_2O$)

# *Ventilator Emergencies*

## High pressure
- If $O_2Sat \leq 80\%$ or hemodynamically unstable, **disconnect from ventilator and bag @ FiO2 100%**; check for causes as per below
- If stable oxygenation and hemodynamics, check ventilator peak and plateau pressures

**Peak (PIP):** max pressure registered with each volume cycled breath
**Plateau:** pressure at end-inspiration (may use 0.5 sec "hold" to measure)

| Increased resistance<br>*Peak pressure elevated* (> 35 cm H$_2$O)<br>*Plateau pressure nml* ($\leq$ 35 cm H$_2$O) | Decreased compliance<br>*Peak and Plateau pressures<br>elevated* (> 35 cm H$_2$O) |
|---|---|
| . Endotracheal tube mucous or plugs<br>. Biting of endotracheal tube<br>. Tracheal obstruction<br>. Bronchospasm | . Tube in main stem bronchus<br>. Asynchronous breathing<br>. Auto-PEEP<br>. Atelectasis, pneumonia, CHF<br>. Pneumothorax |
| **Interventions:**<br>. Check ventilator circuit<br>. Suction<br>. Bronchodilators<br>. Reposition tube<br>. Consider bronchoscopy | **Interventions:**<br>. Stat chest x-ray to determine<br>  underlying cause<br>. Decrease auto-PEEP by<br>  decreasing tidal volume:RR ratio<br>  or temporarily disconnecting from<br>  ventilator circuit |

## Low-pressure
- If $O_2Sat \leq 80\%$ or hemodynamically unstable, **disconnect from ventilator and bag @ FiO2 100%**
- **Causes:**
  - . Endotracheal tube slipped out of trachea→ reintubate
  - . Cuff leak → instill more air into cuff or reintubate
  - . Tracheoesophageal fistula → attempt to reposition tube
  - . Leak within mechanical ventilator circuit

69 Hillberg RE, Johnson DC. Noninvasive ventilation. *NEJM* 1997; 337(24):1/46-52. Brochard L. Noninvasive ventilation for acute respiratory failure. *JAMA* 2002; 288:932-5. Hess DR, Kacmarek RM. *Essentials of Mechanical Ventilation.* McGraw-Hill, New York, 1996.

# Weaning from Mechanical Ventilation

## Optimize before extubation
- Withdraw sedative drugs
- Ensure adequate rest and nutrition
- Prepare patient psychologically
- Diurese to minimize pulmonary edema
- Treat bronchospasm
- Minimize secretions
- Normalize electrolytes affecting muscle function e.g. $PO_4$, $Mg^{++}$, $Ca^{++}$
- Suppress fever with antipyretics
- Treat systemic illness (e.g. infections)
- Institute effective antianginal therapy
- Exclude drug-induced neuromuscular blockade (e.g. aminoglycosides)

## Criteria for starting weaning [70]
- Cause of respiratory failure improved
- Adequate oxygenation: $PaO_2 \geq 60$ mm Hg on $FiO_2 \leq 0.4$ ($PaO_2/FiO_2$ = 150-300) with PEEP $\leq 5$ cm $H_2O$
- Hemodynamic stability: No myocardial ischemia or hypotension
- Temperature < 38° C
- Hemoglobin $\geq$ 8-10 g/dl
- Patient awake or easily aroused

## Predicting successful extubation [71]
- Rapid shallow breathing index (RSBI = respiratory rate÷tidal volume) < 105 during T-piece trial best predicts successful weaning [72]
- Higher values may be compatible with weaning in certain populations (e.g. small, elderly women [73]) or if clinical judgment predicts success

## Conducting a trial of spontaneous breathing
- Give 30 minute trial of T-tube or pressure support ventilation of 7 ± 3 cm $H_2O$
- Consider adding CPAP (5 cm $H_2O$) for patients with obstruction (asthma, COPD)
- Successful trial:
  - $O_2$sat > 90 % or $PaO_2$ > 60 mmHg on $FiO_2$ < 0.4-0.5
  - Increase in $PaCO_2$ < 10 mmHg or decrease in pH < 0.10
  - Respiratory rate < 35
  - RSBI (RR÷TV) <100-105
  - HR < 140 or increased < 20% from baseline
  - SBP 80-160 mmHg or changes < 20% from baseline
  - No signs of increased work of breathing (paradoxical breathing, accessory muscle use) or other signs of distress (diaphoresis, agitation)
- If successful, proceed with extubation
- If unsuccessful, repeat trial daily and gradually withdraw ventilator support (pressure support and T-piece weaning equally efficacious and superior to IMV wean) [74]

70 Frutos-Vivar F, Esteban A. When to wean from a ventilator: An evidence-based strategy. Cleve Clin J Med 2003; 70:389, 392-3
71 Alia I, Esteban A. Weaning from mechanical ventilation. Crit Care 2000; 4:72-80.
72 Yang KL, Tobin MJ. A prospective trial of indexes predicting the outcome of trials of weaning from mechanical ventilation. NEJM 1991; 324:1445-50.
73 Krieger B et al. Serial measurements of the rapid shallow breathing index as a predictor of outcome in elderly medical patients. Chest 1997; 112: 1029-34
74 Esteban A et al. A comparison of four methods of weaning patients from mechanical ventilation. NEJM 1995;332(6):345-50. Esteban A et al. Extubation outcome after spontaneous breathing trials with T-tube or pressure support ventilation. Am J Rep Crit Care Med 1997; 156: 459-65.

# Endocrinology

## *Thyroid Function In Critical Illness* [75]

**Thyroid function tests**

| TSH | Free T4 * | Free T3 * | Interpretation |
|---|---|---|---|
| Nml | Nml | - | Thyroid disease excluded |
| ↓ | Nml | ↓ or Nml | Non-thyroid illness (most common, esp. if TSH > 0.1 μU/mL) vs. subclinical hyperthyroidism(less common) |
| ↓ | ↑ | ↓,↑, or Nml | Non-thyroid illness vs. primary thyrotoxicosis. NTI more likely if free T3 is normal-low and sx are absent. |
| ↓ | Nml | ↑ | T3 thyrotoxicosis |
| ↓ | ↓ | ↓ | Non-thyroid illness (most common) vs. central hypothyroidism (rare) |
| ↑ | Nml | ↓ or Nml | Recovery phase of non-thyroid illness (common)vs. subclinical hypothyroidism (more likely if pattern found early in critical illness) |
| ↑ | ↓ | ↓ - Nml | Primary hypothyroidism |
| ↑-Nml | ↑ | ↑ | Central hyperthyroidism (very rare) |

* Direct measurement or calculated index     Nml = normal

**Non-thyroid illness ("sick euthyroid state")**
- Most common cause of abnormal thyroid function in hospitalized patients (accounts for 80% of abnormal TSH levels)
- TSH usually low-normal, but may rise during recovery phase of illness
- Free and total T4 initially rise (decreased peripheral conversion and increased binding proteins) but become subnormal during severe or prolonged illness
- Total and free T3 characteristically fall due to decreased peripheral conversion
- No apparent benefit to supplementation with levothyroxine or liothyronine

**Etiology of abnormal TSH levels in hospitalized patients** [76]

| TSH level (μU/mL) | Thyroid Disease | NTI * | Glucocorticoid Rx |
|---|---|---|---|
| < 0.1 | 24 % | 41 % | 35 % |
| 0.1-0.34 | 0 % | 73 % | 27 % |
| 0.35-6.8 | - | - | - |
| 6.9-20 | 14 % | 72 % | 14 % |
| > 20 | 50 % | 45 % | 5 % |

* NTI = non-thyroid illness ("sick euthyroid")

**Non-thyroid causes of abnormal TSH**

| Decreased | Increased |
|---|---|
| Acute or chronic illness | Recovery phase of acute illness |
| Glucocorticoids | Cimetidine |
| Caloric restriction | Dopamine antagonists |
| Dopamine or adrenergic agonists | Neuroleptics |
| Opiates | Metoclopramide |
| Phenytoin | |

75 Farwell AP. Sick euthyroid syndrome in the intensive care unit. In: *Irwin and Rippe's Intensive Care Medicine*, 5th ed. Irwin RS, Rippe JM, editors. Philadelphia: Lippincott Williams & Wilkins, 2003.
76 Spencer CA. Clinical utility and cost effectiveness of sensitive thyrotropin assays in ambulatory and hospitalized patients. *Mayo Clin Proc* 1988; 63:1214-22.

# *Myxedema Coma* [77]

## Etiology
- **Underlying thyroid disease**: ◆ Autoimmune ◆ Previous thyroid surgery or ablation (check for neck scars or history of $^{131}I$ administration) ◆ Occasionally caused by 2° hypothyroidism (↓TSH) or drugs (amiodarone, lithium)
- **Acute precipitants:** ◆ Hypothermia (most cases in winter) ◆ Stroke ◆ MI ◆ Infection ◆ Drugs: anesthetics, sedatives, narcotics ◆ Trauma ◆ GI bleed

## Manifestations:
- **Hypothermia:** Mortality increases as temperature falls
- **Neurologic:** ◆ Lethargy→ stupor→ coma (↑ mortality if ↓ consciousness) ◆ "Myxedema madness": depression, paranoia, hallucinations ◆ Hyporeflexia
- **Respiratory:** ◆ ↓ Hypoxic drive → hypoventilation→ hypercapnia ◆ Pleural effusions ◆ Airway obstruction from macroglossia and myxedema infiltrate
- **Cardiac:** ◆ Bradycardia ◆ Hypotension ◆ Pericardial effusion ± tamponade ◆ Systolic/diastolic dysfunction ◆ ECG: block, ↓ voltage, ↑ QT
- **Renal:** ◆ Hyponatremia (impaired water excretion) ◆ Intravascular vol contraction

## Management
- Replace **thyroid hormone**. Give IV initially (PO absorption ↓ from gut edema). Reduce dose if elderly or cardiac ischemia. No randomized studies clarifying optimal preparation and dose. Options: **(1) Levothyroxine (T4):** $T_{1/2}$ ~ 7d, must be converted to T3 for activity. Load 300-600 mcg IV then 50-100 mcg qd. **(2) Liothyronine (T3):** Active hormone, $T_{1/2}$ ~ 1d. Controversial; high doses associated with increased mortality. Rationale for use includes slow-onset of T4 monotherapy and inhibition of T4→T3 conversion by concurrent non-thyroid illness. Load 10-20 mcg PO/IV, then 10 mcg q4-6h until clinical improvement. [78] Doses as low as 2.5 mcg appear to reverse metabolic abnormalities. **(3) Dual therapy:** Give T4 at slightly reduced dose (4 mcg/kg) plus T3 as above
- Concurrent **adrenal insufficiency** common (5-10%) → Initial stress dose IV glucocorticoids (draw cortisol level beforehand or use dexamethasone and perform ACTH stimulation test)
- Expedite mechanical ventilation for **respiratory failure** (progresses rapidly, with high risk for aspiration). Upper airway obstruction possible.
- If **hypotensive** give adequate volume prior to adding vasopressors (dopamine preferred over pure $\alpha$-agonists). Consider tamponade or adrenal insufficiency for refractory hypotension.
- **Hypothermia:** Re-warm passively with blankets and warm room; active re-warming may cause distributive shock
- **Hyponatremia:** Usually corrects with levothyroxine therapy. Avoid rapid correction and use of hypertonic saline unless Na < 120 mEq/L and/or symptoms.
- Search for precipitant; consider empiric antimicrobial therapy
- Adjust drug dosing for reduced drug metabolism

---

77 Wartovsky L. Myxedema coma. In: *Werner and Ingbar's Thyroid: a Fundamental and Clinical Text*, 8<sup>th</sup> ed. Braverman LE, Utiger RD (eds). Philadelphia : Lippincott; 2000; Emerson CH. Myxedema Coma. In: *Irwin and Rippe's Intensive Care Medicine*, 5th ed. Irwin RS, Rippe JM, editors. Philadelphia: Lippincott Williams & Wilkins, 2003.

78 MacKerrow SD et al. Myxedema-associated cardiogenic shock treated with intravenous triiodothyronine. *Ann Intern Med* 1992;117(12):1014-5.

# Thyroid Storm [79]

## Etiology
- **Underlying thyrotoxicosis**: Usually Grave's disease ◆ Other: acute thyroiditis, toxic multinodular goiter, jod-basedow (iodine-induced), factitious (ingestion of thyroxine)
- **Acute precipitants**: Infection ◆ Surgery or trauma ◆ Iodine load ([131]I-therapy, contrast dye, kelp, amiodarone) ◆ Childbirth ◆ Thyroid manipulation or surgery ◆ Psychiatric stress ◆ Withdrawal of antithyroid drugs ◆ Diabetic ketoacidosis ◆ Pulmonary embolism ◆ Stroke ◆ Sympathomimetic drugs (pseudoephedrine)

## Features
- **General**: Fever, tachycardia, diaphoresis (out of proportion to apparent infection)
- **Cardiopulmonary**: ↑ Metabolic demand, ↑ $O_2$ consumption, ↑ cardiac output ◆ Hyperdynamic circulation→ high-output CHF ◆ Myocardial ischemia ◆ Arrhythmias (usually SVT, esp. AF) ◆ Systolic HTN with widened pulse pressure
- **Neurologic**: ◆ Delirium, stupor or coma, seizures ◆ Myopathy > 50% ◆ Ophthalmopathy (Grave's) ◆ Rare complications: aggravated myasthenia gravis or thyrotoxic hypokalemic periodic paralysis (Asian men)
- **GI**: ◆ Vomiting, diarrhea, malabsorption ◆ ↑Gastrin → PUD ◆ Abnormal LFTs
- **Labs**: ↑ glucose, ↑ WBC, ↓ Hct, ↓ platelets, ↓ $K^+$, ↑ $Ca^{2+}$ (may be severe), ↑LFTs

## Treatment
1) **Antithyroid treatment** – effective for hyperfunctioning gland (e.g. Grave's) but not thyroiditis or exogenous thyroid hormone
   - Inhibit new hormone synthesis with **propylthiouracil** (PTU; 200-250 mg PO/NG q4hr) or **methimazole** (20 mg PO/NG q 4 hr). PTU preferred because it blocks peripheral T4→T3 conversion. IV form not available in U.S.; may give as retention enema.
   - Inhibit hormone secretion with **iodine**: SSKI or Lugol's solution (8 gtts PO q 6 hr). **Caution:** Use at least 2 hr after methimazole or PTU (iodine monotherapy can exacerbate thyrotoxicosis). **Iodine allergy:** Lithium carbonate 300 mg PO q 6 hr to keep lithium level ~ 1mEq/L
2) **Block peripheral action and conversion of thyroid hormone**
   - β-adrenergic blockade, e.g. **propranolol** (0.5-1 mg IV/min to total of 2-10 mg, titrated to heart rate; then 20-80 mg PO q4-6 hr)
   - Inhibit peripheral T4→T3 conversion with oral iodinated contrast agent e.g. **iopanoate** (Telepaque®) 1 gm × 8 hr PO load then 500 mg bid) and/or glucocorticoids e.g. **dexamethasone** (2 mg IV/PO q 6 hr) or **hydrocortisone** (100 mg IV q 8 hr). β-blockers & PTU also block T4→T3. High iodine content in iopanoate may substitute for SSKI or Lugol's.
   - If intractable symptoms consider dialysis or plasmapheresis; or enteric binding of thyroid hormone with cholestyramine (4 g PO q 6hr)
3) **Treat underlying illness**, e.g. occult infection, CHF, diabetic ketoacidosis, etc.
4) **General supportive care**
   - Control hyperthermia with acetaminophen, cooling blankets
   - Fluid resuscitation + dextrose for diaphoresis, vomiting, diarrhea, hypoglycemia
   - Parenteral vitamin supplements (e.g. B-complex)
   - Consider empiric glucocorticoids if adrenal insufficiency suspected

---

79  Wartowsky L. Myxedema coma In: *Werner and Ingbar's Thyroid: a Fundamental and Clinical Text*, 8th ed. Braverman LE, Utiger RD (eds). Philadelphia : Lippincott, 2000; Safran MS *et al.* Thyroid storm. In: *Irwin and Rippe's Intensive Care Medicine*, 5th ed. Irwin RS, Rippe JM, editors. Philadelphia: Lippincott Williams & Wilkins, 2003.

# Hyperglycemic Crisis [80]

| Features | Diabetic ketoacidosis (DKA) | Hyperosmolar hyper-glycemic state (HHS) |
|----------|------------------------------|------------------------------------------|
| Type of diabetes | 1 > 2 | 1 << 2 |
| Evolution | Hours to days | Days to weeks |
| Dehydration | Mild-moderate | Moderate to severe |
| Plasma glucose | > 250; usually < 800 | > 600; can be > 1000 |
| Arterial pH | mild 7.25-7.3<br>moderate 7.00-7.24<br>severe < 7.0 | > 7.3<br>(50% have mild anion gap) |
| Serum $HCO_3^-$ (mEq/L) | mild 15-18<br>moderate 10-15<br>severe < 10 | > 15 |
| Ketones | Positive | Trace |
| Serum osmolarity | Variable (usually < 320 mOsm/kg) | > 320 mOsm/kg |
| Stupor or coma | Variable based on severity | Common (25-50% of cases) |
| Mortality | < 5% | 15% |

**Precipitating factors**
- Infection (30-60% of cases) • New onset diabetes (20-25% of DKA)
- Non-compliance or inadequate treatment (15-20% of DKA) • Stroke • MI
- Pancreatitis • Alcohol abuse • Drugs (steroids, thiazide, sympathomimetics)
- Inadequate access to fluids (HHS)

**Clinical manifestations**
- **Symptoms:** • Polyuria/dipsia • Weight loss • Weakness • N/V • Abdominal pain (up to 50% of DKA) • Lethargy • Confusion
- **Signs:** • Poor skin turgor • Kussmaul's respiration (DKA) • Altered mental status (look for other cause if serum osm < 320 mOsm/kg)
- **Labs:** • ↑ anion gap (DKA) • ↑ serum osmolarity • ↑ WBC • ↑ amylase in absence of pancreatitis • Na⁺ and K⁺ variable (Na⁺ falls 1 mEq/L for every 40-60 mg/dl increase in glucose)

**Management**
- Seek precipitating cause.
- **Fluids:** Volume deficit averages 3-6 L in DKA and 8-10 L in HHS.
  - Give 1 L NS within first hour.
  - Subsequent fluid therapy geared toward correction of volume deficit and volume expansion to enhance renal clearance of ketones (DKA). Typical fluid rates are 500 mL/hr x 2-4 hr then 250 mL/hr if mild-moderate deficit; 750-1000 mL/hr x 2-4 hr then 500 mL/hr in hypovolemic shock.
  - After initial volume expansion, assess "corrected" serum sodium (add 1.6 x [Glucose − 100] to measured sodium), serum osmolarity and volume status. If corrected sodium normal or elevated, change fluid to 0.45% NaCl. If corrected sodium low or patient in hypovolemic shock, continue 0.9% NaCl.

80 Kitabchi AE et al. Hyperglycemic crises in patients with diabetes mellitus. *Diabetes Care* 2003; 26 Suppl 1:S109-17. Ennis ED, Kreisberg, RA. Diabetic ketoacidosis and the hyperglycemic hyperosmolar syndrome. In: *Diabetes Mellitus : A Fundamental and Clinical Text*, 3rd ed. LeRoith D et al. editors. Philadelphia: Lippincott Williams & Wilkins, 2003.

- **Insulin**
  - Start with 10 unit IV bolus followed by IV infusion at 0.1 unit/kg/hr.
  - Re-bolus and double rate if glucose does not fall 50-100 mg/dl per hour.
  - Continuous insulin necessary to correct acidosis even after glucose normalizes; when glucose is < 250 mg/dL (DKA) or < 300 mg/dL (HHS), **continue** insulin at lower rate (0.05-0.1 unit/kg/hr) but add D5 to IV fluids to keep glucose 200-250 mg/dL.
  - Subcutaneous short-acting insulin should be given at least one hour before insulin infusion discontinued.
- **Potassium**: Total body depleted but serum levels variable.
  - Add 20-40 mEq KCl to each liter IV fluids once serum K+ < 5.0 mEq/L, as long as urine output is adequate
  - If K+ < 4.0 mEq/L, add 40-60 mEq KCl to each liter IV fluids
  - If K+ < 3.5 mEq/l, give KCl prior to insulin

> **Pearls and nonsense**
> - Mild ketosis is common in HHS and does not indicate DKA. However, ketoacidosis and hyperosmolar state may co-exist in same patient.
> - The goal of therapy is to eliminate acidosis (DKA) and restore normal volume and osmolarity, not to correct glucose.
> - Urine and blood ketone levels fluctuate during illness and correlate poorly with response to treatment.
> - Presenting K+ levels vary, but total body K+ depletion is the rule.

- **Bicarbonate**: Indicated only for severe acidosis (pH < 7.0) or symptomatic hyperkalemia.
  - Give 50-100 mEq $NaHCO_3^-$ diluted in 200-400 mL sterile water with goal of raising pH to 7.15-7.20.
- **Phosphate**: Total body depletion, serum levels variable.
  - However, no value to repletion unless cardiac dysfunction, respiratory depression or serum level < 1.0 mg/dL.
- **Lab monitoring**: • Glucose every 1-2 hr • Electrolytes, $PO_4$ and venous pH (~0.03 units < arterial pH) every 2-6 hours

## Complications
- Hypoglycemia (overdose of insulin) or rebound hyperglycemia (insulin discontinued too soon)
- Profound hypokalemia or hypophosphatemia
- Hyperchloremic (non-anion gap) acidosis following fluid resuscitation
- Non-cardiogenic pulmonary edema from volume overload
- Cerebral edema: Common in first presentation of DKA or in HHS, especially if volume and sodium deficits repleted too rapidly (> 3 mOsm/kg/hr). Mortality > 70% if early signs not detected.

## Glycemic control in critical illness [81]
Reduced morbidity and mortality seen with intensive insulin therapy in post-operative patients, critically ill medical patients and acute MI. Possible mechanism includes tight glycemic control versus anabolic effects of insulin. *For sample intensive insulin protocol see page 192*

---

81   Van den Berghe G *et al*. Intensive insulin therapy in critically ill patients. *NEJM* 2001; 345:1359-1367. Krinsley JS. Association between hyperglycemia and increased hospital mortality in a heterogeneous population of critically ill patients. *Mayo Clin Proc* 2003; 78:1471-8.

# Adrenal Crisis [82]

## Setting
- Sudden extensive adrenal destruction (e.g. hemorrhage or infarction) **or**
- Major physiologic stress (e.g. surgery, infection, trauma) in patient with unrecognized primary adrenal insufficiency **or**
- Inadequate "stress dose" corticosteroids in a patient with known or suspected adrenal insufficiency (e.g. chronic corticosteroid treatment, even at low doses)
- Uncommon in secondary or tertiary (central) adrenal insufficiency because of preserved mineralocorticoid homeostasis. However, severe or sudden pituitary dysfunction (e.g. hemorrhage) may produce hypotension on basis of glucocorticoid deficiency (mineralocorticoid → intravascular volume; glucocorticoid → vascular tone)
- Septic shock itself may cause relative (reversible) adrenal insufficiency

## Etiology of adrenal insufficiency
- **Bilateral adrenal destruction:** • Hemorrhagic (often occult): anticoagulation, coagulopathy, postoperative • Thrombotic: adrenal vein thrombosis after back injury, thrombotic microangiopathy (DIC, HIT) • Metastatic tumor
- **Sepsis:** Meningococcemia (Waterhouse-Friderichsen), *Pseudomonas*
- **Autoimmune adrenalitis:** Idiopathic vs. polyglandular failure syndrome
- **Granulomatous infection:** Tuberculosis, histoplasmosis, other fungi
- **HIV:** HIV itself, CMV, MAC
- **Drugs:** Adrenal suppression (corticosteroids, megestrol, medroxyprogesterone acetate) • Inhibition of cortisol synthesis (ketoconazole, etomidate) • Accelerated cortisol degradation (phenytoin, rifampin, barbiturates)
- **Pituitary apoplexy:** Secondary insufficiency (i.e. glucocorticoid only)

## Manifestations
- **Shock:** Both hypovolemic and distributive. Often out of proportion to severity of acute illness and refractory to fluids and pressors until adrenal hormone replacement given.
- **GI symptoms:** Nausea and vomiting, anorexia; abdominal pain (may mimic acute abdomen)
- **Fever:** Accentuated by low cortisol but occult infection common
- **CNS:** Lethargy, confusion, coma
- **Physical/radiologic findings:** Hyperpigmentation of mucosae, creases, and sun-spared skin (1° insufficiency only) • Small cardiac silhouette on CXR • Calcified or enlarged adrenals on CT
- **Labs:** ↓$Na^+$, ↑$K^+$ (↓aldo), ↑BUN/Cr, ↓glucose, ↑$Ca^{++}$, eosinophilia
- **Secondary adrenal insufficiency** differs in that • ACTH low-normal • No hyperpigmentation • Mineralocorticoid activity preserved (no hyperkalemia) • Hyponatremia from centrally increased ADH • Hypoglycemia common

---

82 Orth DN et al. The adrenal cortex. In: Wilson JD, Foster DW (eds). *Williams Textbook of Endocrinology*, 9th ed. Philadelphia: Saunders, 1998. Longcope CN, Aronin N. Hypoadrenal crisis. In: *Irwin and Rippe's Intensive Care Medicine*, 5th ed. Irwin RS, Rippe JM, editors. Philadelphia: Lippincott Williams & Wilkins, 2003.

## Diagnosis

- **High dose ACTH (cosyntropin) stimulation**: [83] Give 250 mcg IV. Cortisol ≥ 18-21 mcg/dL at baseline or within 60 minutes of injection is highly accurate at ruling out chronic, severe adrenal insufficiency. However, criteria may miss partial or recent onset insufficiency, especially in critically ill patients.
- **Random cortisol level**: [84] In patients with critical illness (especially septic shock), relative adrenal insufficiency may occur and contribute to hypotension, etc. Random cortisol level < 15 mcg/dL is clearly abnormal in critical illness, while random cortisol level > 34 mcg/dL is clearly sufficient. If random cortisol is 15-34 mcg/dL, check ACTH stimulation and consider abnormal if incremental response is < 9 mcg/dL.
- **ACTH level:** Used to differentiate primary (ACTH >> normal) vs. secondary or tertiary disease (ACTH low-normal). Check random sample prior to empiric corticosteroids.

## Therapy

1) Rapid **volume resuscitation** (30-50% of normal intravascular volume, typically 2-3 L NS) titrated to JVP or pulmonary edema. Replace K, glucose prn.
2) Draw baseline cortisol and ACTH level
3) **Dexamethasone** (4 mg IV) to restore vascular tone (will not interfere with ACTH stimulation test)
4) Perform ACTH stimulation test
5) Start **hydrocortisone** 100 mg IV q 6-8h. Taper gradually (e.g. 50% per day) after stabilized. Separate mineralocorticoid repletion not required acutely, but fludrocortisone should be added when total daily hydrocortisone < 100 mg/day.
6) Identify and treat precipitating illness
7) If primary adrenal insufficiency, will need chronic repletion with hydrocortisone (typically 20 mg q AM, 10 mg q PM) and fludrocortisone (0.1 mg qd, titrated to K⁺).

---

[83] Dorin RI *et al.* Diagnosis of adrenal insufficiency. *Ann Intern Med* 2003; 139:194-204.
[84] Annane D *et al.* Effect of treatment with low doses of hydrocortisone and fludrocortisone on mortality in patients with septic shock. *JAMA* 2002; 288:862-871; Cooper MS, Stewart PM. Corticosteroid insufficiency in acutely ill patients. *NEJM* 2003; 348:727-734.

# Hypocalcemia

## Etiology

| | |
|---|---|
| Pseudo-hypocalcemia | • $Ca^{++} \downarrow 0.8$ mg/dl for each 1.0 g/dl $\downarrow$ in serum albumin<br>• Ionized (i.e. biologically active) calcium unaffected |
| Calcium sequestration | • $\uparrow PO_4$ (renal failure, rhabdomyolysis, tumor lysis)<br>• Pancreatitis<br>• Widespread osteoblastic metastasis<br>• "Hungry bone" syndrome after correction of hyperparathyroidism, hyperthyroidism or prolonged metabolic acidosis<br>• Intravascular binding: citrate (banked blood), lactate or lactic acidosis, foscarnet, EDTA, respiratory alkalosis ($\uparrow$ albumin binding) |
| $\downarrow$PTH secretion | • Post-surgical (parathyroidectomy, thyroidectomy, radical neck resection) or XRT<br>• Autoimmune<br>• $\downarrow Mg^{++}$ (< 0.8 mEq/L) or severe $\uparrow Mg^{++}$ (> 5 mEq/L)<br>• HIV<br>• Infiltrative disease (hemachromatosis, metastases) |
| $\downarrow$PTH action | • Congenital (pseudohypoparathyroidism)<br>• $\downarrow Mg^{++}$ (ethanol, diarrhea, diuretics, aminoglycosides) |
| $\downarrow$25-OH vitamin D | • Poor intake or malabsorption<br>• Inadequate sunlight<br>• Liver disease<br>• Anticonvulsants |
| $\downarrow$1,25-OH vitamin D | • Kidney disease |
| Miscellaneous | • Sepsis or toxic shock syndrome<br>• Post-surgical<br>• Fluoride |

## Manifestations

- **Neuromuscular**: Generalized irritability (twitching, paresthesias) progressing to frank tetany (carpopedal spasm, laryngospasm); Trousseau's and Chvostek's signs. Tetany exacerbated by alkalosis, $\downarrow Mg^{++}$, $\downarrow K^+$.
- **CNS**: Fatigue or lethargy; emotional irritability; generalized seizures; papilledema
- **Cardiac**: Prolonged QT (with narrow T); heart block; hypotension; myocardial dysfunction

## Treatment of acute symptomatic hypocalcemia

1) Confirm true hypocalcemia by checking ionized $Ca^{++}$ or correcting for albumin
2) If etiology unclear draw pre-treatment creatinine, $PO_4$, albumin, PTH, 25-OH vitamin D (**not** 1,25-OH vitamin D unless renal disease)
3) In **symptomatic** hypocalcemia, give 1-2 amps 10% **calcium gluconate** (93 mg elemental $Ca^{++}$/10 ml) ) IV in 50-100 ml D5W. Then start drip of 10 amps Ca gluconate in 1 liter D5W at 50 ml/hour. Titrate drip to low-normal serum calcium. Calcium chloride IV used less frequently; must be given via central line. Start oral calcium 500-1000 mg po qid when patient stable.
4) If magnesium deficiency suspected, give empiric infusion of **magnesium sulfate** (2 grams IV over 1 hour) unless serum level elevated, e.g. renal failure
5) If vitamin D deficiency, start 1,25-OH vitamin D (calcitriol) 0.25 mcg po qd x 1 week, then switch to non-hydoxylated form for chronic therapy. Monitor 25(OH)-vitamin D levels.
6) If inadequate 1-alpha hydroxylation (renal failure, PTH deficiency or resistance), start 1,25-OH vitamin D (calcitriol) 0.25 mcg PO qd.

# Hypercalcemia [85]

**Etiology:** 90% of cases caused by **malignancy** (most common in inpatients) and **primary hyperparathyroidism** (most common in outpatients)

| | |
|---|---|
| **Malignancy** | • Usually clinically apparent primary (myeloma, breast, lung, head/neck, renal cell, bladder most common)<br>• Three mechanisms: **(1)** diffuse skeletal metastases **(2)** ectopic production of PTH-like protein (PTH-rP) **(3)** elevated vitamin D metabolites (lymphoma) |
| **Hyperparathyroidism** | • Primary (adenoma, MEN syndrome)<br>• Chronic renal failure with 3° hyperparathyroidism |
| **↑ Vitamin D** | • 25-OH vitamin D: dietary supplements<br>• 1,25-OH vitamin D: granulomatous disease (sarcoid, TB), lymphoma, meds (calcitriol) |
| **Skeletal mobilization** | • Immobilization<br>• Multiple fractures |
| **Medications** | • HCTZ • Lithium • Vitamin A intoxication<br>• Antacids (Milk-alkali syndrome) |
| **Miscellaneous** | • Pheochromocytoma<br>• Adrenal insufficiency<br>• Thyrotoxicosis<br>• Rhabdomyolysis with renal failure<br>• Pseudohypercalcemia (normal ionized calcium but elevated bound fraction to albumin or paraproteins) |

## Manifestations
- **CNS:** confusion, lethargy, psychosis, coma
- **GI:** constipation, anorexia, pancreatitis
- **Cardiac:** ↓ QT, ↑ PR and QRS, ↑QRS voltage, T-wave flattening and widening, notching of QRS, A-V block, cardiac arrest ($Ca^{++}$> 15 mEq/L)
- **Renal:** volume depletion, renal insufficiency, stones, distal RTA

## Treatment of acute symptomatic hypercalcemia
1) Diagnostic studies: ionized calcium, $PO_4$, creatinine, intact PTH, 1,25-OH and 25-OH vitamin D levels
2) Promote urinary calcium excretion with aggressive **saline** infusion (NS 250 mL/hr IV); when volume deficit is repleted follow with loop diuretic (e.g. **furosemide** 20-40 mg IV q2-4 hr) to maintain euvolemia. Initial effect within 2-4 hr. **Dialysis** indicated if intolerance to fluids due to renal insufficiency or CHF.
3) Inhibit bone resorption with **zoledronate** 4 mg IV over 15 minutes or **pamidronate** 60-90 mg IV infused over 4 hr. Onset of action 1-2 days with maximum effect in 4-6 days.
4) For severe hypercalcemia give **calcitonin** 4 units/kg IV q 12 hr x 4 doses; effective within 4-6 hr but tachyphylaxis usually develops over 2-3 days
5) IV glucocorticoids (e.g. **prednisone** 20-40 mg qd) beneficial if hypercalcemia due to lymphoma or granulomatous disease
6) Inhibit GI absorption of calcium with oral PO4 500 mg PO qid (but risk of ectopic calcification if serum PO4 is raised in setting of hypercalcemia)
7) Consider **gallium nitrate** for refractory hypercalcemia (effective but significant toxicities)

---

[85] Bilezekian JP. Management of acute hypercalcemia. *NEJM* 1992; 326:1196-12

# Gastroenterology

## Upper GI Hemorrhage [86]

### Diagnosis
- **Stool color:** [87] 14% of UGI bleeds present with hematochezia (bright red blood per rectum or maroon stool) • Patients with hematochezia have significantly higher transfusion requirements, need for surgery and mortality (14 vs. 8%) compared with melena or brown stool
- **Nasogastric (NG) aspirate:** 90% sensitive in localizing bleeding to UGI tract (high neg predictive value if non-bloody bile in NG aspirate) • No value to large volume lavage • Mortality: clear (6%) < coffee grounds (10%) < red blood (18%)

### Prognosis
- **Pre-endoscopy:** Low risk of rebleeding/complications if **all** of following present: [88]
  - BUN < 18 mg/dl • SBP ≥ 110 mmHg • HR < 100 bpm
  - Hgb > 13 mg/dL (men) or 12 mg/dL (women)
- **Post-endoscopy**

| Re-bleeding risk based on endoscopic findings [89] | | | |
|---|---|---|---|
| **Low Risk** | **Moderate Risk** | **High Risk** | **Highest Risk** |
| • PUD–no SRH<br>• Mallory-Weiss tear, non-bleeding<br>• Erosive disease<br>• Normal | • PUD - black spot or clot<br>• Erosive disease with SRH<br>• Angiodysplasia | • PUD – non-bleeding visible vessel<br>• PUD – other SRH | • Active UGI bleeding<br>• Varices<br>• Malignant lesion |

M-W= Mallory-Weiss   PUD= peptic ulcer disease   SRH= stigmata of recent hemorrhage

| Rockall scoring system [90] | | | | |
|---|---|---|---|---|
| **Score** | **0** | **1** | **2** | **3** |
| **Age (yrs)** | < 60 | 60-79 | ≥ 80 | n/a |
| **Shock** | HR < 100<br>SBP ≥ 100 | HR ≥ 100<br>SBP ≥ 100 | SBP < 100 | n/a |
| **Co-morbidity** | None | n/a | CAD, CHF, other major co-morbidity | Renal failure, liver failure, metastatic ca |
| **Endoscopic Diagnosis** | M-W lesion<br>No lesion/no SRH | All other diagnoses | Malignant lesion of UGIT | n/a |
| **Stigmata of recent hemorrhage** | None or dark spot in ulcer base | n/a | Blood in UGIT, adherent clot, visible vessel | n/a |

SRH= stigmata of recent hemorrhage      UGIT=Upper GI Tract

86  Peter DJ, Dougherty JM. Evaluation of the patient with gastrointestinal bleeding: An evidence based approach. Emerg Med Clin North Am 1999; 17:239-61. Barkun A et al. Consensus recommendations for managing patients with nonvariceal upper gastrointestinal bleeding. Ann Intern Med 2003; 139:843 -857.

87  Wilcox CM et al. A prospective characterization of upper gastrointestinal hemorrhage presenting with hematochezia. Am J Gastro 1997; 92(2): 231-5.

88  Blatchford O et al. A risk score to predict need for treatment for upper-gastrointestinal haemorrhage. Lancet 2000; 356:1318-21.

89  Hay JA et al. Prospective evaluation of a clinical guideline recommending hospital length of stay in upper gastrointestinal tract hemorrhage. JAMA 1997; 278: 2151-56.

90  Rockall TA et al. Selection of patients for early discharge or outpatient care after acute upper gastrointestinal hemorrhage. Lancet 1996; 347: 1138-40.

| Rockall score | % of Patients | Re-bleeding Rate | Mortality | Mortality in patients with re-bleeding |
|---|---|---|---|---|
| 0-2 | 29 % | 4.3 % | 0.1 % | n/a |
| 3-4 | 34 % | 13 % | 3 % | 12 % |
| 5 | 15 % | 17 % | 8 % | 21 % |
| 6 | 9 % | 29 % | 15 % | 29 % |
| 7 | 8 % | 40 % | 20 % | 35 % |
| ≥8 | 5 % | 48 % | 40 % | 53 % |

## Treatment
- **Supportive:** 70-85% of patients stop bleeding without specific treatment
- **Acid suppression:** $H_2$ blockers do not alter course or prognosis • High-dose proton pump inhibitors improve outcomes in moderate risk patients not treated with endoscopic therapy and reduce re-bleeding rate after endoscopic therapy [91]
- **Other medical therapy:** *H. pylori* testing and treatment (see page 67) • Somatostatin and octreotide not indicated in routine management of bleeding, but maybe useful for uncontrolled bleeding in patients awaiting endoscopy or surgery, or in whom surgery is contraindicated
- **Endoscopic therapy:** [92] Not required in majority of patients, but provides valuable prognostic data and may shorten hospitalization • In high risk patients (e.g. bloody NG aspirate) early endoscopic therapy reduces complications (re-bleeding, transfusion, surgery) and possibly mortality • In patients who bleed after initial endoscopic therapy, repeat endoscopic therapy preferable to surgery [93]
- **Surgery:** Required in about 6% of all patients and ¼ of those who re-bleed after initial endoscopic therapy

## Variceal bleeding [94]
- **Prognosis:** • 35-80% of patients with portal hypertension develop varices • 25-35% of patients with varices bleed within 1 yr of diagnosis • 30-50% mortality during first bleeding episode • 70% of patients who survive first bleed will re-bleed, most within 6 months • Mortality rate remains 30-35% for each additional episode of bleeding
- **Treatment:**
  1) Volume resuscitation with saline and PRBC
  2) Platelet transfusion if < 50 K
  3) Correct coagulopathy with vitamin K and FFP
  4) Adequate airway control prior to endoscopy
  5) Octreotide (see Groovy Drugs, page 203)
  6) Transjugular intrahepatic portosystemic shunting (TIPS procedure) should be considered for refractory bleeding
  7) Surgical shunts typically reserved for non-transplant candidates
- **Prevention:** Risk of recurrent bleeding significantly reduced by non-selective β-blocker (propranolol or nadolol, titrated to HR 50-60 bpm or 25% ↓ in baseline HR) or variceal band ligation • Non-selective β-blockers should also be considered prior to first bleed in patients with documented varices (only effective prophylactic therapy)

91  Khuroo M et al. A comparison of omeprazole and placebo for bleeding peptic ulcer. *NEJM* 1997; 336:1054-8. Lau JYW et al. Effect of intravenous omeprazole on recurrent bleeding after endoscopic treatment of bleeding peptic ulcers. *NEJM* 2000; 343: 310-316.

92  Van Dam J, Brugge WR. Endoscopy of the upper gastrointestinal tract. *NEJM* 1999; 341:1738-48.

93  Lau JYW et al. Endoscopic retreatment compared with surgery in patients with recurrent bleeding after initial endoscopic control of bleeding ulcers. *NEJM* 1999; 340: 751-6.

94  Grace ND. Diagnosis and treatment of gastrointestinal bleeding secondary to portal hypertension. *Gastroenterology* 1997; 92(7): 1081-91.

# *Helicobacter Pylori* Infection [95]

## Diagnostic testing and treatment indications:
- **Definite:** Active peptic ulcer disease (PUD) • History of PUD without prior treatment for *H. pylori* • Gastric MALT lymphoma • Atrophic gastritis • Recent resection of gastric cancer • 1° relative of patient with gastric cancer
- **Possible benefit:** Non-ulcer dyspepsia • Gastro-esophageal reflux disease (if on long-term acid suppression) • Chronic NSAID use

| Diagnostic Test | Sensitivity | Specificity | Comments |
|---|---|---|---|
| Histology | 93-96 % [a] | 98-99 % | EGD required |
| Biopsy urease test | 79-99 % [b] | 92-99 % | EGD required |
| Urea breath test | 90-96 % [b] | 88-98 % | Non-invasive. Useful for diagnosis and confirmation of eradication (check > 4 wks after treatment). |
| Serum or whole blood ELISA | 86-94 % | 78-95 % [c] | Unreliable indicator of active infection |
| Stool antigen | 88-98 % [b] | > 90 % | Alternative to urea breath test. Can confirm eradication (check 8 wks after treatment). |

**a:** Reduced sensitivity if taking H2 blocker (H2B) or proton pump inhibitor (PPI)
**b:** Reduced sensitivity if taking H2B, PPI, bismuth or antibiotics; sensitivity also reduced if active or recent bleeding
**c:** Reduced specificity in patients with cirrhosis

| Treatment | Duration | Cure Rate |
|---|---|---|
| PPI [d] *plus* metronidazole 500 mg bid *plus* clarithromycin 500 mg bid-tid [e] | 7-14 d [f] | 80 -90 % |
| PPI [d] *plus* amoxicillin [g] 1000 mg bid *plus* clarithromycin 500 mg bid-tid [e] (PrevPac ®) | 7-14 d [f] | 85-90 % |
| PPI [d] *plus* bismuth subsalicylate (Pepto Bismol ®) 525 mg qid *plus* metronidazole 250 mg qid *plus* tetracycline 500 mg qid | 2 wks | 94-98 % |
| Ranitidine bismuth subsalicylate (RBC) [h] 400 bid *plus* clarithromycin 500 bid *plus* amoxicillin 1000 mg *or* metronidazole 500 mg *or* tetracycline mg 500 bid | 2 wks | 80-90 % |
| Bismuth subsalicylate (Pepto Bismol ®) 525 mg qid *plus* metronidazole 250 mg qid *plus* tetracycline 500 mg qid *plus or* H₂ blocker [i] (x 4 weeks total) | 2 wks | 84-95 % |

**d:** PPI = proton pump inhibitor: omeprazole 20 mg bid *or* lansoprazole 30 mg bid *or* esomeprazole 20 mg bid/40 mg qd *or* pantoprazole 40 mg bid *or* rabeprazole 20 mg qd
**e:** Cure rates higher with clarithromycin 500 mg tid rather than bid
**f:** 2 week rather than 1 week treatment improves cure rate by 7-9%
**g:** Amoxicillin preferred over metronidazole if significant local metronidazole resistance
**h:** Ranitidine bismuth subsalicylate no longer available in U.S.
**i:** Famotidine 40 mg qd/20 mg bid *or* ranitidine/nizatidine 300 mg qd/150 mg bid

---

95 Howden CW, Hunt RH. Guidelines for the management of *Helicobacter pylori* infection. *Am J Gastroenterology* 1998; 93(12) 2330-2338; Suerbaum S, Michetti P. *Helicobacter pylori* infection. *NEJM* 2002; 347:1175-1186.

# *Acute Infectious Diarrhea* [96]

| Pathogen | Comments | Fever | Abd Pain | Bloody Stool | N/V | Fecal WBC |
|---|---|---|---|---|---|---|
| Toxins (staph, B. cereus, C. perfringens) | Incubation < 6 to 24 hr. | - | + | - | ++ | - |
| Salmonella | Community acquired, food-borne | ++ | ++ | + | + | ++ |
| Campylobacter | Community acquired, undercooked poultry | ++ | ++ | + | + | ++ |
| Shigella | Community acquired, person-to-person | ++ | ++ | + | ++ | ++ |
| Shiga toxin-producing E. Coli (e.g. O157:H7) | Food-borne outbreaks, under-cooked beef; bloody stool w/o fever | - | ++ | ++ | + | - |
| C. difficile | Nosocomial, post-antibiotics; marked leukocytosis in 50% | + | + | + | - | ++ |
| Vibrio | Seafood | +/- | +/- | +/- | +/- | +/- |
| Yersinia | Community acquired, food-borne | ++ | ++ | + | + | + |
| E. histolytica | Tropical | + | + | ++ | +/- | +/- |
| Cryptosporidium | Waterborne outbreaks, travel, immune compromise; symptoms > 10 days | +/- | +/- | - | + | - |
| Cyclospora | Travel, food-borne; profound fatigue | +/- | +/- | - | + | - |
| Giardia | Water-borne, day care, IgA deficiency; symptoms > 10 days | - | ++ | - | + | - |
| Norovirus | Winter outbreaks; nursing homes, schools, cruise ships, shellfish | +/- | ++ | - | ++ | - |

++ Common      + Occurs      +/- Variable      - Atypical or not characteristic

## Non-infectious differential diagnosis
• Medications  • Tube feeding  • Inflammatory bowel disease  • Ischemic colitis
• Factitious  • Secretory: villous adenoma, gastrinoma, VIPoma

## Treatment
• Anti-motility agents (loperamide, bismuth subsalicylate) OK to use in typical traveler's or watery diarrhea, but **avoid** if bloody or inflammatory diarrhea (may prolong fever, or predispose to toxic megacolon or hemolytic-uremic syndrome)
• Consider empiric fluoroquinolone if moderate-severe traveler's diarrhea or febrile community acquired diarrhea.  Add erythromycin or azithromycin if suspected fluoroquinolone-resistant Campylobacter infection (e.g. travel to southeast Asia), severely ill or immunocompromised.  **Avoid** antibiotics if bloody stools without fever or other suspicion for shiga-toxin E. coli (may predispose to hemolytic-uremic syndrome)

96  Thielman NM, Guerrant RL. Acute infectious diarrhea. *NEJM* 2004; 350:38-47.

# Treatment of C. Difficile colitis [97]

## Initial therapy
- **First line**: Stop antibiotics if at all possible and observe without treatment if symptoms are mild ♦ If symptoms severe: **metronidazole** 500 mg PO tid
- **Second line**: Vancomycin 125 mg PO qid ♦ No documented benefit over metronidazole; consider if no prompt response to metronidazole in severe infection
- **IV**: **metronidazole** 500 mg IV q 8 hr if NPO; add to PO vanco in severe infection (IV vancomycin is ineffective)
- **Duration**: 10-14 days (longer if receiving long-term antibiotics for other infection)

## Recurrent infections (10-25% of cases) [98]
- **Initial relapse:** Tapering **oral vancomycin** ♦ Confirm diagnosis ♦ Retreat with metronidazole or vancomycin for 10-14 days
- **Multiple relapses:** Tapering **oral vancomycin**

| | |
|---|---|
| Week 1: 125 mg qid | Week 4: 125 mg qod |
| Week 2: 125 mg bid | Weeks 5-6: 125 mg q 3 days |
| Week 3: 125 mg qd | Weeks 7-10: cholestyramine 4 gm PO qid |

- **Alternative therapies:** Colestipol (5 g bid) or **cholestyramine** (4 g tid/qid) with oral vancomycin (2-3 hr apart) ♦ **Vancomycin** (125 mg PO qid) plus **rifampin** (600 mg PO bid) ♦ Reconstitution of bowel flora with *Saccharomyces boulardii*, lactobacillus or stool enemas

## Indications for surgery (required in 1-3% of patients):
♦ Perforation ♦ Severe ileus with toxic megacolon ♦ Refractory septicemia ♦ Failure of medical treatment

# Serum-Ascites Albumin Gradient [99]

- Serum-ascites albumin gradient (SAAG) = serum albumin − ascitic fluid albumin
- SAAG ≥ 1.1 mg/dl predicts presence of **portal hypertension**
- 97% accuracy in classifying etiology (superior to "exudate-transudate" concept)

| SAAG ≥ 1.1 mg/dl<br>*(Portal hypertension present)* | SAAG < 1.1 mg/dl<br>*(Portal hypertension absent)* |
|---|---|
| • Cirrhosis (± co-existent infection or cancer) | • Peritoneal carcinomatosis |
| • Cardiac ascites (CHF, tricuspid regurgitation, constrictive pericarditis or tamponade) | • Peritonitis in absence of cirrhosis (bacterial, TB) |
| • Massive liver metastases | • Nephrotic syndrome |
| • Portal vein thrombosis | • Pancreatic or biliary ascites |
| • Budd-Chiari syndrome | • Malignant chylous ascites |
| • Fulminant hepatic failure | • Bowel infarction or obstruction |
| • Hepatocellular carcinoma | • Hypothyroidism |
| • Acute hepatitis (viral or alcoholic) superimposed on cirrhosis | |

97  Fekety R. Guidelines for the diagnosis and management of *C. difficile*-associated diarrhea and colitis. *Am J Gastroenterology* 1997: 92:739-50. Bartlett JG. Antibiotic-associated diarrhea. *NEJM* 2002; 346:334-339.

98  Tedesco FJ *et al.* Approach to patients with multiple relapses of antibiotic-associated pseudomembranous colitis. *Am J Gastroenterology* 1985; 80:867-8.

99  Runyon BA *et al.* The serum-ascites albumin gradient is superior to the exudate-transudate concept in the classification of ascites. *Ann Int Med* 1992; 117:215-220.

# Viral Hepatitis Serologies

| Scenario | ALT | HAV IgM | HAV IgG | HBsAg | HBc IgM | HBc IgG | HBeAg | HBeAb | HBsAb | HBV DNA | HCV Ab | HCV RNA |
|---|---|---|---|---|---|---|---|---|---|---|---|---|
| Acute HAV infection | ↑↑ | + | − | | | | | | | | | |
| Prior HAV infection or vaccination | Nml | − | + | | | | | | | | | |
| Acute HBV | ↑↑ | | | + | + | − | − | − | − | + | | |
| Acute HBV in "window period" | ↑↑ | | | − | + | − | − | − | − | +/− | | |
| Chronic HBV, active replication | ↑ | | | + | − | + | + | − | − | + | | |
| Chronic HBV, "pre-core" mutant | ↑ | | | + | − | + | − | + | − | + | | |
| Chronic HBV, minimally replicative (carrier) | Nml | | | + | − | + | − | + | − | − | | |
| Prior HBV infection | Nml | | | − | − | + | − | − | +/− | − | | |
| Prior HBV vaccination | Nml | | | − | − | − | − | − | + | − | | |
| Acute HCV | ↑↑ | | | | | | | | | | − | + |
| Chronic HCV | Nml/↑ | | | | | | | | | | + | + |
| False positive HCV or prior infection with eradication | Nml | | | | | | | | | | + | − |

**Notes:** Ab = antibody   Ag = antigen   ALT= alanine aminotransferase   DNA = viral DNA   HAV = hepatitis A virus
HBc = hepatitis B core   HBe = hepatitis B "e"   HBs = hepatitis B surface   HBV = hepatitis B virus
HCV = hepatitis C virus   RNA = viral RNA   Nml = normal

# Bacterial Peritonitis [100]

| Clinical Syndrome | AF PMN Count * | Gram Stain or Culture | Comments |
|---|---|---|---|
| Spontaneous bacterial peritonitis (SBP) | ≥ 250 cells/mm³ | Positive (1 organism) | Accounts for 2/3 of ascitic fluid infections |
| Culture-negative neutrocytic ascites (CNNA) | ≥ 250 cells/mm³ | Negative | Treat as SBP. Differential dx includes TB, peritoneal carcinomatosis, pancreatitis |
| Monomicrobial non-neutrocytic ascites (MNB) | < 250 cells/mm³ | Positive (1 organism) | Treat as SBP if symptoms (fever, abd pain); observe if asymptomatic |
| Secondary bacterial peritonitis | ≥ 250 cells/mm³ | Positive (poly-microbial) | Signs/sx same as SBP, but typically pneumoperitoneum present or fluid meets 2 of 3: 1) protein > 1 g/dL  2) glucose < 50 mg/dL, or 3) LDH > 225 (or > upper limit serum nml) |
| Polymicrobial bacterascites | < 250 cells/mm³ | Positive (polymicrob) | Usually from bowel puncture from tap; observe unless sx |

* AF PMN count = Ascitic fluid polymorphonuclear count

## Etiology/presentation of spontaneous bacterial peritonitis (SBP)
• Most cases in advanced cirrhosis, but can occur in CHF or nephrotic syndrome
• **Risk factors:** Severe liver disease (70% Child-Pugh class C or bili > 2.5 mg/dl) • Ascitic fluid total protein < 1 g/dL • co-existing GI bleeding • UTI • GI bacterial overgrowth • indwelling catheters • previous SBP (70% recurrence at 1 yr)
• **Bacterial flora:** ≥ 60% gram-negative rods (E. coli and Klebsiella) • 25% gram-positive cocci (mostly pneumococcus and other strep) • Enterococci, staph and anaerobes < 5% each (unless secondary peritonitis)
• **Symptoms and Signs:** Fever (69%), abdominal pain (59%), encephalopathy (54%), abdominal tenderness (49%) • 10% asymptomatic
• **Diagnosis:** Ascitic fluid PMN count critical parameter – empiric treatment if ≥ 250 cells/mm³ • Blood culture positive in 30-60% • AF cultures negative in 32-44% (i.e. CNNA) • Higher yield if ascitic fluid inoculated in blood culture bottles

## Treatment, prognosis and prevention of SBP
• **Treatment:** 3rd generation cephalosporin clearly superior to ampicillin plus aminoglycoside [101] • Alternatives: aztreonam, ampicillin-sulbactam, ticarcillin-clavulanate, fluoroquinolones • Duration: 5 days as effective as 10 (if clinically responding) • Cure rate 80-85% • Oral fluoroquinolones may be safe/effective in low risk patients • Albumin infusion (1.5 g/kg at diagnosis, plus 1 g/kg on day 3) during treatment may reduce risk of renal impairment and improve mortality [102]
• **Prognosis:** Related to liver disease (survival 30% at 1 yr, 20% at 2 yr)
• **Prophylaxis:** [103] Consider empiric oral antibiotic (e.g. norfloxacin 400 mg qd or trimethoprim-sulfa DS qd) in cirrhotic patients with acute GI bleeding (rx for 7 days), AF protein levels < 1 g/dL (rx during hospitalization) or prior SBP (rx indefinitely)

100 Such J, Runyon B. Spontaneous bacterial peritonitis. Clin Inf Dis 1998; 27:669-676; Mowat C, Stanley AJ. Spontaneous bacterial peritonitis. Aliment Pharmacol Ther 2001; 15:1851-9.

101 Felisart J et al. Cefotaxime is more effective than ampicillin-tobramycin in cirrhotics with severe infections. Hepatology 1985; 5:457.

102 Sort P et al. Effect of intravenous albumin on renal impairment and mortality in patients with cirrhosis and spontaneous bacterial peritonitis. NEJM 1999; 341:403-409.

103 Soriano G et al. Selective intestinal decontamination prevents spontaneous bacterial peritonitis. Gastroenterology 1991; 100:477-481. Gines P et al. Norfloxacin prevents spontaneous bacterial peritonitis recurrence in cirrhosis. Hepatology 1990; 12(4 Pt1):716-24.

# Jaundice[104]

Skin pigment change generally seen with serum bilirubin > 2.5 mg/dL

| Major Lab Abnormality | Etiology | Examples | Evaluation |
|---|---|---|---|
| None | "Pseudo-jaundice" | • Carotenemia<br>• Normal pigmentation | • Assess vegetable intake |
| Isolated increase in unconjugated (indirect) bilirubin | Increased bili load or production, or decreased bili conjugation | • Hemolysis<br>• Transfusion<br>• Hematoma resorption<br>• Gilbert syndrome | • Transfusion load*<br>• Blood smear<br>• Haptoglobin<br>• Direct Coomb's<br>• CT abdomen-pelvis for hematoma |
| Increase in transaminases and direct (conjugated) bilirubin | Hepatocellular injury | • Drug injury<br>• Hypotension<br>• Hypoxemia<br>• Acute hepatitis (viral, ethanol, autoimmune)<br>• Wilson's disease<br>• Non-alcoholic steatohepatitis<br>• Veno-occlusive disease<br>• Budd-Chiari<br>• Worsening of pre-existing liver disease | • R/O drug injury<br>• Assess tissue perfusion (Doppler ultrasound)<br>• Hepatitis serologies<br>• Liver biopsy |
| Increase in alkaline phosphatase ± direct (conjugated) bilirubin | Cholestatic injury | • Drug injury<br>• "Benign post-operative" **<br>• Sepsis<br>• TPN | • R/O drug injury<br>• Amylase, lipase<br>• US or CT scan<br>• ERCP or MRCP if ducts are dilated<br>• Liver biopsy |
| | Biliary obstruction (intra- vs. extra-hepatic) | • Choledocholithiasis<br>• Pancreatitis<br>• Biliary stricture (benign or malignant)<br>• Hepatic metastasis<br>• Sarcoidosis #<br>• PBC #, PSC<br>• AIDS cholangiopathy | |

\*     Each unit PRBCs contains ~250 mg bilirubin
\*\*   Mild elevations in bilirubin (2-4 mg/dL) seen in ¼ of post-surgical patients [105]
\#    Injury often at level of portal triad; radiographic evidence of obstruction often absent
Bili = bilirubin     R/O = rule out     US = ultrasound
PBC = primary biliary cirrhosis     PSC = primary sclerosing cholangitis

104 Pasha TM, Lindor KD. Diagnosis and therapy of cholestatic liver disease. Med Clin North Am 1996;
    80:995-1019; Hawker F. Liver dysfunction in critical illness. Anaesth Intensive Care 1991; 19:165-81.
105 Becker SD, Lamont JT. Postoperative jaundice. Semin Liver Dis 1988; 8:183-90.

# Surgical Risk in Liver Disease [106]

| Modified Child-Pugh Score [107] | 1 point | 2 points | 3 points |
|---|---|---|---|
| Encephalopathy # | None | Grade I-II | Grade III-IV |
| Ascites | Absent | Slight | Moderate |
| Bilirubin (mg/dL) - non-cholestatic | < 2 | 2-3 | >3 |
| cholestatic * | < 4 | 4-10 | > 10 |
| Albumin (g/dL) | > 3.5 | 2.8-3.5 | < 2.8 |
| INR | < 1.7 | 1.7-2.3 | > 2.3 |

\# Encephalopathy: (I) mild confusion or slowing; no asterixis (II) drowsy, asterixis present (III) marked confusion, somnolence; asterixis present (IV) unresponsive or responsive only to painful stimuli; no asterixis

\* e.g. primary biliary cirrhosis

## Modified Child-Pugh Class

| Class | Child Pugh Score | Peri-operative mortality[108] | Description | Survival (%) 1 yr | Survival (%) 2 yr |
|---|---|---|---|---|---|
| A | 5-6 | 10 % | Near-normal response to all operations, normal regenerative ability. Increased risk of complications if portal hypertension present. | 100 | 85 |
| B | 7-9 | 31 % | Moderate liver impairment. Tolerates non-cardiac surgery with pre-op preparation. Limited regeneration; sizable resections contraindicated. | 80 | 60 |
| C | ≥ 10 | 76 % | Poor response to all operations regardless of preparatory efforts. Liver resection contraindicated regardless of size. | 45 | 35 |

## Contraindications to elective surgery
• Acute alcoholic or viral hepatitis • Fulminant hepatic failure • Severe chronic hepatitis • Child-Pugh class C • PT prolongation > 3 seconds despite vitamin K • Platelet count < 50 K • Co-existing renal failure, cardiomyopathy or hypoxemia

## Optimizing medical therapy
• Adequate nutrition
• Correct PT (≤ 3 seconds of normal) with vitamin K, FFP or recombinant human factor VIIa
• Maintain platelet count > 50 K
• Treat prolonged bleeding time with ddAVP (see page 179)
• Prophylactic ß-blocker for varices
• Correct hypokalemia and metabolic alkalosis
• For encephalopathy: Use lactulose with target 3-4 bowel movements/day; avoid narcotics and sedatives
• For ascites: Salt restriction and potassium-sparing ± loop diuretic

---

106 Patel T. Surgery in the patient with liver disease. *Mayo Clin Proc* 1999; 74:593-9; Friedman LS. The risk of surgery in patients with liver disease. *Hepatology* 1999; 29:1617-23.

107 Pugh RN et al. Transection of the oesophagus for bleeding oesophageal varices. *Br J Surg* 1973;60:646-9.

108 Garrison RN. Clarification of risk factors for abdominal operations in patients with hepatic cirrhosis. *Ann Surg* 1984; 199: 648-55.

# Pancreatitis[109]

## Diagnosis
- **Amylase and lipase:** Value > 3x normal supports clinical diagnosis ♦ Value < 3x normal non-specific (differential diagnosis includes perforated ulcer, mesenteric ischemia, renal failure) ♦ Lipase probably better test; no value to measuring both ♦ Absolute values do not correlate with disease severity or prognosis ♦ Serial measurements do not predict clinical response or prognosis
- **ALT:** > 80 unit/mL highly specific for gallstone pancreatitis
- **Abdominal ultrasound:** Indicated to assess for gallstones or bile duct dilatation
- **Dynamic contrast CT scan:** Perform at 72 hr in severe pancreatitis to assess for presence and degree of necrosis

## Prognosis
- **Organ failure:** Most important indicator of severity. Defined by any of following: SBP < 90, $PaO_2$ < 60 mmHg, creatinine > 2 mg/dL, or GI bleeding > 500 mL/24hr
- **Hemoconcentration:** Hct > 44% predicts pancreatic necrosis
- **APACHE-II score:** see page 46; most sensitive/specific for severity
- **Ranson criteria** [110]

| Upon arrival | At 48 hours after admission |
|---|---|
| • Age > 55 yrs | • Hct < 30% or fall >10% |
| • WBC > 16,000 | • Serum calcium < 8 mg/dL |
| • Blood glucose > 200 mg/dL | • BUN increase > 5 mg/dL |
| • Serum LDH > twice normal | • $PaO_2$ < 60 mm Hg |
| • Serum AST > 6x normal | • Base deficit > 4 mEq/L |
| | • Estimated fluid sequestration > 6 liters |
| | • Massive volume resuscitation |

| Ranson factors | Mortality (%) | % Dead or > 7d in ICU |
|---|---|---|
| 0-2 | 0.9% | 3.7% |
| 3-4 | 16% | 40% |
| 5-6 | 40% | 93% |
| 7-8 | 100% | 100% |

## Treatment
- **Supportive care:** Fluid resuscitation, pain control, nutritional support if NPO >1week
- **Urgent ERCP:** Indicated in severe gallstone pancreatitis. Sphincterotomy should be performed if stones demonstrated. [111]
- **Prophylactic broad-spectrum antibiotics:** Indicated in necrotizing pancreatitis associated with organ failure [112]
- **Percutaneous aspiration:** Indicated to exclude superinfection in patients with necrotizing pancreatitis who fail to show clinical improvement
- **Surgical intervention:** ♦ Gallstones (cholecystectomy should be performed after resolution of episode; increased mortality if performed within first 48 hr) ♦ Abscess or super-infected necrosis ♦ Sterile necrosis with prolonged organ failure (i.e. 4-6 weeks) ♦ Symptomatic pseudocyst that fails conservative treatment and is not amenable to endoscopic or percutaneous drainage

109 Banks P. Practice guidelines in acute pancreatitis. *Am J Gastroenterology* 1996; 92(3):377-386.
110 Ranson JH et al. Prognostic signs and the role of operative management in acute pancreatitis. *Surg Gynecol Obstet* 1974; 139:69-81.
111 Fan S-T et al. Early treatment of acute biliary pancreatitis by endoscopic papillotomy. *NEJM* 1993; 328:228-232.
112 Sainio V et al. Early antibiotic treatment in acute necrotising pancreatitis. *Lancet* 1995; 346:663-7.

# Nutrition Support [113]

## Nutritional requirements
- **Calories** (Kcal/kg/day, max 2500/day): 20-25 (mild stress); 25-30 (typical ICU patient); 30-40 (severe stress or BMI < 20), 15-20 (BMI > 30)
- **Protein** (g/kg/day, max 150 g/day): normal 0.8; illness/injury 1.0-1.5; uremia (not dialyzed) 0.8-1.0; dialysis:1.2-1.5; hepatic encephalopathy 0.5
- **Fluid:** typically 30 ml/kg/d
- **Nitrogen balance** = Protein intake (grams) / 6.25 - (urine urea nitrogen + 4) (6.25 reflects that protein ≈ 16% N; 4 reflects obligatory N loss in skin/stool) Goal = 0; Moderate stress 0-5; Severe stress > 5

| Timing to initiate feeding | Enteral | Parenteral |
|---|---|---|
| Well nourished, non-hypercatabolic | 7-10 days | 14-21 days |
| Malnourished *or* hypercatabolic | 1-5 | 1-10 |
| Malnourished *and* hypercatabolic | 1-3 | 1-7 |

## Parenteral nutrition components

| Component | Typical values | Comments |
|---|---|---|
| Volume | 2 liters/day | 1.5 liters/day if wt < 60 kg |
| Rate | Start 1 liter/day (42 ml/hr); can increase to goal on day 2 if stable | To prevent hypoglycemia do not stop abruptly (hang D10 if needed or cut rate in half during surgery/procedures) |
| Dextrose | 10-30% solution (D10-D30) | D25 typical via dedicated central line. Max in other lines: femoral - D15; non-dedicated central - D10; peripheral line - D5. 3.4 Kcal/g (340 Kcal/L D10) |
| Protein | 30-70 grams/liter (3-7% amino acid soln) | 4 Kcal/g (200 Kcal in 1 liter 5% soln) |
| Lipids | 200 g/l (20% solution); may give separately | 9 Kcal/g. 20% lipid solution (contains glycerol and phospholipids) provides 2 Kcal/mL. Total dose = 20-30% of total Kcal. Decrease dose if ↑ triglycerides, ↑ PO4. |
| Electrolytes | K+ 30 mEq/L, Na+ 30 mEq/L, Mg++ 4 mEq/L, Ca++ 4 mg/l, PO4 15 mmol/l | Add acetate (HCO3) if hyperchloremic acidosis; additional phosphate for severe malnourishment |
| Vitamins | Standard multivitamin (10 mL MVI-12 or MVI-13) plus trace minerals (Zn, Cu, Mn, Se, Cr) | |
| Optional | H2 blocker, vitamin K, insulin | |

[113] Kirby DF *et al.* American Gastroenterological Association technical review on tube feeding for enteral nutrition. *Gastroenterology* 1995; 108:1282-301; Koretz RL *et al.* AGA technical review on parenteral nutrition. *Gastroenterology* 2001; 121:970-1001.

## Enteral feeding commercial products

| Type | Example Products | Kcal/mL | Protein (g/L) | mOsm/L |
|---|---|---|---|---|
| Standard polymeric * | Osmolite HN Plus | 1.2 | 45-55 | 360-450 |
| Standard polymeric w/fiber | Jevity Plus, Fibersource HN | 1.2 | 45-55 | 360-450 |
| Polymeric reduced protein | Jevity, Osmolite, Isocal HN, Ultracal | 1.06 | 35-42 | 300 |
| High protein & calories | Ensure Plus HN, Boost Plus | 1.5 | 63 | 650 |
| Fluid restricted | TwoCal HN, Magnacal, Nutren 2.0 | 2.0 | 84 | 690-720 |
| Elemental ** | Criticare HN, Vital HN, Vivonex TEN | 1.0 | 38-42 | 500-650 |
| Liver disease | Nutrihep | 1.5 | 40 | 690 |
| Renal | Nepro | 2.0 | 70 | 635 |
| Pulmonary | Pulmocare, Respalor | 1.5 | 60-75 | 475-580 |

\* Appropriate for most patients
** For patients with malabsorption (e.g. short bowel, IBD)

- **Gastric Feeding:** Start with full strength @ 30 mL/hr, advance 20 mL q 8 hr to goal ◆ Check residual volume q 4 hr, continue if < 150 mL, hold 1 hr if > 150 mL
- **Jejunostomy Feeding:** Start with full strength @ 20 mL/hr, advance 20 mL q 8 hr to goal ◆ Follow clinical exam to assess tolerance (do not check residuals) ◆ Do not bolus feed via jejunostomy tube
- **Intermittent/Bolus feeding:** Start with full strength @ 120 mL q 4 hr
  ◆ Advance 60 mL q 2-3 boluses to goal
- **General:**
  - Elevate head of bed 30°
  - Consider jejunostomy feeding if patient develops recurrent aspiration with gastric feeding
  - If patient develops diarrhea consider
    1) Decreasing rate, then titrating upward at slower pace
    2) Evaluating for *C. difficile* or bacterial overgrowth
    3) Eliminating GI irritants including magnesium and sorbitol (in elixir meds)
    4) Use of a low-fat, peptide-containing formula
    5) Adding fiber or kaolin-pectin
- **Avoid** using blue food dye [114]

---

[114] Maloney JP *et al.* Systemic absorption of food dye in patients with sepsis. *NEJM* 2000; 343:1047-8

# Hematology

## *Hemolytic Anemia*

**Mechanistic classification**
- **Intrinsic (RBC defect)**
  - **Acquired:** paroxysmal nocturnal hemoglobinuria; liver disease; vitamin E deficiency
  - **Hereditary:** unstable hemoglobin (thalassemias); membrane defects (spherocytosis); metabolic defect (G6PD deficiency); blood group Ag deficiencies
- **Extrinsic**
  - **Antibody-mediated**
    - **Warm-antibody immune hemolytic anemia** (usually IgG, rarely IgM): idiopathic (50-70%); lymphoproliferative disorder; SLE or other rheumatic disorder; infection (HIV, EBV); congenital immunodeficiency; solid tumor (rare)
    - **Drugs: autoantibody, hapten, or immune complex mechanisms**
      - Antibiotics: Penicillins, cephalosporins, sulfa drugs, rifampin
      - Analgesics: NSAIDs
      - Psychiatric agents: Tricyclic antidepressants, phenothiazines
      - Cardiovascular agents: α-methyldopa, procainamide, thiazide diuretics
      - Endocrine agents: Sulfonylureas
      - Others: Methotrexate, 5-FU
    - **Cold agglutinin disease** (usually IgM): •Acute: mycoplasma infection, EBV •Chronic: idiopathic; lymphoproliferative disorders
    - **Paroxysmal cold hemoglobinuria** (polyclonal IgG: "Donath-Landsteiner" antibody): •Acute: viral syndromes (rarely in adults) •Chronic: idiopathic; CLL; secondary/tertiary syphilis
  - **Mechanical trauma:** • Microangiopathic: TTP/HUS, DIC, malignant hypertension, eclampsia •Physical (e.g. "march" hemoglobinuria, cardiopulmonary bypass) or heat (e.g. burns) • Cardiac valvular stenosis or prosthesis
  - **Direct infection or toxin-effect:** • Infections: malaria, babesiosis, Bartonella, clostridia, sepsis • Snake and spider venoms • Copper toxicity including Wilson's disease • Osmotic: hypotonic infusions, freshwater drowning
  - **Other:** Splenomegaly; hypophosphatemia; hemolytic transfusion reactions

**Diagnosis**
- **Smear:** Spherocytes (immune-mediated hemolysis or hereditary); reticulocytes (active marrow); schistocytes (microangiopathic hemolysis); RBCs with inclusions (e.g. malaria); "bite" cells (G6PD deficiency)
- **Haptoglobin:** Low level is accurate indicator of intravascular hemolysis, but may be elevated in inflammation (acute phase reactant); absent (ahaptoglobinemia) in 4-10% of African-Americans
- **Reticulocyte Production Index:** RPI = % retics x (Hct÷45) ÷ reticulocyte maturation time (days); maturation time is 1 day at Hct 45%, 1.5 days at 35%, 2 days at 25%, 2.5 days at 15%. RPI > 2 suggests active hemolysis and adequate marrow response
- **Coombs** (direct anti-globulin test): Confirms antibody-mediated process; pattern may suggest specific antigen
- **Cold agglutinins or paroxysmal cold hemoglobinuria-specific antibody:** If symptoms related to cold exposure

## G6PD deficiency[115]

- X-linked disorder (heterozygous females may have ≥ 50% affected RBCs)
- Minority of patients have chronic hemolysis; majority develop acute hemolysis in response to **infections** (pneumonia, UTI, viral hepatitis, salmonella), **metabolic stress** (e.g. DKA), or **drugs**. Fresh fava beans (**favism**) trigger attacks primarily in boys < 5 y.o. of Mediterranean descent.

| Drugs *Unsafe* in G6PD Deficiency | Drugs Generally *Safe* in G6PD Deficiency |
|---|---|
| dapsone • methylene blue nalidixic acid naphthalene (mothballs) nitrofurantoin • primaquine sulfamethoxazole | acetaminophen • ascorbic acid • aspirin chloramphenicol • chloroquine • colchicine diphenhydramine • isoniazid • L-DOPA PABA • phenytoin • probenecid • procainamide pyrimethamine • quinidine quinine • streptomycin sulfisoxazole • trimethoprim • vitamin K |

# *Iron-Deficiency Anemia*[116]

## Iron absorption and transport
- Absorbed by duodenal crypt cells near gastroduodenal junction
- Only 10-20% absorbed from 10-20 mg/d ingested
- Absorption ↑ by acid, citrate and ascorbate, ↓ by achlorhydria, tannate (tea), $PO_4$
- Transferrin binds Fe once translocated across gut epithelium
- Excess iron stored as **ferritin** in reticuloendothelial system; ferritin levels reflect total body iron stores, but may be falsely elevated (acute phase reactant) by inflammation or infection

## Natural history
1) Storage depletion (decreased marrow stores and ferritin levels) without anemia
2) Abnormal erythropoiesis: microcytosis, hypochromia
3) Anemia and thrombocytosis

## Clinical Manifestations
- Symptoms: pallor, fatigue; pica for ice, starch, clay, tomatoes
- Heme: microcytic, hypochromic anemia; thrombocytosis
- GI: glossitis, stomatitis; esophageal webs (Plummer-Vinson); atrophic gastritis
- Spooning of fingernails (koilonychia)
- Impaired cognitive function

## Etiology
- **GI loss:** [117] 40% upper GI source (ulcers, esophagitis, AVM, cancer), 3 % small intestine, 22% colon (cancer, AVM, large polyps); 34% with no identifiable source, and 5% with lesions in both upper and lower GI tract. Only ~50% with identifiable source have heme positive stools.
- **Non-GI loss:**   Genitourinary bleeding; intravascular hemolysis (paroxysmal nocturnal hemoglobinuria, cardiac valves); lung (hemosiderosis, bronchiectasis); severe trauma; surgical blood loss; repeated phlebotomy; elective blood donation
- **Increased utilization:** EPO administration
- **Physiologic loss:** Menstruation, pregnancy, lactation
- **Decreased intake:** Primary malabsorption (e.g. celiac sprue, lead poisoning); s/p gastrectomy (↓ transit time); s/p duodenal/jejunal resection; high gastric pH (achlorhydria, acid blockade; also may be caused by iron deficiency itself)

---

115 Beutler E. Glucose-6-Phosphate dehydrogenase deficiency. *N Engl J Med* 1991; 324(3):170-4; Reutler E. G6PD deficiency. *Blood* 1994; 84:3613.
116 Andrews NC. Disorders of iron metabolism. *NEJM* 1999; 341:1986-95.
117 Rockey DC. Occult gastrointestinal bleeding. *NEJM* 1999; 341:38-46.

## Assays of iron stores
- **Direct**: Bone marrow biopsy; diagnosis requires absence of stainable iron
- **Indirect**: Serum markers of iron stores [118]

| Condition | Fe (mcg/dl) | TIBC (mcg/dl) | Fe/TIBC (transferrin saturation) | Ferritin (ng/ml) | Soluble transferrin receptor[119] |
|---|---|---|---|---|---|
| Normal | 60-150 | 250-450 | 20-50% | 40-200 | 10-30 nM/L |
| Iron Deficiency | ↓ | ↑ | < 15 % spec 65% sens 80% | < 30 spec 98% * sens 92% | ↑ |
| Iron Overload | ↑ | ↓ | > 50% women > 60% men (90% sens) | > 300 women > 400 men (sensitive but not specific) | |
| Anemia of Chronic Dz | Nml/↓ | Nml/↓ | Typically ↓ | ↑ | Nml |

Fe= iron    TIBC= total iron binding capacity
* Specificity for Fe-deficiency is lower in presence of underlying inflammation or infection

## Differential diagnosis of hypochromia and microcytosis[120]
- Anemia of chronic disease: May be difficult to exclude co-existing Fe deficiency (consider bone marrow bx with iron stain if serum markers non-diagnostic)
- Sideroblastic anemia: Confirmed by bone marrow biopsy with iron stain
- Thalassemia: Hb electrophoresis diagnostic in β-thal but usually normal in α-thal. Review of previous CBCs should show consistently low MCV (often < 70 fL). Free erythrocyte protoporphyrin (FEP) should be normal (elevated in Fe deficiency) and RBC count should be normal-high (low in Fe deficiency).

## Iron supplementation
- Avoid enteric coated products
- Absorption increased if given with vitamin C (250 mg)
- Take on empty stomach and avoid giving with antacids
- If achlorhydria or acid suppression consider iron polysaccharide
- Reticulocytosis begins at 5-7d, max 10d
- Hb should rise 2 g/dl over three weeks
- Failure to respond: wrong diagnosis, noncompliance, loss exceeds replacement, bone marrow suppression, malabsorption; consider intravenous supplementation

118 Guyatt GM et al. Laboratory diagnosis of iron deficiency anemia. J Gen Int Med 1992;7:145-53.
119 Mast AE et al. Clinical utility of the soluble transferrin receptor and comparison with serum ferritin in several populations. Clin Chem 1998; 44:45-51.
120 Griner PF. Microcytosis. In: Diagnostic Strategies for Common Medical Problems, 2nd ed. Black ER (ed.) Philadelphia: American College of Physicians; 1999: 575-584.

# Megaloblastic Anemias[121]

## Etiology
- **Vitamin B12 (cobalamin) deficiency**: ♦ Inadequate diet (vegan) ♦ Increased requirements ♦ Deficiency of gastric intrinsic factor: gastrectomy, pernicious anemia, inherited ♦ Malabsorption: ileitis, bowel resection, tapeworms, bacterial overgrowth, lowered intestinal pH (Zollinger-Ellison), pancreatic insufficiency, drugs (colchicine, neomycin, sustained release KCl, cholestyramine), alcohol

| **Non-megaloblastic macrocytosis** |
|---|
| • Reticulocytosis |
| • Ethanol |
| • Liver disease |
| • Hypothyroidism |
| • Hyperlipidemia |
| • Spurious or artifactual (cold agglutinins, ↓Na+, ↑ glucose) |
| • Pure RBC aplasia |

- **Folate deficiency**: ♦ Increased requirements: pregnancy, hemolytic anemia, hyper- or myeloproliferative syndromes, sickle cell ♦ Malabsorption: sprue, extensive small bowel disease/resection/fistulae, anticonvulsants, oral contraceptives
- **Drug-induced suppression of DNA synthesis**: ♦ Folate antagonists: trimethoprim, methotrexate, pyrimethamine, EtOH ♦ Inhibitors of nucleoside synthesis: anti-neoplastic (5-FU, ara-C, hydroxyurea, alkylating agents); antiviral (nucleoside analogues); immunomodulators (6-MP, azathioprine) ♦ Nitrous oxide
- **Congenital**: Lesch-Nyhan; orotic aciduria; folate metabolism; B12 transport
- **Erythroleukemia** (M6 AML)
- **Myelodysplastic syndromes** (e.g. 5q⁻ syndrome)

## Diagnosis[122]
- **MCV**: May be normal; <110 fL: non-specific; 115-130 fL: 50% have B12/folate deficiency; > 130 fL: most have B12/folate deficiency unless taking hydroxyurea
- **Peripheral smear**: Evidence of megaloblastic "arrest" with hypersegmented neutrophils (98% sensitive for megaloblastic anemia) and macro-ovalocytes (egg shaped, not elliptocytes)
- **Serum B12**: Low level (100-250 pg/ml) supports but does not prove deficiency
- **Serum folate**: Poor correlation with tissues levels; **RBC folate** better test but may be artifactually low in B12 deficiency
- **Methylmalonic acid**: Elevated in 98% of confirmed cases of B12 deficiency (normal level rules out); **homocysteine** elevated in both folate & B12 deficiency
- **Intrinsic factor antibody**: Highly specific but present in only 50% of cases of pernicious anemia; recent B12 injection or radioisotopes may cause false (+)
- **Marrow**: Discordance of nuclear/cytoplasmic maturation, evident in most mature cells. Hypercellular, erythroid population in marrow. Intramedullary hemolysis with ineffective erythropoiesis. Giant band forms and metamyelocytes.
- **Schilling test**: (1) Supraphysiologic B12 IM to saturate B12 binding sites (2) Oral administration of dual-labeled B12 (IF-bound and unbound with different isotopes) (3) Urinary measurement of radiolabeled B12 excretion. *Normal:* Both isotopes excreted in urine. *Pernicious anemia:* Only IF-bound B12 excreted in urine. *Malabsorption:* Neither isotope excreted. Can repeat after tetracycline 250 mg qid x 10 days; if normalizes, suggests bacterial overgrowth.

---

121 Carmel R, Rosenblatt DS. Disorders of cobalamin and folate metabolism. In *Blood : Principles and Practice of Hematology*, 2nd edn. Handin RI et al, editors. Philadelphia, Pa.: Lippincott Williams & Wilkins, 2003.

122 Lancet JE, Rapoport AP. Macrocytosis. In: *Diagnostic Strategies for Common Medical Problems*, 2nd ed. Black FR (ed.) Philadelphia. American College of Physicians; 1999: 585-595.

# Heparin-Induced Thrombocytopenia[123]

- **Type I:** Non-immune mechanism ♦ Platelets rarely < 100K ♦ Occurs in ~ 30% of patients given heparin ♦ Onset 1-2 days after heparin exposure ♦ Resolves spontaneously without complications
- **Type II:** Immune-mediated platelet activation ♦ Less common than type I ♦ Platelets usually < 100K ♦ Onset typically 4-8 days after heparin exposure, but may be delayed up to 3 weeks after heparin d/c'd, more rapidly if prior exposure ♦ Persists until all heparin stopped, including LMWH & heparin-coated catheters
- **HIT with thrombosis syndrome (HITTS):** HIT type II with thrombotic or thromboembolic complications (30-50% of cases)

## Clinical manifestations (Type II) [124]

- **Early:** Increasing heparin resistance ♦ Erythematous plaques or skin necrosis at heparin injection site ♦ "Pseudo-embolism": fever, dyspnea, ↑ HR or BP, cardio-pulmonary arrest, or transient global amnesia 5-30 min after heparin bolus
- **Thrombocytopenia:** Typically 30-70K or 50% decrease from baseline (consider alternative diagnosis if platelets < 20K)
- **Thromboembolism ("white clot syndrome"):** Venous > arterial by 4:1 ♦ Events commonly occur at site of pre-existing pathology (surgery, vascular device) ♦ **Venous:** DVT, PE, limb gangrene, cerebral sinus thrombosis ♦ **Arterial:** limb ischemia, stroke, MI, graft closure, mesenteric or renal infarction ♦ **Other:** intracardiac thrombus, prosthetic valve thrombosis, A-V fistula occlusion
- **Hemorrhage:** Uncommon unless infarcted tissue (e.g. adrenal)

## Diagnosis

1) Timing: onset 4-8 day after heparin exposure, or within 8-10 hours if previous heparin exposure [125]
2) Resolves after d/c of heparin
3) Exclusion of other causes
4) Confirmatory testing with serotonin release assay or ELISA (highly sensitive, less specific) or heparin-induced platelet aggregation (highly specific, less sensitive). Negative result on two tests usually excludes diagnosis.

### Differential diagnosis

- Sepsis ♦ DIC/TTP ♦ HELLP
- Immune: ITP, SLE, post-transfusion
- Ethanol ♦ Splenomegaly
- Infections: HIV, EBV, hepatitis
- Drugs: chemo, quinidine, NSAIDs, sulfa, GP IIb/IIIa inhibitors
- Marrow suppression
- Pseudothrombocytopenia (platelet clumping): examine smear, re-draw in citrate or heparin containing tube

## Treatment (HIT Type II or HITTS)

1) Discontinue **all** heparin (including LMW heparin and line flushes) – platelet count should rise in 24-48 hr, with return to normal by 4-5 days.
2) Avoid platelet transfusion – may induce thromboembolic complications.
3) Given high risk of late thromboembolic complications, consider prophylactic anti-coagulation with lepirudin (*page 194*) or argatroban (*page 175*) unless patient at high risk of bleeding.
4) If established HITTS, use lepirudin or argatroban as anticoagulant. Treatment should continue until thrombosis resolves and platelet count normalizes, or therapeutic level of warfarin attained.
5) In acute HITTS, do not give warfarin without concomitant therapy with lepirudin or argatroban -- may predispose to venous limb gangrene. Delay starting warfarin until platelet count >100K.

---

123 Brieger DB *et al.* Heparin-induced thrombocytopenia. *JACC* 1998; 31:1449-59. Warkentin TE. Heparin-induced thrombocytopenia: Pathogenesis and management. *Br J Haematol* 2003; 121:535-55.

124 Warkentin TE. Clinical presentation of HIT. *Semin Hematol* 1998; 35(4) Suppl 5:9-16.

125 Warkentin TE, Kelton JG. Temporal aspects of heparin-induced thrombocytopenia. *NEJM* 2001; 344:1286-1292.

# Blood Products[126]

| Product | Vol (ml) | Indications | Comments |
|---|---|---|---|
| Whole Blood (WB) | 400-500 | • Massive transfusion in acute blood loss | • RBCs plus plasma<br>• Rarely used |
| Packed Red Blood Cells (PRBCs) *see next page for specific types* | 250-350 | • Increase $O_2$-carrying capacity if evidence/risk of end-organ ischemia<br>• Maintain volume and $O_2$ capacity in acute blood loss<br>• **Not** indicated solely to maintain "target" Hb/Hct or for volume repletion (isovolemic anemia well-tolerated if no cardiac, pulmonary or cerebro-vascular disease) | • Massive transfusion may cause hypo-thermia, low $Ca^{++}$, high $K^+$, dilutional thrombocytopenia<br>• In critically ill patients, "restrictive" transfusion practice (i.e. at Hb of 7-9 mg/dl vs 10-12 mg/dl) may reduce mortality[127]<br>• In acute MI, transfusion to Hct 30-33% may reduce mortality [128] |
| Platelet Concen-trates (PCs) | 200-250 (per 5-6 unit pool) | • Bleeding & plts < 100K<br>• Procedure & plts < 50K<br>• Prophylactic if plts < 10K<br>• Bleeding & qualitatively abnormal platelets (e.g. uremia, ASA)<br>• Serious bleeding after GP IIb/IIIa inhibitor therapy | • 6-unit pool should raise count 50-60 K, less if alloimmunized.<br>• May support platelets in patients refractory to SDPs<br>• Contraindicated in consumptive coag-ulopathy (HIT, HUS/TTP, HELLP) |
| Single-Donor Platelets (SDPs) | 200-250 | • Same as platelet concentrates but fewer donor exposures (allo-immunization, infection) | • No data to support routine use to *prevent* alloimmunization [129] |
| Fresh Frozen Plasma (FFP) | 200-250 | • Bleeding if multiple factor deficiency (massive transfusion, liver disease)<br>• DIC or TTP<br>• Reversal of warfarin<br>• Factor XI deficiency | • Contains factors II, VII, IX, X, XI, XII, and XIII<br>• Dose: 15 ml/kg for massive transfusion, 3-5 ml/kg to reverse warfarin (titrate to PT) |
| Cryo-precipitate | 100-200 (per 10 unit pool) | • Replacement of fibrinogen when acutely depleted (<100 mg/dl) or qualitatively abnormal<br>• Serious bleeding after thrombolytic therapy<br>• Factor VIII or vWF replacement if concentrate not available | • Contains factor VIII, vWF, fibronectin and fibrinogen<br>• Fibrinogen in 10-unit pool = 4 units FFP (but roughly 20% the volume) |

126 Churchill WH. Transfusion therapy. In: *Scientific American Medicine*. Federman D (ed.) New York: Scientific American, Inc.; March 2001.

127 Hebert PC *et al.* A multicenter, randomized, controlled clinical trial of transfusion requirements in critical care. *NEJM* 1999; 340:409-17.

128 Wu W-C *et al.* Blood transfusion in elderly patients with acute MI *NEJM* 2001; 345.1230-1236.

129 TRAPS Group. Leukocyte reduction and UVB irradiation to platelets to prevent allo-immunization and refractoriness to platelet transfusions. *NEJM* 1997; 337:1861-9.

**Types of Red Cells:**
• **Packed red cells (PRBCs):** Most plasma removed; for general use.
• **Leukopoor:**[130] Most WBCs removed; used if prior febrile transfusion reactions or multiple transfusions. May prevent CMV infection. • **Washed:** Plasma virtually removed; used if prior allergic reactions. • **Irradiated:** Hematopoietic progenitor cells killed to prevent graft-versus-host disease; for related donors or patients with suppressed marrow. • **Emergency release** (i.e. no crossmatch): O-negative in women of childbearing age, O-positive in all others (if O-negative not available); immune reaction in 5% if ABO-compatible but antibody screen incomplete.

# Transfusion Risks[131]

| Adverse Outcome * | Risk per Unit Transfused |
|---|---|
| Hepatitis B | 1: 220,000 |
| Hepatitis C | 1: 600,000 |
| HTLV 1 or 2 | 1: 600,000 |
| HIV 1 or 2 | 1: 1,800,000 |
| Bacterial contamination – platelets | 1: 25,000 |
| Bacterial contamination – red blood cells | 1: 250,000 |
| Fatal hemolytic transfusion reaction | 1: 500,000 |
| Fatal acute lung injury (ARDS) | 1: 3,000,000 |

* Emerging risks include variant Creutzfeldt-Jakob, West Nile virus, and *T. cruzi*

# Transfusion Reactions[132]

**Acute Hemolytic:** 1-4 events/million units transfused ♦ Preformed antibodies against major RBC antigens cause acute intravascular hemolysis ♦ *Symptoms*: fever, chills, back pain, N/V, hypotension, renal failure, DIC *Treatment*: Stop transfusion immediately ♦ Give diphenhydramine, acetaminophen ± hydrocortisone 50-100 mg IV ♦ Maintain urine output with alkalinized IVF ♦ Alert blood bank and send back product plus samples for Coombs, bilirubin, LDH, free Hb, DIC screen.
**Delayed Hemolytic:** 1/1000 units transfused ♦ 1-25 days post-transfusion ♦ Sx similar to acute reaction but often less severe ♦ *Treatment:* Same as acute reaction if warranted by sx **Non-hemolytic febrile:** Common (1-2 events/100 units transfused) ♦ Platelets > PRBCs ♦ Onset ≤ 5 hr of transfusion ♦ Fever may be only 1-2 ° F > normal ♦ Other symptoms: chills, resp distress (usually self-limited) ♦ Differential dx: hemolytic reaction, sepsis, contaminated blood product *Treatment:* Stop transfusion & send back to blood bank ♦ Blood cultures ♦ Antipyretics ± meperidine 50-75 mg IV ♦ Consider leukocyte-reduced products if patient has had ≥ 2 febrile reactions **Allergic:** Most common reaction (3-4 events/100 units transfused) ♦ Immune response to plasma proteins ♦ *Symptoms*: pruritus, urticaria, bronchospasm, anaphylaxis (more likely if recipient is IgA-deficient) *Treatment:* Diphenhydramine ♦ Unnecessary to stop transfusion if mild, but consider slowing infusion ♦ If severe or recurrent reactions use washed RBCs
**Transfusion-related acute lung injury (TRALI):** ARDS-like condition ♦ 1-10 events/100,000 units transfused, with 3-5% mortality ♦ Bilateral pulmonary infiltrates within 4 hr of transfusion ♦ Diagnosis of exclusion (assess for CHF, sepsis) ♦ *Treatment:* Same as ARDS, usually responds within 24 hours
**Post-transfusion purpura (PTP):** Rare, severe thrombocytopenia 5-10 d post-transfusion (usually RBC transfusion) ♦ Due to anti-platelet alloantibodies

130 Heddle NM, Blajchman MA. The leukodepletion of cellular blood products in the prevention of HLA-alloimmunization and refractoriness to allogeneic platelet transfusions. *Blood* 1995; 85:603-6.
131 Goodnough LT *et al.* Transfusion Medicine. *NEJM* 1999; 340(6):438-447. Busch MP *et al.* Current and emerging infectious risks of blood transfusions. *JAMA* 2003; 289:959-62.
132 Churchill WH. Ibid.

# Coagulation Disorders [133]

## Causes of a prolonged PT or aPTT

| | aPTT Normal | aPTT Prolonged |
|---|---|---|
| **PT Normal** | *If bleeding* <br>• Platelet disorder (quantitative or qualitative) <br>• von Willebrand disease <br>• Factor XIII deficiency <br>• Non-specific vascular | See diagram next page <br>*Inherited* <br>• Deficiency of vWF or factors VIII, IX, XI or XII * <br>*Acquired* <br>• Heparin or direct thrombin inhibitor (lepirudin, argatroban) <br>• Lupus anticoagulant (LAC) * <br>• Inhibitor of vWF or factors VIII, IX, XI or XII * |
| **PT Prolonged** | *Inherited* <br>• Factor VII deficiency <br>*Acquired* <br>• Vitamin K deficiency <br>• Warfarin (iatrogenic, or self-inflicted) <br>• Liver disease <br>• Inhibitor of factor VII (very rare) | *Inherited* <br>• Deficiency of prothrombin, fibrinogen or factors V or X <br>• Combined factor deficiency <br>*Acquired* <br>• Liver disease <br>• DIC <br>• Excessive heparin/warfarin <br>• Inhibitor of prothrombin (LAC), fibrinogen or factors V or X (X associated with amyloidosis) |

* Most lupus anticoagulant and factor XII deficiency not associated with clinical bleeding

## Acquired inhibitors
### Factor VIII inhibitors [134]
- **Etiology:** Pregnancy or postpartum ♦ Drug reactions ♦ Connective tissue disease or antiphospholipid antibody syndrome ♦ Malignancy (solid tumors)
- **Clinical:** Prolonged aPTT, normal PT ♦ May cause severe bleeding from GU and GI tracts and into soft tissues (hematomas) ♦ Alternatively, may have hypercoagulable state (e.g. antiphospholipid antibody syndrome)
- **Work-up: (1)** Exclude heparin (prolonged thrombin time, normal reptilase time; aPTT should correct with protamine) **(2)** Mixing studies (aPTT should not correct) **(3)** Rule out lupus anticoagulant **(4)** Quantify inhibitor with Bethesda assay
- **Treatment for bleeding:** ♦ Control bleeding with ddAVP or recombinant factor VIII for low-titer inhibitor, otherwise, use porcine factor VIII (if no porcine inhibitor), activated prothrombin complex concentrate (Autoplex, FEIBA) or recombinant factor VIIa concentrate ♦ Prednisone ± cyclophosphamide or intravenous immunoglobulin (IVIG) to eliminate inhibitor

### Factor II (prothrombin) inhibitors
- **Etiology:** Most commonly seen in patients with antiphospholipid antibody syndrome who present with bleeding
- **Clinical:** PT and aPTT prolonged ♦ ± LAC ♦ Bleeding may be severe
- **Treatment:** FFP ♦ Other treatments listed for acquired factor VIII inhibitors

133 Coutre S. Acquired inhibitors of coagulation. In: *UpToDate*, v. 11.3. Rose, BD (Ed), UpToDate, Wellesley, MA, 2003.
134 Bossi P et al. Acquired hemophilia due to factor VIII inhibitors in 34 patients. *Am J Med* 1998; 105:400-8.

*Factor V inhibitors*
- **Etiology:** Most arise after exposure to fibrin glue or bovine thrombin
- **Clinical:** Prolonged aPTT and PT but normal thrombin time • Bleeding variable
- **Diagnosis:** Mixing/inhibitors studies
- **Treatment for bleeding:** • Platelet transfusions and plasma exchange
  • Immunosuppression not usually needed

## Evaluation of an isolated prolonged aPTT

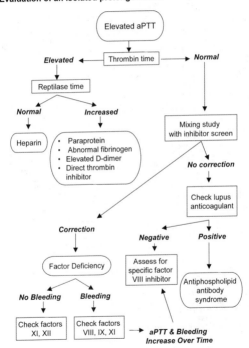

# Infectious Disease

## Duke Criteria for Endocarditis[135]

### Criteria for diagnosis of infective endocarditis (IE)

| | |
|---|---|
| **Definite** | • **Pathologic criteria**:<br>(1) Micro-organisms (demonstrated by culture or histology in a vegetation, embolized vegetation or intracardiac abscess) **or**<br>(2) Pathologic lesions (vegetation or intracardiac abscess confirmed by histology showing active endocarditis) **OR**<br>• **Clinical criteria**: 2 major **or** 1 major plus 3 minor **or** 5 minor |
| **Possible** | • **Clinical criteria**: 1 major plus 1 minor **or** 3 minor |
| **Rejected**<br>(negative predictive value ≥ 92%) [136] | • Firm alternate diagnosis explaining evidence of IE **or**<br>• Resolution of endocarditis syndrome with antibiotic therapy for ≤ 4 days **or**<br>• No pathologic findings of IE at surgery or autopsy (after antibiotic therapy for ≤ 4 days) **or**<br>• Does not meet criteria for possible IE |

**Major Criteria**

1) Positive blood cultures for IE
   - 2 separate blood cultures with organisms *typical* for IE *
   - Persistently positive blood cultures with organism *consistent* with IE (2 drawn > 12 hr apart; or all of 3 or majority of ≥ 4 separate cultures, with 1st and last drawn ≥ 1 hr apart)
   - Single positive blood culture for *Coxiella burnetii* or Ab titer > 1:800
2) Evidence of endocardial involvement
3) Echocardiogram positive for IE: **
   Oscillating intracardiac mass# **or** abscess **or** new partial dehiscence of prosthetic valve
4) New valvular regurgitation †

**Minor Criteria**

1) Predisposing heart condition or IVDU
2) Fever ≥ 38.0°C (100.4°F)
3) Vascular phenomena: Major arterial emboli, septic pulmonary infarcts, mycotic aneurysm, intracranial hemorrhage, Janeway lesions, conjunctival hemorrhages
4) Immunologic phenomena: Osler nodes, glomerulonephritis, Roth spots, rheumatoid factor
5) Microbiologic evidence: Positive blood culture for organism that causes IE but not meeting major criteria **or** serologic evidence of active infection with organism consistent with IE

---

\* Typical organisms include viridans streptococci, *S. bovis*, HACEK group, *S. aureus*; or community-acquired enterococci in the absence of a primary focus

\*\* Transesophageal echocardiogram (TEE) recommended in patients with prosthetic valves; in those rated at least "possible IE" by clinical criteria; or complicated IE (paravalvular abscess); transthoracic echocardiogram (TTE) first study in other patients

\# Mass on valve or supporting structures or in the path of regurgitant jets or on implanted material, in the absence of an alternative anatomic explanation

† Increase or change in preexisting murmur **not** sufficient

135 Durack DT et al. New criteria for diagnosis of infective endocarditis. *Am J Med* 1994; 96: 200-9; Li JS et al. Proposed modifications to the Duke criteria for the diagnosis of infective endocarditis. *Clin Infect Dis* 2000; 30:633-8.

136 Dodds GA et al. Negative predictive value of the Duke criteria for infective endocarditis. *Am J Cardiol* 1996; 77: 403-7.

# Surgery for Infective Endocarditis [137]

| Level of Evidence | Indication for Surgery | |
|---|---|---|
| | Native Valve | Prosthetic Valve |
| Strong (Class I) | • Acute aortic or mitral regurgitation with CHF despite treatment<br>• Perivalvular abscess*<br>• Bacteremia > 1 week on treatment without other source<br>• Fungal endocarditis | • PVE < 2 months post-op<br>• CHF resistant to treatment<br>• Fungal PVE<br>• *Staph* not responding to treatment<br>• Perivalvular leak<br>• Resistant organism or poor treatment response |
| Conflicting (Class II) | • Recurrent emboli on appropriate treatment<br>• Resistant organism, with poor response or CHF<br>• Mobile, left sided vegetation > 1 cm | • Persistent bacteremia<br>• Recurrent emboli on treatment |

PVE: Prosthetic valve endocarditis
\* Conduction abnormality may be first manifestation of perivalvular abscess

# Streptococcal Endocarditis Risk [138]

## Probability of endocarditis from streptococcal bacteremia

| Streptococcal species | Endocarditis: Nonendocarditis | Streptococcal species | Endocarditis: Nonendocarditis |
|---|---|---|---|
| *S. mutans* | 14.2:1 | Misc streptococci | 1:1.3 |
| *S. bovis* # | 5.9:1 | *S. bovis II* | 1:1.7 |
| Dextran-forming *mitior* | 3.3:1 | *S. anginosus* | 1:2.6 |
| *S. Sanguis* | 3.0:1 | Group G streptococci | 1:2.9 |
| *S. mitior* | 1.8:1 | Group B streptococci | 1:7.4 |
| Unclassified viridans | 1.4:1 | Group A streptococci | 1:32.0 |
| *Enterococcus faecalis* | 1:1.2 | | |

# Consider colonoscopy to exclude malignancy in cases of *S. bovis* and *Clostridia septicum* bacteremia

137  Mauri L et al. Infective endocarditis. *Curr Probl Cardiol* 2001; 26(9):562-610.
138  Parker MT, Ball LC. Streptococci and aerococci associated with systemic infection in man. *J Med Microbiol* 1976;9:275-302.

# *Bacterial Endocarditis Prophylaxis*[139]

## Endocarditis Prophylaxis Recommended

| High Risk | Moderate Risk |
|---|---|
| • Prosthetic cardiac valves<br>• Prior endocarditis<br>• Complex cyanotic congenital heart disease (single ventricle, tetralogy of Fallot, transposition of great vessels)<br>• Surgically constructed systemic-pulmonary shunts or conduits | • Most other congenital cardiac disease (not otherwise listed)<br>• Rheumatic and other acquired valvular heart disease<br>• Hypertrophic cardiomyopathy<br>• MVP **with** regurgitation or thickened leaflets (by echo or exam) |

## Endocarditis Prophylaxis *NOT* Recommended

| | |
|---|---|
| • Isolated secundum ASD<br>• Surgical repair of ASD, VSD or PDA<br>• Previous CABG<br>• MVP **without** regurgitation | • Previous Kawasaki or rheumatic heart disease w/o valve dysfunction<br>• Pacemakers and ICDs<br>• Physiologic or functional murmurs |

Selected procedures and endocarditis prophylaxis

| Procedure | Prophylaxis | No Prophylaxis |
|---|---|---|
| Dental | • extractions<br>• implants<br>• periodontal procedures<br>• root canal surgery<br>• subgingival surgery<br>• orthodontic bands<br>• intraligamentary injections<br>• cleaning when bleeding is anticipated | • restorative dentistry<br>• routine cleaning (no bleeding)<br>• local anesthetic injections<br>• intra-canal endodontic surgery<br>• placement of removable appliances<br>• suture removal<br>• orthodontic appliance adjustment |
| Respiratory tract | • tonsillectomy/adenoidectomy<br>• surgery involving mucosa<br>• rigid bronchoscopy | • endotracheal intubation<br>• flexible bronchoscopy (± bx) #<br>• tympanostomy tubes |
| GI tract § | • sclerotherapy for varices<br>• esophageal stricture dilation<br>• ERCP with biliary obstruction<br>• biliary tract surgery<br>• surgery involving mucosa | • trans-esophageal echo #<br>• endoscopy ± biopsy# |
| GU tract | • prostate surgery<br>• cystoscopy<br>• urethral dilatation | • vag hysterectomy or delivery #<br>• C-section<br>• sterilization*<br>• urethral catheterization*<br>• therapeutic abortion or D&C*<br>• IUDs*<br>• circumcision |
| Cardiac | • open heart surgery including valve replacement and implantation of synthetic material | • cardiac catheterization<br>• PTCA or stent placement<br>• ICDs or pacemakers |

# Prophylaxis optional for high risk patients
§ Recommended for high risk patients; optional for moderate risk patients
* Prophylaxis unnecessary in **uninfected tissue**

[139] Dajani AS *et al.* Prevention of Bacterial Endocarditis. Recommendations by AHA. *JAMA* 1997; 277:1794-1801. Durack DT. Prevention of infective endocarditis. *NEJM* 1995;332(1):38-44.

## Antibiotic Regimens for patients at risk

### Dental, Oral, Respiratory and Esophageal Procedures

| | |
|---|---|
| Standard | Amoxicillin 2 g PO 1 hr before procedure |
| NPO | Ampicillin 2 g IV or IM, 30 min before procedure |
| PCN-allergic | Clindamycin 600 mg *or* cephalexin/cefadroxil 2 g *or* azithro/clarithromycin 500mg, PO 1 hr prior to procedure |
| PCN-allergic/NPO | Clindamycin 600 mg *or* cefazolin 1 g, IV 30 min prior to procedure |

### GU or GI (excluding esophageal) Procedures

| | |
|---|---|
| High risk Standard | Ampicillin 2 g IM/IV *plus* gentamicin 1.5 mg/kg (up to 120 mg) IM/IV within 30 min of starting procedure, *plus* ampicillin 1 g IM/IV *or* amoxicillin 1 g PO 6 hours later |
| High risk PCN-allergic | Vancomycin 1 g IV over 1-2 hr *plus* gentamicin 1.5 mg/kg (up to 120 mg) Complete infusion within 30 min of starting procedure |
| Moderate risk Standard | Amoxicillin 2 g PO 1 hr before procedure *or* ampicillin 2 g IV/IM 30 min before procedure |
| Moderate risk PCN allergic | Vancomycin 1 g IV over 1-2 hr Give within 30 minutes of starting procedure |

# Rheumatic Fever: Jones Criteria [140]

| Major manifestations | Minor manifestations | Evidence of antecedent group A strep infection [d] |
|---|---|---|
| • Carditis [a]<br>• Polyarthritis [b]<br>• Sydenham's chorea<br>• Erythema marginatum<br>• Subcutaneous nodules [c] | • Fever<br>• Arthralgia<br>• ↑ ESR<br>• ↑ C-reactive protein<br>• Prolonged PR interval | • Positive throat culture or rapid streptococcal antigen test<br>• Elevated or rising streptococcal antibody (ASO) titer |

**a:** Almost always with murmur of valvulitis
**b:** Almost always migratory unless aborted with NSAIDS; large joints; almost never deforming; almost always dramatic response to salicylates < 48h
**c:** Over joint extensor surfaces, occiput, vertebral spinous processes
**d:** Note streptococcal skin infections are not associated with rheumatic fever

## Diagnosis
- High probability of acute rheumatic fever if evidence of antecedent group A streptococcal infection *plus* the presence of two major manifestations or of one major and two minor manifestations
- Exceptions to Jones criteria: (1) Isolated chorea (2) indolent carditis (3) history of rheumatic fever with one major or two minor manifestations and evidence of recent group A streptococcal infection

140 Guidelines for the diagnosis of rheumatic fever: Jones Criteria, updated 1992. *Circulation* 1993; 87(1):302.

# Life-threatening Rashes [141]

| Epidemiology | Manifestations | Diagnosis | Prognosis/Rx |
|---|---|---|---|
| **Rocky Mountain Spotted Fever (RMSF)**<br><br>• *Rickettsia rickettsii*<br>• Tick-borne<br>• Occurs in almost all US states, but most cases in Southeast<br>• Most cases spring/summer | • Fever, myalgia, headache<br>• **Rash:** typically starts day 4 on wrists/ ankles, spreads to palms/soles then centrally. Initially pink-red macules that blanch; evolves to petechiae, purpura and gangrene of digits, nose and genitals<br>• 10% "spotless"<br>• Atypical rash in deeply pigmented patients | • Clinical diagnosis<br>• No early lab clues<br>• Triad of fever, rash & tick bite in only 60-70%<br>• Late serology confirmatory<br>• DFA of skin biopsy 70% sensitive, 100% spec<br>• ?PCR | • Mortality 5-25% (higher with delayed diagnosis)<br>• **Rx:** doxycycline (IV or PO); chloramphenicol in pregnancy or young child |
| **Meningococcal Sepsis**<br><br>• *N. meningitidis*<br>• Transmission via respiratory droplets (close contact)<br>• Most cases winter/spring<br>• Patients usually < 20 y.o. | • Fever, headache, N/V, confusion, meningeal signs<br>• **Rash:** petechial, scattered on trunk/ extremities; evolves to palpable purpura ("gun-metal gray" with necrotic center). Petechiae clustered at pressure points.<br>• **Purpura fulminans:** cutaneous DIC with hemorrhagic bullae | • Gram stain/cx of blood, CSF, skin<br>• Gram stain of petechiae 70% sensitive<br>• Cx of skin bx may remain (+) after antibiotics given | • Mortality 10-20%<br>• **Rx:** PCN G IV<br>• Contacts: rifampin, ciprofloxacin or ceftriaxone |
| **Staphylococcal Toxic Shock Syndrome (STSS)**<br><br>• *Staph aureus* (toxin-producing)<br>• Most cases non-menstrual<br>• Associated with flu, childbirth, tracheitis, wound infection, nasal packing<br>• 40% recurrence | • Fever, malaise, myalgia, N/V, diarrhea<br>• Prominent confusion<br>• **Rash:** sunburn-like, diffuse macular erythroderm followed by desquamation of hands and feet in 5-14 days. Also causes conjunctival injection, oral-genital mucosal hyperemia, and "strawberry" tongue | • Isolation of *S. aureus* from blood unusual<br>• Diagnostic criteria:<br>1) fever or ↓BP<br>2) typical rash<br>3) multi-organ involvement<br>4) exclusion of other causes | • Mortality 10-15% (5% in menstrual cases)<br>• **Rx:** anti-staph antibiotic, supportive care, removal of source<br>• Concurrent clindamycin may reduce toxin release<br>• Possible role for IVIG |

---

141 Drage L. Life-threatening rashes: dermatologic signs of four infectious diseases. *Mayo Clin Proc* 1999; 74:68-72.

| Epidemiology | Manifestations | Diagnosis | Prognosis/Rx |
|---|---|---|---|
| **Streptococcal Toxic Shock Syndrome**<br><br>• Group A strep<br>• Soft tissue infections most common<br>• Most patients 20-50 y.o. and otherwise healthy | • Fever, hypotension, severe local pain<br>• **Rash:** highly variable: localized erythema, diffuse erythroderm or violaceous bullae<br>• Pain >> physical findings<br>• Can occur after blunt trauma or muscle strain | • Bacteremia in 60%, but open biopsy often necessary<br>• Diagnostic criteria: isolation of group A strep, ↓BP and multi-organ involvement | • Mortality 30-70%<br>• **Rx:** PCN G plus aggressive surgical exploration and debridement<br>• Concurrent clindamycin may reduce toxin release |

## Bacterial vs. Viral Meningitis[142]

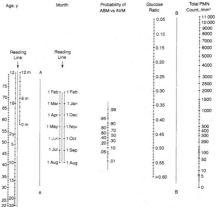

**Directions:** to estimate probability of acute bacterial (ABM) vs. acute viral meningitis (AVM): **(1)** Place ruler on reading lines for patient age and month of presentation; mark intersection on line A **(2)** Repeat for glucose and CSF neutrophil count on line B **(3)** Place ruler on the marks on lines A and B and read probability of ABM vs. AVM.
Derived from data 1969-80. No prospective validation to date; several retrospective validations have been published.[143] **Note:** Data from population at low risk for TB meningitis; assess risk of TB independent of nomogram. Data from northern hemisphere.

---

142 Spanos A *et al.* Differential diagnosis of acute meningitis: an analysis of the predictive value of initial observations. JAMA 1989; 262(19):2700-7. Copyright 1989, American Medical Association, reproduced with permission.

143 J Gen Intern Med 1994; 9:8-12; Eur J Clin Microbiol Infect Dis 1995; 14: 267-74.

# Bacterial Meningitis in Adults[144]

Data from review of 493 episodes in 445 adults at referral center 1962-1988

| Finding | Community–Acquired | Nosocomial |
|---|---|---|
| Total cases | 296 episodes in 275 patients (60% of total) | 197 episodes in 175 patients (40% of total) |
| Recurrent cases | 38 episodes in 17 patients | 41 episodes in 19 patients |
| Predisposing factors | Otitis media (26%) Sinusitis (12%) Pneumonia (15%) Immunocompromise (19%) Diabetes (10%) Alcoholism (18%) CSF leak (8%) | Recent neurosurgery (68%) Neurosurgical device (32%) Immunocompromise (31%) Recent head injury (13%) CSF leak (13%) |
| Predisposing factors for recurrent meningitis | CSF leak (76%) History of head trauma or neurosurgery (47%) | Neurosurgical procedure (100%) CSF leak (47%) |
| Causative organism (in single episodes) | Strep pneumonia (38%) N. meningitidis (14%) Listeria (11%) Streptococci (7%) Staph aureus (5%) H. influenza (4%) Gram neg bacilli (4%) Culture negative (13%) | Gram neg bacilli (38%) Streptococci (9%) Staph aureus (9%) Coag neg staph (9%) Mixed species (7%) Strep pneumonia (5%) H. influenza (4%) Culture negative (11%) |
| Clinical findings (in community acquired cases) | Fever, nuchal rigidity and abnormal mental status | 66% |
| | Fever | 95% |
| | Nuchal rigidity | 88% |
| | Abnormal mental status | 78% |
| | Seizures | 23% |
| | Focal neurologic findings | 28% |

| *Cerebrospinal Fluid (CSF) Findings* | | | | |
|---|---|---|---|---|
| Opening pressure (cm $H_2O$) | 0-139: | 9% | 0-139: | 23% |
| | 140-299: | 52% | 140-299: | 52% |
| | > 300-399: | 39% | > 300: | 26% |
| WBC per $mm^3$ | 0-99: | 13% | 0-99: | 19% |
| | 100-4999: | 59% | 100-4999: | 62% |
| | > 5000: | 28% | >5000: | 20% |
| % PMNs | 0-19: | 2% | 0-19: | 2% |
| | 20-79: | 19% | 20-79: | 31% |
| | > 80%: | 79% | > 80%: | 66% |
| Protein (mg/dl) | 0-45: | 4% | 0-45: | 6% |
| | 46-199: | 40% | 46-199: | 42% |
| | >200: | 56% | >200: | 52% |
| Glucose <40 mg/dl | 50% | | 45% | |
| Gram-stain, Cx (+) | 60%, 73% | | 46%, 83% | |

- Overall fatality rate = 25% (19% meningitis-related)
- No significant change in mortality rate over time
- 98% of patients who died had at least one of three risk factors: (1) age > 60 (2) onset of seizures within 24 hr of admission (3) obtunded mental status on admission

144 Durand M et al. Acute bacterial meningitis in adults – A review of 493 episodes. *NEJM* 1993;328(1):21-28.

# Community-Acquired Pneumonia [145]

## Etiology

| Pathogen | % cases | Pathogen | % cases |
|---|---|---|---|
| Strep pneumoniae # | 20-60 | Chlamydia pneumoniae | 4-6 |
| H. influenza | 3-10 | Mycoplasma + | 1-6 |
| Staph aureus | 3-5 | Influenza/Viruses * | 2-15 |
| Gram-negative rods * | 3-10 | Aspiration * | 6-10 |
| Legionella | 2-8 | Unknown | ~ 40 |

\# Accounts for 2/3 of bacteremic cases     * Higher rate in nursing home population
+ Most common *identifiable* cause of "walking" pneumonia in healthy young outpatients

**Diagnostic evaluation: Inpatients**
- **CXR:** Confirms pneumonia in < 25% of patients with lower respiratory tract sx
- **Sputum gram stain and culture:** Utility of gram stain controversial, but high quality specimen (<10 epithelial cells and >25 PMNs per low powered field) with gram positive diplococci is 50% sensitive and 90% specific for pneumococcal pneumonia
- **Labs:** CBC w/diff, chemistry panel including glucose, sodium, LFTs, renal function (see PORT score) • HIV test (if at risk) • Pre-treatment blood cultures x 2 (positive in 11% of patients with CAP)
- **If failure to improve after initial treatment:** • Serologies/PCR for mycoplasma and chlamydia • Legionella culture/urinary antigen • HIV
- ***Severely ill patients:*** • ABG • Sputum culture and urine antigen for Legionella (especially if local outbreak)
- ***Immunocompromised patients:*** • Induced sputum for AFB, fungal, PCP
- Rapid viral antigens (DFA) including influenza, RSV, parainfluenza, adenovirus
- Consider early bronchoscopy if failure to respond to treatment
- Routine serologies for Chlamydia and Mycoplasma **not** recommended

**Diagnostic evaluation: Outpatients**
- CXR • CBC, chemistry panel

## Prognosis in community acquired pneumonia (PORT Score) [146]

| Characteristic | Score | Exam Findings | Score |
|---|---|---|---|
| Age | Age | Altered mental status | + 20 |
| Female Gender | - 10 | Resp rate ≥ 30 | + 20 |
| Nursing home resident | + 10 | SBP < 90 | + 20 |
| **Co-existing Illness** | | Temp < 35° or ≥ 40° C | + 15 |
| Malignancy | + 30 | Pulse ≥ 125 | + 10 |
| Liver disease | + 20 | **Laboratory/CXR findings** | |
| CHF | + 10 | Arterial pH < 7.35 | + 30 |
| Cerebrovascular disease | + 10 | BUN ≥ 30 mg/dl | + 20 |
| Renal disease | + 10 | Na+ < 130 mmol/L | + 20 |
| **Exclusion criteria:** | | Glucose ≥ 250 mg/dl | +10 |
| • Age <18 • HIV or AIDS | | Hct < 30 % | +10 |
| • 1° diagnosis other than pneumonia | | PaO₂ < 60 mmHg | +10 |
| • Previous admission within 7 days | | Pleural effusion | +10 |

---

145 Mandell LA *et al.* Update of practice guidelines for the management of community-acquired pneumonia in immunocompetent adults. *Clin Infect Dis* 2003; 37:1405-33. Halm EA, Teirstein AS. Clinical practice. Management of community-acquired pneumonia. *NEJM* 2002; 347:2039-45.

146 Fine MJ *et al.* A prediction rule to identify low-risk patients with community acquired pneumonia. *N Eng J Med* 1997; 336:243-50.

| PORT Score | Class | Mortality (%) | Admit Rate (%) [a] | ICU Admit (%) | Median Stay (days) | Recommended Site of Care |
|---|---|---|---|---|---|---|
| ≤ 50 [b] | I | 0.1 | 5.1 | 4.3 | 5.0 | Outpatient |
| ≤ 70 | II | 0.6 | 8.2 | 4.3 | 6.0 | Outpatient |
| 71-90 | III | 0.9 | 16.7 | 5.9 | 7.0 | Inpatient (brief) |
| 91-130 | IV | 9.3 | 20.0 | 11.4 | 9.0 | Inpatient |
| > 130 | V | 27.0 | n/a | 17.3 | 11.0 | Inpatient |
| Total | | 5.2 | 7.4 | 9.2 | 7.0 | |

**a:** Subsequent admission rate if initially treated as outpatient (no increased mortality)
**b:** Class I - age 50 or less and **no** co-existent illnesses or exam findings

## Treatment [147]

| Outpatients | Empiric Antibiotic Selection |
|---|---|
| Healthy outpatient | • Macrolide [a] or doxycycline<br>• If recent antibiotics: fluoroquinolone [b] alone, or advanced macrolide [c] plus high-dose amoxicillin (1 g tid) or amoxicillin-clavulanate (2 g bid) |
| Outpatient with co-morbidities (e.g. COPD, diabetes, ESRD, CHF, cancer) | • Advanced macrolide [c] or fluoroquinolone [b]<br>• If recent antibiotics: fluoroquinolone alone or advanced macrolide [c] plus β-lactam [d] |
| Suspected aspiration | • Amoxicillin-clavulanate or clindamycin |
| Influenza with bacterial superinfection | • β-lactam [d] or fluoroquinolone [b] |
| Nursing home resident | • Fluoroquinolone [b] alone, or advanced macrolide [c] plus amoxicillin/clavulanate |

| Inpatients | Empiric Antibiotic Selection |
|---|---|
| General medical ward | • Fluoroquinolone [b] alone, or advanced macrolide [c] plus β-lactam [e] *(consider recent antibiotic exposure)* |
| ICU | • β-lactam [e] plus either an advanced macrolide [c] or fluoroquinolone [b]<br>• PCN allergy: fluoroquinolone [b] +/- clindamycin |
| Risk for *Pseudomonas* [f] | • Anti-pseudomonal agent [g] plus:<br>(1) ciprofloxacin, or<br>(2) a macrolide [a] or a fluoroquinolone [b] plus an aminoglycoside (AG) [h]<br>• PCN allergy: aztreonam + fluoroquinolone [b] +/- AG |

**a:** Azithro-, clarithro- or erythromycin
**b:** Levo-, gati-, gemi- or moxifloxacin
**c:** Azithro- or clarithromycin
**d:** High-dose amoxicillin (1 g tid), high-dose amoxicillin/clavulanate (2 g bid), cefpodoxime, cefprozil, or cefuroxime
**e:** Cefotaxime, ceftriaxone, ampicillin/sulbactam, or ertapenem
**f:** Risk factors for pseudomonas include severe structural lung disease (e.g., bronchiectasis), recent antibiotics, recent hospitalization (especially ICU)
**g:** Piperacillin, piperacillin/tazobactam, imipenem, meropenem, or cefepime
**h:** Data suggests elderly patients do worse with aminoglycoside

---

147 Mandell LA et al. Update of practice guidelines for the management of community-acquired pneumonia in immunocompetent adults. *Clin Infect Dis* 2003; 37:1405-33.

**Additional considerations**
- Mortality increased in patients with delay > 8 hr from hospital admission to initial antibiotics
- No controlled trials on optimal duration of treatment but atypical infections (*Chlamydia, Mycoplasma* or *Legionella*) may relapse if treated < 2 weeks
- Consider influenza and pneumococcal vaccine upon discharge
- Consider follow-up chest x-ray to ensure resolution, with caveat that mean persistence of radiographic infiltrate is 8-12 weeks for patients > 50 y.o. (4-8 weeks if < 50 y.o)

# *Occupational HIV Exposure*[148]

### Risk after occupational exposure to HIV-infected blood[149]
- Average risk for seroconversion after percutaneous exposure to HIV-infected blood: ~ 0.3%
- Mucous membrane exposure to HIV-infected blood: ~ 0.09%
- Non-intact skin exposure to blood, or exposure to fluids other than HIV-infected blood: Unknown, but presumably < 0.09%
- Risk increases with exposure to larger quantity of blood, including **(1)** deep injury **(2)** visible blood on device causing injury **(3)** device previously placed in source-patient's vein or artery. Risk also increased if source-patient has advanced HIV disease (i.e. high viral load). **Note**: Undetectable HIV viral load in source patient does not exclude possibility of transmission.
- HIV also transmittable by semen, vaginal secretions, and any fluid grossly contaminated with blood
- Unclear risk with CSF, peritoneal, pleural, synovial, pericardial and amniotic fluids
- Negligible risk with saliva, tears, sweat, breast milk, non-bloody urine or feces

### HIV seroconversion in health care personnel (HCP)
- 81% have syndrome compatible with 1° infection (median 25 days postexposure)
- Median time of exposure to seroconversion = 46 days
- 95% seroconvert by 6 months
- Post-exposure prophylaxis with ZDV reduces risk of seroconversion by ~80%

### Management of potential exposures to HIV
1) Evaluate exposed HCP within hours (rather than days)
2) Rapid HIV test of source patient -- no further testing or treatment warranted if test is negative, unless source patient has signs/symptoms consistent with acute HIV
3) Obtain baseline HIV status of exposed HCP (also HBsAg, HBsAb, HCV Ab)
4) Decide about postexposure prophylaxis (PEP) based on exposure type and medical status of source patient (*see next page*)
5) Consider pregnancy testing, HBV postexposure prophylaxis, Td

---

148 Updated U.S. Public Health Service guidelines for the management of occupational exposures to HBV, HCV, and HIV and recommendations for postexposure prophylaxis. *MMWR* 2001;50(No. RR-11); Gerberding JL. Occupational exposure to HIV in health care settings. *NEJM* 2003; 348:826-833.
149 Cardo DM *et al.* A case-control study of HIV seroconversion in health care workers after percutaneous exposure. *NEJM* 1997; 337:1485-90.

### Percutaneous Injuries - Recommended Postexposure Prophylaxis (PEP)

| Percutaneous Exposure Type | Infection status of source patient | | | | |
|---|---|---|---|---|---|
| | HIV Class 1 * | HIV Class 2 ** | Unknown HIV status | Unknown source | HIV negative |
| Less severe # | Recommend 2 drugs | Recommend 3 drugs | Generally withheld; consider 2 drugs if source has HIV risk factor | Generally withheld; consider 2 drugs in setting where HIV exposure is likely | No treatment |
| More severe † | Recommend 3 drugs | Recommend 3 drugs | | | |

\* HIV class 1: asymptomatic HIV infection or low viral load
\*\*HIV class 2: symptomatic HIV, AIDS, acute seroconversion, or known high viral load
\# Solid needle, superficial injury
† Large-bore hollow needle, deep puncture, visible blood on device, needle in vessel

### Mucous Membrane and Non-intact Skin* Exposures - Recommended (PEP)

| Exposure Type | Infection status of source patient | | | | |
|---|---|---|---|---|---|
| | HIV Class 1 ** | HIV Class 2 # | Unknown HIV status | Unknown source | HIV negative |
| Small volume † | Consider 2 drugs | Recommend 2 drugs | Generally withheld; consider 2 drugs if source has HIV risk factor | Generally withheld; consider 2 drugs in setting where HIV exposure is likely | No treatment |
| Large volume ‡ | Recommend 2 drugs | Recommend 3 drugs | | | |

\* Follow-up indicated only if open wound, dermatitis, abrasion, etc.
\*\*HIV class 1: asymptomatic HIV infection or low viral load
\# HIV class 2: symptomatic HIV, AIDS, acute seroconversion, or known high viral load
† e.g. few drops     ‡ e.g. major blood splash

| PEP Regimen | Examples | Duration |
|---|---|---|
| 2 drug (basic): 2 NRTIs | • ZDV (300 mg bid) + 3TC (150 mg bid)<br>• 3TC (150 mg bid) + d4T (40 mg bid)<br>• d4T (40 mg bid) + ddl (250 mg qd *) | 4 weeks |
| 3 drug (expanded): 2 NRTIs plus PI or NNRTI | **2 drug regimen plus:**<br>• indinavir (800 mg tid) or<br>• nelfinavir (750 mg tid or 1250 mg bid) or<br>• efavirenz (600 mg qhs) or<br>• abacavir (300 mg bid) | 4 weeks |

NRTI: nucleoside reverse transcriptase inhibitor     PI: Protease inhibitor
NNRTI: non-nucleoside reverse transcriptase inhibitor    * delayed-release capsule

## Additional considerations
- Start prophylaxis ASAP, ideally within 1-2 hr
- Health care personnel begun on PEP should have follow-up HIV serology at 6, 12 & 26 wks
- National Clinician's Post-exposure Hotline: 1-888-448-4911 or www.ucsf.edu/hivcntr or Needlestick! Online: www.needlestick.mednet.ucla.edu
- Consider expert consultation if:
  - > 24-36 hr interval from exposure to evaluation
  - Unknown source (e.g. needle in laundry)
  - Known or suspected pregnancy in exposed person (should not preclude initiating treatment). Antiviral Pregnancy Registry: 1-800-258-4263
  - Known or suspected antiretroviral resistance in source patient (e.g. clinically progressive HIV, rising viral load, or declining CD4 count on treatment)
  - Significant side effects from PEP regimen (~50% incidence, higher if 3 drug regimen)

# Acute HIV Infection[150]

## Clinical presentation
- Acute illness 2-4 wks after exposure (range: 6 days-10 months)
- Average duration of symptoms 22 days (range: 3 days-10 wks)
- 80-90% individuals symptomatic
- Most patients seek care (17% hospitalized) but diagnosis usually missed; clinicians should maintain a high level of suspicion when evaluating a mono-like illness

## Common symptoms
- Fever (96%) • Adenopathy (74%) • Pharyngitis (70%) • Rash (maculo-papular) or oral-genital ulcers (70%) • Arthralgia/myalgia (54%) • Diarrhea (32%) • Headache/aseptic meningitis (32%) • Nausea/vomiting (27%) • Thrush (12%)
- **Note:** *Presence of more severe or prolonged symptoms (fever, thrush) correlates with more rapid progression to AIDS*

## Differential diagnosis:
- EBV • CMV • Viral hepatitis • Enterovirus infection • 2° syphilis • Toxoplasmosis • HSV with erythema multiforme • Drug reaction • Behcet's • SLE

## Laboratory features
- **Hematologic:** Lymphopenia followed by lymphocytosis • Mild or no atypical lymphocytosis • Thrombocytopenia • Elevated transaminases • Depressed CD4
- **HIV antibody:** Usually negative; median time to conversion 3-4 wks with > 95% positive at 6 months
- **Confirmation:** HIV RNA (viral load) should be markedly elevated (usually > 100 K); confirm by antibody at 1-3 months
- **Genotypic resistance testing:** Given high rate of resistant strains, all patients with acute HIV should have genotypic resistance test performed to guide therapy

## Management
- Supportive care
- Referral to HIV specialist
- Probable long-term benefit with early institution of triple drug therapy

---

150 Kahn KO, Walker BD. Current Concepts: Acute HIV type 1 infection. *NEJM* 1998; 339(1) 33-37.

# Complications of HIV Infection[151]

| CD4 Count | Common Clinical Syndromes[152] | |
|---|---|---|
| | *Infectious* | *Non-Infectious* |
| > 500 | • Acute retroviral syndrome<br>• Vaginal candidiasis<br>• Non-HIV infections | • Lymphadenopathy<br>• Guillain-Barré syndrome<br>• Aseptic meningitis |
| 200-500 | • Bacterial pneumonia/sinusitis<br>• Pulmonary TB<br>• Oral/esophageal candidiasis<br>• Herpes zoster<br>• Cryptosporidiosis<br>• Kaposi's sarcoma<br>• Oral hairy leukoplakia | • B-cell or Hodgkin's lymphoma<br>• Anemia<br>• Immune thrombocytopenic purpura<br>• Cervical cancer/dysplasia<br>• Mononeuritis multiplex |
| 50-200 | • *P. carinii* pneumonia#<br>• Disseminated HSV<br>• Toxoplasmosis#<br>• Cryptococcosis<br>• Disseminated histoplasmosis or coccidioidomycosis<br>• Chronic cryptosporidiosis<br>• Microsporidiosis<br>• Miliary or extrapulmonary TB#<br>• Progressive multi-focal leukoencephalopathy (PML) | • Wasting<br>• HIV-associated dementia<br>• CNS lymphoma<br>• Cardiomyopathy<br>• Peripheral neuropathy<br>• Myelopathy/polyradiculopathy<br>• Immunoblastic lymphoma |
| < 50 | • Disseminated CMV<br>• Disseminated *M. avium* # | |

# If prophylaxis given opportunistic infection unlikely unless CD4 < 50-100

## HIV: Pulmonary disease [153]

| Very Common | Somewhat Common | Uncommon |
|---|---|---|
| • *P. carinii* #<br>• *S. pneumoniae*<br>• *H. influenza*<br>• Staph aureus<br>• TB | • *Pseudomonas*<br>• Enteric gram-negatives<br>• Histoplasmosis<br>• *Cryptococcus*<br>• CMV<br>• Aspergillus<br>• Kaposi's sarcoma<br>• Lymphoma<br>• CHF<br>• LIP* (mostly children) | • Nocardia<br>• *Legionella*<br>• *M. avium* complex<br>• *Toxoplasma*<br>• *Coccidioides*<br>• *Cryptosporidia*<br>• *Rhodococcus*<br>• 1° pulmonary HTN |

# PCP highly unlikely if patient compliant with trimethoprim-sulfa prophylaxis
* LIP = lymphocytic interstitial pneumonitis

151 Sax PE. Opportunistic infections in HIV disease: Down but not out. *Infect Dis Clin North Am* 2001; 15:433-55.; Bartlett JG, Gallant JE. *Medical Management of HIV Infection.* Baltimore: Johns Hopkins University, 2003.

152 Hanson DL. Distribution of CD4+ T lymphocytes at diagnosis of acquired immunodeficiency syndrome-defining and other human immunodeficiency virus-related illnesses. *Arch Int Med* 1995; 155(14):1537-1542.

153 Murray JF, Mills J. Pulmonary infectious complications of HIV infection. *Am Rev Resp Dis* 1990; 141:1356-72, 1582-98; Hirschtick RE *et al.* Bacterial pneumonia in persons infected with the human immunodeficiency virus. *NEJM* 1995; 333: 845-51.

| Radiographic Finding | Pulmonary Pathogen/Disease |
|---|---|
| Diffuse infiltrate | • PCP • TB (in advanced disease) • Histoplasmosis • Lipoid interstitial pneumonia • Coccidioidomycosis • Less common: CMV, HSV, influenza, toxoplasmosis |
| Focal consolidation | • Bacterial pneumonia • Kaposi's sarcoma • Cryptococcosis |
| Nodules or mass lesions | • TB • Cryptococcus • Histoplasmosis • *M. avium* complex • Kaposi's • PCP • Aspergillus • Lymphoma • Toxoplasmosis |
| Hilar/mediastinal adenopathy | • TB • *M. avium* complex • Histoplasmosis • Coccidioidomycosis • Lymphoma • Kaposi's sarcoma |
| Pneumothorax | • PCP (esp. if treated with aerosolized pentamidine) |
| Normal | • PCP • TB • Cryptococcosis • *M. avium* complex |
| Cavitary lesions | • Bacterial pneumonia • TB • Atypical mycobacteria • Cryptococcosis • Histoplasmosis • Coccidioidomycosis • Aspergillus • *Nocardia* • *Rhodococcus* |
| Pleural effusion | • Bacterial pneumonia • Kaposi's • TB • Cryptococcosis • PCP • Low albumin • CHF • Aspergillus |

## HIV: Neurologic disease [154]

| Very Common | Somewhat Common | Rare |
|---|---|---|
| • Cryptococcus | • TB | • Nocardia * |
| • Toxoplasmosis * | • Cytomegalovirus | • Histoplasmosis |
| • Adverse drug reaction | • Bacterial brain abscess * | • *Coccidioides* |
| • Psychiatric illness | | • *Aspergillus* * |
| • HIV encephalopathy | | • Listeria |
| • Progressive multifocal leukoencephalopathy * | | • Varicella |
| • CNS lymphoma * | | • Herpes simplex * |
| | | • Syphilis |

* Usually focal lesions on CT/MRI

**Comments:**
• Nodular or ring-enhancing lesions on CT/MRI are usually toxoplasmosis or lymphoma; single lesion favors lymphoma. Less common lesions include TB, Cryptococcus, Nocardia, Aspergillus.
• Non-enhancing lesion: HIV, progressive multifocal leukoencephalopathy (PML), CMV most common
• Serum cryptococcal antigen nearly 100% sensitive
• Prior (+) toxoplasma IgG helpful (although negative serology does not exclude active infection)

## HIV: Chronic* diarrhea [155]

| Very Common | Somewhat Common | Rare |
|---|---|---|
| • Microsporidia | • Giardia | • Amebiasis |
| • Cryptosporidia | • Cytomegalovirus | • *Isospora belli* |
| • *M. avium* complex | • GI lymphoma | • Strongyloides |
| • Medication side effects | • *C. difficile* | • Cyclospora |
| • AIDS enteropathy (50%) | | • Kaposi's sarcoma |

* Causes of acute diarrhea include *Salmonella, Shigella, Campylobacter, C. difficile* and viruses

154 Simpson DM, Tagliati M. Neurologic manifestations of HIV infection. *Ann Int Med* 1994; 121:769-785.
155 DuPont HL, Marshall GD. HIV-associated diarrhea and wasting. *Lancet* 1995; 346:352-356.

## HIV: Undifferentiated fever [156]

| Very Common | Somewhat Common | Rare |
|---|---|---|
| • M. avium complex | • Histoplasmosis | • Extrapulmonary |
| • Early Pneumocystis carinii | • Lymphoma | Pneumocystis carinii |
| • Cytomegalovirus | • Sinusitis | • Cryptococcus |
| • TB | • Central line infection | • Atypical mycobacteria |
| • Undetermined (?HIV itself) | • Bacterial endocarditis | • Toxoplasma |
| | • Drug fever | • Bartonella |
| | • Miscellaneous viral (hepatitis B, hepatitis C, varicella, herpes simplex) | • Coccidioides |

### Comments:
- 88% of fever in patients with HIV are due to occult infections
- Multiple causes of fever are common

### Pearls and nonsense [157]
- People with HIV die of AIDS-related diseases, not low CD4 counts
- Minor illnesses occur, but in proportion to the CD4 count
- Most HIV-related conditions are suppressed – not cured – and tend to relapse unless the CD4 count rises on antiviral therapy
- Drug reactions are common
- All patients on antiviral therapy should be on at least 3 agents in combination, with a goal of reducing the HIV viral load to below the limit of detection
- Strict adherence to medications ("every dose, every day") should be emphasized
- Antiretroviral therapy should not be stopped unless absolutely necessary
- Updated treatment guidelines at: http://www.aidsinfo.nih.gov/guidelines

[156] Armstrong WS, Katz JT, Kazanjian PH. HIV-associated fever of unknown origin: a study of 70 patients in the U.S. and review. *Clin Inf Dis* 1999; 28:341-5.
[157] Special thanks to Drs. Paul Sax and Joel Katz for these words of wisdom

# *Infections after Transplantation*[158]

**Timing of common infections after marrow transplant**

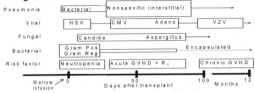

**Viral infections after marrow transplant**

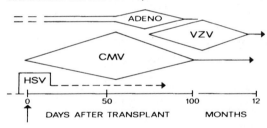

**Solid-organ transplant infections in the first year**

| Type | Infection per pt | Infection mortality | Bacter- emia | Symptom atic CMV | Invasive fungus | Site most common |
|------|-----------------|--------------------|-------------|-----------------|----------------|------------------|
| Renal | 0.98 | 0 | 5% | 5% | 0 | UTI 41% |
| Heart | 1.36 | 15% | 13% | 5% | 8% | Lung 27% |
| Heart-Lung | 3.19 | 45% | 19% | 32% | 23% | Lung 57% |
| Liver | 1.86 | 23% | 23% | 5% | 16% | Abd,GI 23% |

158 Meyers JD. Infections in marrow transplant recipients; and Ho M *et al.* Infections in solid organ transplant recipients. In: *Principles and Practice of Infectious Disease*, 3rd ed. Mandell *et al* (eds). New York: Churchill-Livingstone, 1990. Reproduced with permission.

## Infections after solid organ transplants[159]

| Time | Typical Infections | Comments |
|------|--------------------|----------|
| 0 – 1 months | **Conventional nosocomial** *Viral*: HSV, onset of HBV/HCV *Bacterial*: wound or catheter infections, nosocomial pneumonia *Fungal*: Candida | 90% of infections related to surgical wound (high risk of contaminating allograft if donor or recipient has active infection) |
| 1 – 6 months (or patients with chronic rejection) | **Unconventional or opportunistic** *Viral*: CMV, EBV, VZV, influenza, RSV, adenovirus *Bacterial*: Nocardia, Listeria, TB *Fungal*: Aspergillus, Cryptococcus, Candida *Parasitic*: PCP, Strongyloides, toxoplasma, leishmania, trypanosoma | Opportunistic infections more common if co-infection with immune-modulating viruses (CMV, EBV) or more intense immunosuppression (i.e. for rejection) |
| > 6 months | **Community-acquired or persistent** *Bacterial*: typical respiratory infections *Viral*: CMV retinitis or colitis, HPV, post-transplant lymphoproliferative disorders (CMV and EBV-related) *Fungal*: Histoplasma, Coccidioides | 80% of patients doing well w/ minimal immuno-suppression; 10% with chronic viral infections; 10% with chronic rejection requiring high intensity immunosuppression |

## Fever & pulmonary infiltrates in solid-organ transplant patients

| Radiographic Abnormality | Acute Illness | Subacute or Chronic |
|--------------------------|---------------|---------------------|
| Consolidation | • Bacteria (incl. legionella) • Thromboembolism • Hemorrhage • Pulmonary edema | • Fungi, Nocardia • Tumor • Viruses, PCP, radiation, drug reactions |
| Peribronchovascular abnormality | • Pulmonary edema • Leukoagglutinin reaction • Bacteria • Viruses (influenza) | • Viruses, PCP • Radiation • Drug reactions • Nocardia, tumor, fungi, TB |
| Nodular infiltrate (≥1 defects > 1 cm² with well-defined borders) | • Bacteria (incl. legionella) • Pulmonary edema | • Fungi • Nocardia, TB • PCP • PTLD |

## CNS infection in transplant recipients

| Pattern | Etiology |
|---------|----------|
| Acute meningitis | Bacterial esp. Listeria, West Nile virus |
| Subacute/chronic meningitis | Cryptococcus (also TB, Listeria, Histoplasma, Nocardia, Strongyloides, Coccidioides, PTLD, HHV 6) |
| Focal brain infection | Aspergillus, listeria, toxoplasma, nocardia, PTLD |
| Progressive dementia | PML, HSV, CMV, EBV, demyelination due to drug reaction |

PTLD = EBV-associated post-transplant lymphoproliferative disease
PML = progressive multifocal leukoencephalopathy

---

159 Fishman JA, Rubin RH. Infections in organ-transplant recipients. *NEJM* 1998; 338(24):1741-51.

# Neurology

## *Common Stroke Syndromes*[160]

### Ischemic Stroke Localization

| Syndrome | Arteries | Common Findings |
|---|---|---|
| Anterior Circulation | Internal carotid, middle cerebral, anterior cerebral | **Left:** Aphasia, right limb/face weakness<br>**Right:** Left visual neglect, denial of deficit, left limb/face weakness, poor visuospatial function |
| Posterior Circulation | Posterior cerebral | **Left:** Right hemianopsia, large lesions may include inability to read but not write and spell<br>**Right:** Left hemianopsia |
| Brainstem-cerebellum | Vertebral, basilar | Vertigo, cranial nerve findings especially extraocular movement palsies, quadriparesis, ataxia, nystagmus, crossed signs (ipsilateral cranial nerve palsies and contralateral limb weakness or sensory loss), coma |
| Lacunar motor stroke | Penetrating artery in pons or internal capsule | Pure hemiparesis |
| Lacunar sensory stroke | Penetrating artery in thalamus or posterior limb of internal capsule | Pure hemisensory symptoms |

### Common aneurysm sites

| Location (junction or bifurcation) | Signs of leak or rupture |
|---|---|
| Internal carotid-posterior communicating artery | • Ipsilateral 3rd nerve palsy |
| Anterior communicating artery | • Bilateral leg weakness, numbness and Babinski reflex |
| Middle cerebral bifurcation | • Contralateral face or hand weakness, aphasia (left) or visual neglect (right) |
| Basilar bifurcation | • Bilateral vertical gaze palsies, Babinski sign, coma |
| Vertebral-posterior inferior communicating artery junction | • Vertigo, lateral medullary syndrome |

---

160 Chung C-S, Caplan LR. Neurovascular Disorders. In: *Textbook of Clinical Neurology*. Goetz CG, Pappert EJ, editors. Philadelphia: W.B. Saunders, 1999.

## Common signs of hypertensive intracranial hemorrhage

| Location | Motor/sensory | Pupils | Eye Movements | Other |
|---|---|---|---|---|
| Putamen or internal capsule (40%) | Contralateral hemiparesis and sensory loss | Normal | Conjugate gaze paresis to opposite side ("eyes look toward lesion") | Aphasia (left), neglect (right) |
| Caudate (8%) | Transient contralateral hemiparesis | Ipsilateral Horner's * | Conjugate gaze paresis to opposite side * | Agitation, poor memory |
| Lobar (15%) | May include hemiparesis, aphasia | Normal | Conjugate gaze paresis to opposite sign | May include confusion, aphasia (left), hemianopsia, neglect (right) |
| Thalamus (20%) | Contralateral sensory>motor loss | Small, poorly reactive, uni- or bilateral | Upgaze paralysis (eyes down and in), ipsilateral conjugate gaze paresis * | Somnolence, aphasia (left), or neglect (right) |
| Pons # | Quadriparesis | Small, reactive | Absent horizontal gaze, ocular bobbing | Coma |
| Cerebellum (8%) | Ipsilateral ataxia, no paralysis | Ipsilateral pupil smaller * | Prominent nystagmus | Vomiting, postural instability |

* Variable finding    # Typical findings for large or bilateral lesions

# *Early Management of Stroke*[161]

## Initial assessment
- Assess ABCs and vital signs
- Provide $O_2$, protect airway
- Establish onset of symptoms: **3 hour** window for thrombolytic therapy (best results if given within 90 minutes; up to 6 hr for intra-arterial therapy)
- Obtain IV access, EKG and send initial studies (CBC, platelets, lytes, PT/PTT, glucose, liver/kidney function, type and screen); consider toxicology screen and hypercoagulable work-up in young patients without apparent risk factors
- C-spine if trauma or comatose
- Check glucose and treat if indicated
- Focused general PE and neurological exam, including level of consciousness (Glasgow Coma Score – *see page 118*) and stroke severity
- Assess for co-existing acute cardiovascular disease (MI, aortic dissection) or unusual cause of stroke (*see page 106* )
- **Urgent non-contrast head CT** or **diffusion-weighted MRI** to assess if stroke is ischemic or hemorrhagic – goal is completion within 25 min of arrival and interpretation within 45 min
  - CT generally preferred for availability & rapid diagnosis of intracranial bleeding
  - CT is 50% sensitive for ischemic changes within 6 hr of stroke
  - Diffusion weighted MRI is > 90% sensitive and turns positive earlier than CT
  - Perform CT angiogram (if available) to assess for large vessel thrombosis

---

[161] Adams HP, Jr. *et al.* Guidelines for the early management of patients with ischemic stroke: A scientific statement from the Stroke Council of the American Stroke Association. *Stroke* 2003; 34:1056-83.

## General treatment

- **Do not treat hypertension** unless BP > 220/120 mmHg, intracranial bleeding, or acute MI or aortic dissection. If SBP > 220 or DBP 120-140, aim for 10-15% reduction with labetalol or nicardipine; consider nitroprusside if DBP > 140. If considering thrombolysis, ensure SBP to ≤ 185 and DBP≤ 110 with labetalol (10 mg IV, may repeat x1) or nitropaste 1-2″.
- Replete fluid deficit (may improve cerebral perfusion) but avoid hypotonic fluids
- Treat seizures with lorazepam (0.1 mg/kg IV at 2 mg/min) or phenytoin (20 mg/kg IV at ≤ 50 mg/min); infuse slowly to avoid drug-induced hypotension. *For status epilepticus see page 107.*
- If febrile assess for infection/meningitis; sterile fever may be seen. Maintaining normothermia with antipyretics or cooling blankets may improve stroke outcome.
- Management of elevated intracranial pressure (ICP) in deteriorating patient, regardless of etiology:
  - Elevate head of bed 30°
  - Induce hyperosmolar intravascular state while maintaining euvolemia. Give **mannitol** IV 1 gm/kg (50-100 gm) followed by 0.25 gm/kg (15-25 gm) q6h. Check $Na^+$ and osmolality q6h and hold if Na>152 mEq/L and/or osmolarity > 305 mOsm/l. If fluid overloaded (or risk of CHF) give **furosemide** IV q6h or as needed.
  - Intubate and **hyperventilate** until $pCO_2$ 25-30 mm Hg. Decreasing $pCO_2$ by 5-10 mmHg will lower ICP by 20-30 within hours; however, useful only as temporizing measure because pH equilibrates in several hours
  - Steroids (e.g. dexamethasone 10 mg IV followed by 6 mg IV Q6hr) work only for *vasogenic* edema (e.g. tumors) and not for *cytotoxic* edema (e.g. strokes)
  - Consult neurosurgery early for possible ventriculostomy or surgical decompression

## Treatment of acute ischemic stroke [162]

- Intravenous thrombolytic therapy with **tPA** should be considered for patients with ischemic stroke (i.e. CT without evidence of hemorrhage), duration of symptoms ≤ 3 hr and no contraindications – *see thrombolytic therapy on page 210.*
- Angiographic intra-arterial thrombolytic therapy appears beneficial within 6 hours, particularly with documented occlusion of middle cerebral or basilar artery
- Aspirin not a contraindication to thrombolytics, but all antiplatelet and anticoagulant agents should be withheld for 24 hr after thrombolysis
- Patients not receiving thrombolysis should receive aspirin

## Treatment of bleeding complications from thrombolytic therapy

- 6% average rate (3-16% range) of symptomatic intracerebral hemorrhage in clinical trials; higher rate when used in patients who fall outside current guidelines
- Clinical deterioration after thrombolysis should be assumed to represent intracerebral bleeding until proven otherwise → **stop tPA infusion immediately** (and heparins if used) and obtain **stat head CT** (non-contrast)
- Check CBC, PT, PTT, platelets, fibrinogen
- Give 6-8 units cryoprecipitate and/or FFP plus 10 units single donor platelets to reverse thrombolytic effect
- Neurosurgical consultation for early decompression

---

162 Meschia JF et al. Thrombolytic treatment of acute ischemic stroke. Mayo Clin Proc 2002; 77:542-51.

## Acute subarachnoid hemorrhage [163]

- Diagnosis:
  - CT 92% sensitive within 24 hr of event
  - Perform lumbar puncture if suggestive history and negative head CT, or presentation > 72 hr after event
  - Xanthochromia does not appear until 4 hr after event, and reaches max at 1 wk
- Consult neurosurgeon
- Treatment of hypertension generally avoided unless patient alert (in which case BP lowering may reduce risk of re-bleeding)
- Nimodipine 60 mg PO q 6 hr reduces vasospasm and improves outcomes
- Analgesics and sedatives as needed; consider empiric anticonvulsants
- Urgent angiography and consideration of surgery (4% chance of recurrent bleeding within 24 hr, and cumulative 20% rebleeding risk at 2 weeks)

## Acute hypertensive intracerebral hemorrhage

- Type and crossmatch 4 units PRBCs, 4-6 units cryoprecipitate or FFP and 1 unit single-donor platelets for emergency use
- Use labetalol or nitroprusside to lower SBP to 140-160 mmHg (or pre-stroke BP)
- Neurosurgical decompression indicated for large cerebellar or intracerebral hemorrhage, especially if associated hydrocephalus or deteriorating level of consciousness
- Ventriculostomy indicated for basal ganglia hemorrhage associated with hydrocephalus

# *Unusual Causes of Stroke* [164]

| Condition | History or PE | Evaluation |
|---|---|---|
| Carotid or vertebral artery dissection | Neck injury or pain, Horner's syndrome ipsi- to dissection, contralateral to stroke | MRI (including T1 axial images of neck), MR angio, contrast angio |
| Aortic dissection | Chest or back pain | TEE, MRI, Chest CT |
| Paradoxical emboli | Co-existing DVT or PE, ASD or VSD findings | Echo with bubble contrast |
| Cardiac source emboli | A-fib, LV dysfunction, recent MI, rheumatic heart disease | Echo (preferably TEE) |
| Endocarditis (bacterial or marantic) | Fever, IVDU, end-stage cancer, heart murmur | Blood cultures, echo |
| Cholesterol emboli | Recent angiography, livedo, ischemic digital lesions | Retinal exam, eosinophilia/uria, ↓complement |
| Venous sinus thrombosis | Postpartum, OCPs, hypercoagulability | MR venogram, angiography |
| CNS vasculitis | SLE, Behçet's, recent ophthalmic zoster | Angiography, brain or meningeal biopsy |
| Antiphospholipid antibody syndrome | Raynaud's, recurrent spontaneous abortion, prior thromboembolism | Anticardiolipin antibody, lupus anticoagulant |
| Thrombotic thrombo-cytopenic purpura | Thrombocytopenia, azotemia, purpura, fever | Blood smear, renal or skin biopsy |
| Drug-induced vasospasm | Drug abuse (cocaine, amphetamines) | Tox screen, angiography |

163 Stieg PE, Kase CS. Intracranial hemorrhage: diagnosis and emergency treatment. *Neurol Clin N Am* 1998; 16: 373-89.

164 Sigurdsson AP, Feldman E. Stroke. In: *Hospitalist Neurology*. Samuels M (ed). Butterworth-Heinemann, Boston, 1999.

# Status Epilepticus[165]

**Definition:** Persistent seizure or repeated seizures without full recovery between episodes; operationally defined as seizure lasting > 5 minutes, or two seizures between which there is incomplete recovery of consciousness

## Etiologies:
- ***Acute structural injury***: Trauma, tumor, stroke, hemorrhage, anoxia
- ***Remote structural injury***: Head trauma, prior stroke or neurosurgery, AVM
- **CNS infection**: Encephalitis, meningitis
- ***Toxic***: Penicillins, imipenem, fluoroquinolones, metronidazole, isoniazid, cyclic antidepressants, lithium, antipsychotics, lidocaine, meperidine, theophylline, cyclosporine, cocaine (often dose-related or with renal or hepatic insufficiency)
- ***Drug withdrawal***: Ethanol, opiates, barbiturates, benzodiazepines (flumazenil)
- ***Metabolic***: Hypo- or hyperglycemia; electrolytes ($\downarrow Na^+$, $\downarrow Ca^{++}$, $\downarrow Mg^{++}$); hyperosmolar state; hypoxia; uremia
- ***New-onset or inadequately controlled chronic epilepsy***: change in anticonvulsant drug levels (drug interactions, noncompliance, altered absorption); intercurrent infection or metabolic abnormality; ethanol excess or withdrawal

## Complications
- Neuronal death after 30-60 minutes of continuous seizure activity (even with little or no motor activity, e.g. paralyzed for airway management)
- Mortality rate up to 35%, depending on underlying etiology
- Other: Rhabdomyolysis, aspiration, metabolic/lactic acidosis, respiratory failure, neurogenic pulmonary edema

## Choice of initial drug therapy
- Randomized trial[166] showed roughly equal efficacy of lorazepam vs. phenobarbital vs. phenytoin vs. diazepam followed by phenytoin
- Benzodiazepines often given first due to rapid onset and ease of delivery; limited by sedation/respiratory depression
- Lorazepam and diazepam have similar onset (3 vs. 2 min) but diazepam has shorter $T_{1/2}$ by redistributing out of CNS; diazepam may also be given PR
- Benzodiazepines and phenytoin incompatible through same IV
- Fosphenytoin (a water-soluble prodrug of phenytoin) may be given more rapidly than phenytoin, although time to onset of clinical effect is similar

## Suggested management algorithm[167]

| Time | Intervention |
|---|---|
| 0-5 min | • Assess ABCs; cardiac monitor • Give $O_2$, intubate if necessary<br>• Obtain history and perform PE including neuro exam<br>• Start IV and draw blood for lytes (including Mg$^{++}$/Ca$^{++}$), glucose, CBC, renal/liver function, tox screen and anticonvulsant drug levels<br>• Check fingerstick glucose; give thiamine 100 mg IV prior to dextrose<br>• Treat hyperthermia promptly with antipyretics or cooling blankets<br>• **Lorazepam** 0.1 mg/kg IV at 2 mg/min<br>• Call for EEG monitoring |
| 5-25 min | *If seizures continue:*<br>• **Phenytoin** 20 mg/kg IV at 50 mg/min **or** **fosphenytoin** 20 mg/kg PE* IV at 150 mg/min<br>• Monitor EKG and vital signs |

165 Lowenstein DH, Alldredge BK. Current concepts: status epilepticus. *NEJM* 1998; 338: 970-6.
166 Treiman DM *et al.* A comparison of four treatments for generalized convulsive status epilepticus. *NEJM* 1998; 339: 792-8.
167 Working Group on Status Epilepticus. Treatment of convulsive status epilepticus. *JAMA* 1993; 270: 854-59. Lowenstein DH, Alldredge BK. Current concepts: status epilepticus. *NEJM* 1998; 338: 970-6.

| Time | Intervention |
|---|---|
| 25-30 min | *If seizures continue:*<br>• **Phenytoin** additional 5-10 mg/kg IV at 50 mg/min **or fosphenytoin** additional 5-10 mg/kg PE* IV at 150 mg/min |
| 30-50 min | *If seizures continue:*<br>• **Phenobarbital** 20 mg/kg IV at 50-75 mg/min **or**<br>• Consider proceeding directly to anesthesia with **midazolam** or **propofol** (see below) if **(1)** patient already in ICU or **(2)** severe systemic disturbance (e.g. hyperthermia) or **(3)** seizures have continued for > 60-90 minutes |
| 50-60 min | *If seizures continue:*<br>• **Phenobarbital** additional 5-10 mg/kg IV at 50-75 mg/min |
| > 60 min | *If seizures continue, begin anesthesia in ICU with:*<br>• **Midazolam** 0.2 mg/kg IV followed by 75-100 mcg/kg/hr **or propofol** 1-2 mg/kg IV followed by 2-10 mg/kg/hr<br>• Adjust dosing to EEG response<br>• Therapeutic levels may require intubation and pressor support |

\* Fosphenytoin dispensed in phenytoin equivalents (PE)

# *Alcohol Withdrawal Syndromes*[168]

**Normal ethanol clearance** $\cong$ 20 mg/dl/hour; more rapid in chronic alcoholics. Symptoms may occur prior to ethanol level reaching zero.

| Syndrome | Timing * | % pts# | Symptoms |
|---|---|---|---|
| Minor or early withdrawal | Onset 8 hr<br>Peak 24-36 hr | ≥ 80% | • Irritability/agitation but **no** delirium<br>• Sleep disturbance, hypervigilance<br>• ↑HR, ↑BP, ↑T°, tremor |
| Hallucinosis | Onset 8 hr<br>Peak 24-72 hr | 25% | • Visual > auditory hallucinations<br>• Sensorium typically intact<br>• Does **not** predict DTs |
| Withdrawal seizures | Onset 8-24 hr<br>Peak 24 hr | 25% | • Generalized tonic-clonic seizures (partial seizures suggest alternative diagnosis)<br>• May occur singly or in clusters, but status epilepticus uncommon<br>• More common in patients with prior history of seizures |
| Delirium tremens (DTs) | Onset 48 hr<br>May occur up to 2 wks | 5% | • Occurs in chronic alcoholics only, rare if age < 30 yrs<br>• Often precipitated and/or masked by medical illness<br>• Delirium and clouded consciousness<br>• Hyperadrenergic state (↑HR, ↑BP, ↑T°, tremor, sweating)<br>• Mortality 1- 5% (historically 20%)<br>• Complications: arrhythmias, sepsis, aspiration, volume depletion, electrolyte disturbances |

\* Timing since last drink of alcohol
# % of pts with **chronic** alcoholism admitted to hospital not given prophylactic treatment

168 Turner RC *et al*. Alcohol withdrawal syndromes: a review of pathophysiology, clinical presentation and treatment. *J Gen Intern Med* 1989;4:432-44.

## Differential diagnosis

- Drug withdrawal: barbiturate, benzos, amphetamine, narcotics
- Metabolic: hypoglycemia, ketoacidosis, thyroid storm, hepatic encephalopathy
- Infection: sepsis, meningitis • Toxic: methanol, ethylene glycol • Psychiatric

## Management[169]

- Monitoring (by experienced personnel), ICU as needed
- Quiet, well-lit room; avoid restraints if possible
- **Benzodiazepines** most effective and well-studied treatment
  - Reduce sx/signs of withdrawal, and decrease incidence of seizure and DTs
  - Typically given prophylactically although randomized studies[170] suggest that symptom-driven dosing is equally effective, but with lower total doses of medications, less sedation and shorter duration of treatment. Prophylactic dosing may be more appropriate for medically unstable patients or patients with history of withdrawal seizures or DTs.
  - Longer-acting agents (chlordiazepoxide, diazepam) more effective in preventing seizures and may result in "smoother" withdrawal, but may also cause excessive sedation in elderly or patients with liver disease when compared to shorter-acting agents (lorazepam or oxazepam)
  - Typical regimens:

| Drug | Dose for severe sx | Fixed dose regimen * |
|---|---|---|
| Chlordiazepoxide | 50-100 mg PO q 1 hr | 50 mg q 6 hr x 4 doses, then 25 mg q 6 hr x 8 doses |
| Diazepam | 10-20 mg PO/IV q 1 hr | 10 mg q 6 hr x 4 doses, then 5 mg q 6 hr x 8 doses |
| Lorazepam | 2-4 mg PO/IV/IM q 1hr | 2 mg q 6 hr x 4 doses, then 1 mg q 6 hr x 8 doses |
| Oxazepam | 30-60 mg PO q 1 hr | 30 mg q 6 hr x 4 doses, then 15 mg q 6 hr x 8 doses |

\* Shorter-acting benzodiazepines should be tapered by 30-50% per day after 48 hours; longer acting agents will "self-taper"

- Hyperadrenergic symptoms warrant treatment with β-blockers (e.g. atenolol 25-100 mg PO qd-bid, titrated to HR) or clonidine (0.1-0.3 mg PO bid)
- All alcoholics should also receive thiamine (100 mg IV qd x 3 days) plus folate
- Hypoglycemia, ↓Mg and ↓$PO_4$ common, especially if malnourished
- Seizures: Benzodiazepines (e.g. lorazepam 2 mg IV) significantly reduce risk of recurrence.[171] Can also consider prophylactic phenytoin (e.g. 100 mg PO tid) if high risk of withdrawal seizures.

## Other alcohol-related neurologic syndromes

- **Wernicke's** encephalopathy: Triad of ataxia, confusion and ophthalmoplegia/ nystagmus. Caused by thiamine deficiency. Risk of irreversible deficits if not treated promptly. Dextrose may exacerbate symptoms if given prior to thiamine.
- **Korsakoff's** psychosis: chronic dementia with severe memory impairment and confabulation out of proportion to other cognitive deficits. Sensorium usually intact. Also caused by thiamine deficiency; may occur with/without Wernicke's.
- Cerebellar degeneration/ataxia
- Central pontine myelinolysis
- Polyneuropathy

169 Mayo-Smith MF *et al.* Pharmacological management of alcohol withdrawal: a meta-analysis and evidence-based practice guideline. *JAMA* 1997; 278: 144-51.

170 Saitz R *et al.* Individualized treatment for alcohol withdrawal: a randomized double-blind controlled trial. *JAMA* 1994; 272: 519-23. Jaeger TM *et al.* Symptom-triggered therapy for alcohol withdrawal syndrome in medical inpatients. *Mayo Clin Proc* 2001; 76:695-701.

171 D'Onofrio G *et al.* Lorazepam for the prevention of recurrent seizures related to alcohol. *NEJM* 1999; 340: 915-9.

# Guillain-Barré Syndrome[172]

## Etiology
- **Infection:** 2/3 of patients with URI or gastroenteritis 1-3 wks prior to onset of symptoms ($\oplus$ *C. jejuni* serology in up to 40%; also CMV, EBV, VZV, HIV, mycoplasma, Lyme) • **Other:** vaccines, SLE, Hodgkin's, sarcoidosis

## Clinical features
- **Symptoms:** • Fine paresthesias of toes and fingertips, followed by ascending weakness that evolves over hours to days (legs → arm/face → oropharynx) • Back and leg pain common although sensory findings minimal or absent • **Miller-Fisher variant:** Ophthalmoplegia, ataxia and areflexia with minimal weakness (5% of cases); associated with *C. jejuni*
- **Physical findings:** • Hypo/areflexia • More-or-less symmetric weakness • Autonomic dysfunction in up to 50% including tachycardia or arrhythmias (major cause of morbidity/mortality), labile or orthostatic BP, bladder/bowel dysfunction

| Clinical feature | Frequency (%) | |
|---|---|---|
| | Initial | Full illness |
| Paresthesias | 70 | 85 |
| Weakness – arms | 20 | 90 |
| legs | 60 | 95 |
| face | 35 | 60 |
| oropharynx | 25 | 50 |
| Ophthalmoplegia | 5 | 15 |
| Sphincter dysfxn | 15 | 5 |
| Ataxia | 10 | 15 |
| Areflexia | 75 | 90 |
| Pain | 25 | 30 |
| Sensory loss | 40 | 75 |
| Respiratory failure | 10 | 30 |
| CSF prot > 55 mg/dl | 50 | 90 |

- **Time course:** • Weakness typically progresses over 1-3 weeks, followed by plateau for 2-4 weeks, then gradual recovery over months (progression over > 6 weeks suggests alternative diagnosis, e.g. chronic demyelinating neuropathy) • Mechanical ventilation required in 25-33% (high risk if vital capacity diminishes acutely or is <18 ml/kg)
- **Prognosis:** • 15% recover fully • 65% with lasting minor deficits • 5-10% with permanent disability • 3-8% mortality (respiratory failure, sepsis, PE, cardiac arrest) • Worse prognosis with ↑ age, rapidly progressive disease, pre-existing pulmonary disease, persistent EMG abnormalities, or mechanical ventilation > 1 month

## Diagnosis
- Clinical diagnosis based on characteristic symptoms and physical findings
- **Nerve conduction** studies 95-99% sensitive and highly specific
- **CSF** may be normal initially but after 1 wk 90% should show mildly ↑ protein
- **Alternative diagnosis** suggested by: • Sensory abnormalities w/o weakness • Sensory level • Persistent asymmetric findings • Significant weakness with normal electrophysiologic studies • CSF: protein > 250 mg/dl or WBC > 50/mm³
- **Differential diagnosis:** • Spinal cord compression • HIV, Lyme or neoplastic meningitis • Transverse myelitis • Myasthenia gravis • Vasculitic neuropathy • Polymyositis • Metabolic neuropathy • Multiple sclerosis • Heavy metal poisoning • Neurotoxic fish poisoning • Botulism • Poliomyelitis • Tick paralysis

## Treatment
- Supportive care including round-the-clock vital capacity and cardiac monitoring
- Improved outcomes with plasma exchange or immune globulin (0.4 g/kg IV qd x 5 days)
- Glucocorticoids provide minimal benefit when added to immune globulin [173]

172 Ropper AM. The Guillain-Barré syndrome. *NEJM* 1992; 326:1130-36. Hahn AF. Guillain-Barré syndrome. *Lancet* 1998; 325: 635-41.

173 van Koningsveld R et al. Effect of methylprednisolone when added to standard treatment with intravenous immunoglobulin for Guillain-Barré syndrome: randomised trial. *Lancet* 2004; 363:192-6.

# Herpes Simplex Encephalitis

## Pathogenesis and epidemiology
- Most common cause of severe encephalitis in U.S.
- Focal encephalitis (usually temporal lobes) with edema and necrosis
- Almost all HSV-1; 2/3 of cases follow 1° or recurrent oropharyngeal infection
- Occurs across age spectrum, usually in immunocompetent hosts
- Even with appropriate diagnosis and treatment, mortality approaches 30% and up to half of survivors have permanent deficits

## Clinical features [174]
- Acute presentation with fever (95%), altered mental status (97%), depressed consciousness, and focal neurological findings (85%) including cranial nerve palsies, hemipareses, visual field cut, ataxia and dysphasia
- Focal seizures (~50%) and behavioral symptoms (>70%) are common
- CSF: Lymphocytic pleocytosis, ↑ erythrocytes, ↑ protein. Low glucose, or normal protein and WBC < 5 /hpf argues for alternative diagnosis.[175]

## Differential diagnosis [176]
- Other viruses: West Nile, togaviruses (St. Louis, Western equine, Eastern equine, California), cytomegalovirus, Epstein-Barr, mumps, adenovirus, influenza, echovirus, progressive multifocal leukoencephalopathy (PML), lymphocytic choriomeningitis (LCM), measles (SSPE)
- Other infectious: Abscess, subdural empyema, Cryptococcus, TB, rickettsiae, toxoplasmosis, meningococcus
- Other: Tumor, vascular disease, toxic encephalopathy, subdural hematoma, SLE, adrenal leukodystrophy

### Diagnosis
- **Brain biopsy** is gold standard but invasive
- **CSF PCR** for HSV DNA is 98% sensitive and 94-100% specific. Test turns positive within 24 hr of onset of symptoms and remains positive ≥ 1 wk after initiation of treatment. May also be positive with HSV meningitis (benign/recurrent).
- **Other CSF tests**: Culture is insensitive (<10%). Rise in CSF antibody titer may confirm atypical cases but negative early in infection.
- **Imaging**: Typically shows temporal lobe lesions with hemorrhage or mass effect. Often unilateral. MRI more sensitive/specific than CT.
- **EEG**: Focal findings in > 80 %

## Treatment
- Initiate **acyclovir**, 10 mg/kg IV q 8 hr if herpes simplex encephalitis is suspected. Give slowly after volume resuscitation to avoid renal toxicity.
- Duration 14 to 21 days; relapses reported.
- Possible benefit to long-term (3 month) treatment with oral famciclovir or valaciclovir following completion of IV acyclovir [177]

---

174 Whitley RJ et al. Herpes simplex encephalitis. Clinical assessment. JAMA 1982; 247:317-20.

175 Tang YW et al. Effective use of polymerase chain reaction for diagnosis of central nervous system infections. Clin Infect Dis 1999; 29:803-6.

176 Whitley RJ et al. Diseases that mimic herpes simplex encephalitis. Diagnosis, presentation, and outcome. NIAD collaborative antiviral study group. JAMA 1989; 262:234-9.

177 Crumpacker CS et al. Case 26-2003 - a 50-year-old Colombian man with fever and seizures. NEJM 2003; 349:789-796.

# Cerebrospinal Fluid Data[178]

## Total protein in CSF from 4200 patients

| CSF protein range (mg/dL) | < 45 | 45-75 | 75-100 | 100-500 | >500 | Average (mg/dL) |
|---|---|---|---|---|---|---|
| **Diagnosis** | *Percent of patients with each disease* | | | | | |
| Purulent meningitis | 2 | 4 | 8 | 64 | 22 | 418 |
| Aseptic meningitis | 46 | 25 | 9 | 21 | - | 77 |
| Brain abscess | 27 | 45 | 9 | 18 | - | 69 |
| TB meningitis | 1 | 12 | 15 | 68 | 5 | 200 |
| Neurosyphilis | 46 | 29 | 11 | 13 | - | 68 |
| Acute ethanol | 92 | 6 | 2 | - | - | 32 |
| Uremia | 58 | 25 | 15 | 2 | - | 57 |
| Myxedema | 24 | 55 | 6 | 16 | - | 71 |
| Epilepsy (idiopathic) | 90 | 10 | - | - | - | 31 |
| Brain tumor | 31 | 25 | 12 | 31 | 1 | 115 |
| Cord tumor | 14 | 11 | 8 | 39 | 28 | 425 |
| Cerebral trauma | 54 | 18 | 9 | 15 | 4 | 100 |
| Multiple sclerosis | 68 | 24 | 6 | 3 | - | 43 |
| Polyneuritis | 51 | 16 | 8 | 21 | 5 | 74 |
| Poliomyelitis | 47 | 28 | 10 | 15 | - | 70 |
| Cerebral thrombosis | 66 | 26 | 4 | 3 | - | 46 |
| Cerebral hemorrhage | 14 | 17 | 13 | 38 | 18 | 270 |

## Hypoglycorrhachia syndromes (CSF/serum glucose < 0.5)

- **Infectious:** ◆ acute bacterial meningitis ◆ TB meningitis ◆ fungal meningitis ◆ amebic/helminthic meningitis (*Naegleria, Cysticerca, Trichinella*) ◆ acute syphilitic meningitis and generalized paresis ◆ specific viruses: lymphocytic choriomeningitis, mumps, herpes simplex/zoster meningitis (uncommon)
- **Rheumatologic:** ◆ meningeal sarcoidosis ◆ rheumatoid meningitis ◆ SLE myelopathy
- **Hypoglycemia**
- **Other:** ◆ leptomeningeal carcinomatosis ◆ subarachnoid hemorrhage ◆ chemical meningitis after intrathecal infusion, myelogram, spinal anesthesia, etc.

## Lumbar fluid changes in 99 patients with brain abscess

| Pressure (cm H₂O) | | | Protein (mg/dL) | | |
|---|---|---|---|---|---|
| | < 200 | 38% | | < 50 | 29% |
| | 200-300 | 35% | | 50-100 | 38% |
| | > 300 | 26% | | > 100 | 33% |

| WBCs (per mm³) | | | Glucose (mg/dL) | | |
|---|---|---|---|---|---|
| | <5 | 29% | | > 40 | 79% |
| | 5-100 | 38% | | < 40 | 21% |
| | > 100 | 33% | | | |

---

[178] Merritt HH, Fremont-Smith F. *The Cerebrospinal Fluid*. Philadelphia: Saunders, 1938

## Admission CSF findings in 35 patients with TB meningitis[179]

| Finding | | Total | Died |
|---------|---|-------|------|
| WBCs (per mm³) | < 50 | 3 | 1 |
| | 51-200 | 12 | 2 |
| | 201-1,000 | 19 | 7 |
| | > 1,000 | 1 | 1 |
| PMNs (%) | 0 | 5 | 2 |
| | 1-25 | 20 | 5 |
| | 26-50 | 5 | 1 |
| | 51-75 | 4 | 3 |
| | > 75 | 1 | 0 |
| AFB Smear | + | 7 | 1 |
| | - | 25 | 10 |
| | Unknown | 3 | 0 |

| Finding | | Total | Died |
|---------|---|-------|------|
| Glucose (mg/dL) | 0-20 | 14 | 5 |
| | 21-40 | 12 | 4 |
| | 41-60 | 7 | 1 |
| | > 60 | 2 | 1 |
| Protein (mg/dL) | 0-50 | 5 | 3 |
| | 21-100 | 7 | 1 |
| | 101-200 | 13 | 4 |
| | > 200 | 10 | 3 |
| TB culture | + | 26 | 8 |
| | - | 8 | 3 |
| | Unknown | 1 | 0 |

## Muscle Innervation[180]

| Muscle | Nerve | Root * |
|--------|-------|--------|
| Trapezius | Spinal accessory | **C3-4** |
| Deltoid | Axillary | **C5**-6 |
| Brachioradialis | Radial | **C5-6** |
| Ext carpi radialis longus | Radial | **C6-7** |
| Triceps | Radial | C6,**7**,8 |
| Extensor digitorum | Posterior interosseus | **C7**-8 |
| Biceps brachii | Musculocutaneous | **C5-6** |
| Flexor carpi radialis | Median | **C6-7** |
| Abductor pollicis brevis | Median | **C8**,T1 |
| Opponens pollicis | Median | **C8**,T1 |
| Flexor digit profundus 1&2 | Anterior interosseus | C7-**8**,T1 |
| Flexor digit profundus 3&4 | Ulnar | C7-**8**,T1 |
| Flexor carpi ulnaris | Ulnar | C7-**8**,T1 |
| Interossei | Ulnar | **C8**,T1 |
| Abductor digiti minimi | Ulnar | **C8**,T1 |
| Iliopsoas | Femoral | L2,**3**,4 |
| Quadriceps femoris | Femoral | L2,**3,4** |
| Adductors | Obturator | L2,**3**,4 |
| Gluteus med/minimus | Superior gluteal | L4,**5**,S1 |
| Gluteus maximus | Inferior gluteal | **L5**, S1,2 |
| Hamstrings | Sciatic | **L5**, S1,2 |
| Gastrocnemius/soleus | Tibial | **S1**,2 |
| Flexor digitorum | Tibial | **L5**,S1 |
| Interossei | Med/lateral plantar | L5, **S1**,2 |
| Tibialis anterior | Deep peroneal | **L4,5** |
| Extensor digitorum | Deep peroneal | L4,**5** |

* Bold denotes predominant root

179 Hinman AR. Tuberculous meningitis at Cleveland Metropolitan General Hospital, 1959-63. *Am Rev Respir Dis* 1967;95:670-3. Adapted with permission, American College of Chest Physicians. Cited in Fishman, *ibid*, p 272.

180 *Aids to the Examination of the Peripheral Nervous System*. 4th ed. Brain, ed. W.B. Saunders, 2000. *Localization in Clinical Neurology*, 4th ed. Brazis PW *et al*, editors. Philadelphia: Lippincott Williams & Wilkins, 2001.

# Spinal & Peripheral Nerves[181]

**Spinal root and selected peripheral nerve lesions**

| Root | Disc | Muscles | Weakness | Reflex loss |
|------|------|---------|----------|-------------|
| C4 | C3-4 | Trapezius, scalene | Shoulder shrugging | None |
| C5 | C4-5 | Deltoid, biceps, brachioradialis | Should abduction, external rotation of arm, elbow flexion | Biceps, brachioradialis |
| C6 | C5-6 | Brachioradialis, biceps, pronator teres, extensor carpi radialis | Elbow flexion, arm pronation, finger and wrist extension | Biceps, brachioradialis |
| | | Radial nerve injuries produce similar findings except brachioradialis function is normal | | |
| C7 | C6-7 | Triceps, pronator teres, extensor digitorum | Elbow extension , finger and wrist extension | Triceps |
| C8 | C7-T1 | Flexor digitorum, flexor/abductor pollicis, interossei | Long flexors of fingers, intrinsics of hand (finger abduction, palmar abduction of thumb) | Finger flexor |
| | | Ulnar nerve injuries similar but also weaken thumb adductor | | |
| T10 | T9-10 | | Beevor's sign (sit-up → umbilicus pulled upwards) | |
| L2 | L1-2 | Iliopsoas | Hip flexion | Cremaster |
| L3 | L2-3 | Iliopsoas, adductors | Hip flexion, thigh adduction | Knee jerk |
| L4 | L3-4 | Quadriceps, sartorius, tibialis anterior | Knee extension, ankle dorsiflexion and inversion | Knee jerk |
| | | Femoral nerve injury limited to knee extension; associated hip flexion and adduction weakness localizes to plexus | | |
| L5 | L4-5 | Glutei, hamstrings, tibialis, extensor hallux/digiti, peronei | Thigh adduction and internal rotation, knee flexion, plantar and dorsiflexion of ankle and toes | None |
| | | Deep peroneal nerve weakness limited to ankle/toe extensors; posterior tibial nerve lesions weaken foot inversion | | |
| S1 | L5-S1 | Gluteus maximus, hamstrings, soleus, gastrocnemius, extensor digitorum, flexor digitorum | Hip extension, knee flexion, plantar flexion of ankle and toes | Ankle jerk |
| S2 | S1-2 | Interossei | Cupping and fanning of toes | |

[181] *Aids to the Examination of the Peripheral Nervous System.* 4th ed. Brain, ed. W.B. Saunders, 2000. *Localization in Clinical Neurology*, 4th ed. Brazis PW et al, editors. Philadelphia: Lippincott Williams & Wilkins, 2001.

## Anterior aspect: Peripheral segments on left
## Spinal segments on right [182]

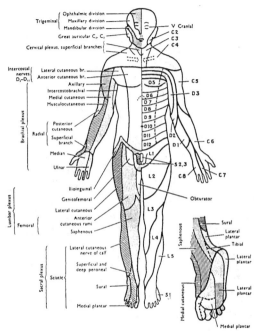

*Key*
C: cervical
D: dorsal (thoracic)
L: lumbar
S: sacral

[182] Figures reproduced from *Brain's Diseases of the Nervous System*, 10th ed. Walton J (ed.). Oxford: Oxford University Press, 1993, p 47, by permission of Oxford University Press.

Posterior aspect: Spinal segments on left, Peripheral on right

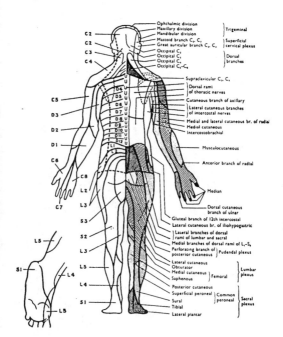

## *Visual Acuity Screen*[183]

| | Distance Equivalent |
|---|---|
| **9 6** | 20/800 |
| **8 7 3** | 20/400 |
| **2 8 4 3**   **O X X** | 20/200 |
| **6 3 8 5 2**   **X O O** | 20/100 |
| **8 7 4 5 9**   **O X O** | 20/70 |
| **6 3 9 2 5**   **X O X** | 20/50 |
| 4 2 8 3 6 5   O X O | 20/40 |
| 3 7 4 2 5 8   X X O | 20/30 |
| 9 3 7 8 2 6   X O O | 20/25 |
| 4 2 8 7 3 9   O O X | 20/20 |

Hold card in good light 14 inches from eye. Record vision for each eye separately with and without glasses. Presbyopic patients should read through bifocal segment. Check myopes with glasses only.

Pupil Diameter (mm)

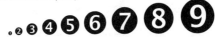

---

183 Adapted with permission from J.G. Rosenbaum MD, Pocket Vision Screen, Beachwood, Ohio.

# Folstein Mini-Mental State[184]

| Area | Points | Task |
|---|---|---|
| Orientation | 5 | Year, Season, Date, Day, Month |
| | 5 | State, County, Town, Hospital, Floor |
| Registration | 3 | Patient recites three consecutive objects named (e.g. ball, flag, tree) |
| Attention, Calculation | 5 | Serial 7's (5 responses: 93-86-79-72-65); alternatively spell "WORLD" backwards |
| Recall | 3 | Three objects registered above, 5 minutes later |
| | 2 | Name a pencil and watch |
| | 1 | Repeat "No ifs, ands, or buts." |
| Language | 3 | 3-stage command: "Take a paper in your right hand, fold it in half, and put it on the floor." |
| | 1 | Read and obey, "Close your eyes." |
| | 1 | Write a sentence |
| | 1 | Copy design below |
| Level of consciousness | 0 | Assess along continuum: Alert-Drowsy-Stuporous-Comatose |

**CLOSE YOUR EYES**

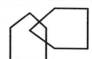

**Interpretation:** Score 0-23 (or score of 23-29 with altered mental status) suggests cognitive dysfunction. No identifiable pathology in 1/3. Excellent for evaluating hospitalized or medically ill patient; less useful in evaluation or staging of dementia.

# Glasgow Coma Scale[185]

| | | | | Score | Mortality in Head Injury |
|---|---|---|---|---|---|
| Best Motor Response | Obeys | 6 | | 3-5 | >60% |
| | Localizes | 5 | | 6-8 | 12% |
| | Withdraws | 4 | | 9-12 | 2% |
| | Abnormal flexion | 3 | | | |
| | Extends | 2 | | | |
| | Nil | 1 | | | |
| Verbal Response | Oriented | 5 | | | |
| | Confused conversation | 4 | | | |
| | Inappropriate words | 3 | | | |
| | Incomprehensible sounds | 2 | | | |
| | Nil | 1 | | | |
| Eye Opening | Spontaneous | 4 | | | |
| | To speech | 3 | | | |
| | To pain | 2 | | | |
| | Nil | 1 | | | |

184 Folstein MF *et al.* Mini-mental state: a practical method for grading the cognitive state of patients for the clinician. *J Psychiatric Res* 1975;12:189.
185 Teasdale GM, Jennet B. Assessment of coma and impaired consciousness: a practical scale. *Lancet* 1974;2(872):81-4. Jennett B *et al.* Predicting outcome in individual patients after severe head injury. *Lancet* 1976(17968):1031-4.

# Hypoxic-Ischemic Coma: Prognosis[186]

## Patients with virtually *no chance* of regaining independence [§]

| Time | Exam Findings |
|------|---------------|
| Initial | Pupils[†]: no light response |
| 1 d | Motor response: no better than flexor *and* <br> Spontaneous eye movements: neither orienting nor roving-conjugate |
| 3 d | Motor response: no better than flexor |
| 1 wk | Motor response: not obeying commands *and* <br> Spontaneous eye movements: were neither orienting nor roving conjugate at initial exam |
| 2 wk | Oculocephalic response: not normal *and* <br> Eye opening: was not spontaneous at day 3 and not improved at least two grades(none→other→roving-disconjugate→roving-conjugate→orienting) at 2 wks *and* Motor response: not obeying commands at day 3 |

## Patients with *best chance* of regaining independence

| Time | Exam Findings |
|------|---------------|
| Initial | Pupillary light reflex: present *and* <br> Motor response: flexor or extensor *and* <br> Spontaneous eye movements: roving-conjugate or orienting |
| 1 day | Motor response: withdrawal or better *and* <br> Eye opening: improved at least 2 grades |
| 3 day | Motor response: withdrawal or better *and* <br> Spontaneous eye movements: normal |
| 1 wk | Motor response: obeying commands |
| 2 wk | Oculocephalic response: normal |

| Level of consciousness 1 day after insult * | Best 1-yr recovery (%) # | | |
|---|---|---|---|
| | A | B | C |
| **106 *Comatose* patients at day 1** | | | |
| (1) Spontaneous eye movement: roving-conjugate or better | 63 | 16 | 21 |
| (2) Not (1) *and* initial motor response: withdrawal or better | 82 | 0 | 14 |
| (3) Not (2) *and* oculovestibular: any response | 100 | 9 | 0 |
| (4) None of above | 98 | 0 | 2 |
| **47 *Vegetative* patients at day 1** | | | |
| (1) Motor response: withdrawal or better | 38 | 19 | 42 |
| (2) Not (1) & spontaneous eye movement: roving or better | 82 | 18 | 0 |
| (3) None of above | 100 | 0 | 0 |
| **15 *Conscious* patients at day 1** | | | |
| (1) Pupillary reflex: present initially & spontaneous eye movement: roving-conj or better & oculovestibular: nml | 0 | 0 | 100 |
| (2) Not (1) | 86 | 0 | 14 |

§ Prognosis same as for categories "A" and "B" from bottom table

† Use caution when interpreting pupillary responses and oculomotor findings in first 24 hr (resuscitation drugs may alter findings)

* **Coma** = no eye opening, no comprehensible words; commands not obeyed
**Vegetative**= eyes open to noise or pain, but no comprehensible words; commands not obeyed **Conscious** = comprehensible words or commands obeyed

# **Outcome categories:** (A) no recovery, persistent vegetative state (B) severe disability (C) moderate disability, good recovery

---

186 Levy D *et al.* Predicting outcome from hypoxic-ischemic coma. *JAMA* 1985;253(10):1420.

# Brain Death[187]

**Definition:** Irreversible loss of brain function, including brainstem
**Usual etiologies**: Head injury, sub-arachnoid or intracerebral hemorrhage, encephalitis. **In ICU**: Hypoxic-ischemic coma (after resuscitation), ischemic strokes with edema and herniation, massive edema 2° to fulminant hepatic failure.

## Diagnostic criteria (*all must be present*)

**A. Prerequisites**: **(1)** Clinical or CT/MRI evidence of an acute, irreversible CNS catastrophe of known etiology compatible with clinical diagnosis of brain death **(2)** No severe, complicating medical conditions (electrolytes, acid-base, endocrine) **(3)** No drug intoxication or poisoning **(4)** Core temperature ≥ 32° C

**B. Coma or unresponsiveness**: No motor responses of limbs to painful stimuli (e.g. nail-bed or supraorbital pressure); excludes spinal reflexes (e.g. Babinski)

**C. Absence of brainstem reflexes:**
   **1)** Pupils: no response to bright light; may be mid-position to dilated (4-9 mm)
   **2)** Ocular movement: no eye movements with head-turning (test only if c-spine is stable) and no eye deviation with 50 ml ice water in each ear (head of bed at 30°, observe for 1 min, with 5 min between sides)
   **3)** Facial sensation and motor response: no corneal reflex; no jaw reflex; no grimacing to deep pressure on nail bed, supra-orbital ridge and TMJ
   **4)** Pharyngeal and tracheal reflexes: no gag with tongue blade, no cough with vigorous bronchial suctioning

**D. Apnea** – procedure:
   **1)** Prerequisites: core temp ≥ 36.5° C, SBP ≥ 90 mmHg, euvolemic or (+) fluid balance x 6 hr, $PCO_2$ normal (or ≥ 40 mmHg), $PO_2$ ≥ normal
   **2)** Connect a pulse-oximeter and disconnect ventilator
   **3)** Deliver 100% $O_2$ @ 6 lpm into trachea (optimally at level of carina)
   **4)** Observe for respiratory movements (chest excursions producing tidal vols)
   **5)** Measure arterial $PO_2$, $PCO_2$, and pH at **8 min** and reconnect ventilator
   **6)** Test is **positive** (confirmatory) if respiratory movements are absent and $PCO_2$ is ≥ 60 mmHg (or increased by 20 mmHg over baseline)
   **7)** If respiratory movements observed, test is **negative** and should be repeated
   **8)** If during test patient develops SBP < 90 mmHg, significant $O_2$ desaturation or cardiac arrhythmias, draw immediate ABG. Test is **positive** if $PCO_2$ is ≥ 60 mmHg (or ↑ by 20 mmHg); otherwise, test is indeterminate and confirmatory testing should be considered.

## Pitfalls in diagnosis of brain death (consider confirmatory testing)

Severe facial trauma • Pre-existing pupillary abnormalities • Toxic levels of drugs affecting neuromuscular or ocular function (sedatives, aminoglycosides, tricyclics, anticholinergics, anticonvulsants, chemotherapeutic agents, neuromuscular blockers) • Chronic $CO_2$ retention (COPD, sleep apnea, morbid obesity)

## Observations compatible with brain death (i.e. diagnosis still valid)

• Respiratory-like movements (shoulder elevation, back arching) *without* tidal volumes • Sweating, blushing, tachycardia • Normal BP without pressors • Spinal reflexes (e.g. Babinski) or spontaneous limb movements

## Confirmatory laboratory testing

Consider repeat clinical evaluation in all patients after 6 hr. If clinical testing cannot be reliably performed or evaluated, confirmatory testing is **desirable** but not mandatory. Options include: angiography (absence of cerebral blood flow), EEG, trans-cranial Doppler, technetium brain scan, or somatosensory evoked potentials.

---

187 American Academy of Neurology. Practice parameters for determining brain death in adults. *Neurology* 1995; 45:1012-1014. Wijdicks EFM. The diagnosis of brain death. *NEJM* 2001; 344:1215-1221.

# Oncology

## *Leukemia, Acute Myelogenous*[188]

| FAB Classification | | % Cases | Comments |
|---|---|---|---|
| M0 | Myeloblastic with minimal differentiation | 3 | Maybe confused with ALL (but no CALLA, B & T cell markers), CD13+ or CD33+ |
| M1 | Myeloblastic without maturation | 15-20 | |
| M2 | Myeloblastic with maturation | 25-30% | |
| M3 | Promyelocytic | 5-10% | DIC common |
| M4 | Myelomonocytic | 20% | Tissue infiltration (gums, skin, hepatosplenomegaly, brain) |
| M4 eo | Myelomonocytic with > 5% eosinophils | 5-10% | Associated with long remission |
| M5 | Monocytic (a: undiff; b: differentiated) | 10% | Tissue infiltration (gums, skin, hepatosplenomegaly, brain) |
| M6 | Erythroleukemia | 3-5% | Common as secondary AML after myelodysplasia |
| M7 | Megakaryocytic | 3-12 | Myelofibrosis and pancytopenia common; most common form of AML in Down's syndrome |

## Adverse prognostic factors

- Age > 60 yrs (3/4 of cases; 50% achieve complete remission, 20% survive > 2 yrs)
- Secondary AML (alkylating agent, MDS, congenital syndromes) • WBC > 20k
- Elevated LDH • Female • Delayed response to induction chemotherapy

## Prognosis by cytogenetics [189]

| Category | Cytogenetics or Clinical Characteristics | 5-year Survival | Relapse Rate |
|---|---|---|---|
| Favorable | • Cytogenetics:  t(8;21); t(15;17); inv(16), t(16;16) or del(16q) <br> • FAB type M3 | 70 % | 33 % |
| Intermediate | • Neither favorable nor unfavorable | 48 % | 50 % |
| Unfavorable | • Cytogenetics:  monosomy chromosome 5 or 7, del(5q), abn (3q26), or complex karyotype <br> • Resistant disease after the first course of chemotherapy and no good risk features | 15 % | 78 % |

[188] Lowenberg B *et al*. Acute myeloid leukemia. *NEJM* 1999; 341(14):1051-1062. Gilliland DG, Tallman MS. Acute myelogenous leukemia. In *Blood : Principles and Practice of Hematology*, 2nd ed. Handin RI *et al*, editors. Philadelphia, Pa.: Lippincott Williams & Wilkins, 2003.

[189] Wheatley K *et al*. A simple, robust, validated and highly predictive index for the determination of risk-directed therapy in acute myeloid leukaemia derived from the MRC AML 10 trial. *Br J Haematol* 1999; 107:69-79.

**Therapy**
- **Pre-induction**
  - Control blast crisis (WBC> 50-100k) with hydroxyurea
  - Leukostasis (WBC> 50-100k associated with headache, retinal hemorrhages, altered mentation, dyspnea or priapism) may warrant leukapheresis
  - Prevent chemo-induced tumor lysis syndrome (hyperuricemia, ↑ K⁺, ↓ Ca⁺⁺, ↑phosphate, acidosis, renal failure) with pre-treatment hydration and allopurinol
  - Neutropenia: protective isolation
  - Fever and neutropenia: empiric broad-spectrum antibiotic therapy
  - DIC (especially in M3 AML): FFP and cryoprecipitate replacement of factors and fibrinogen
- **Intensive induction:** With anthracycline (e.g. daunorubicin) plus cytarabine. Complete remission in 70-80% in patients < 60 yrs and 50% of older patients.
- **Post-induction treatment:** (75% relapse if no post-induction therapy given)
  1) **Allogeneic bone marrow transplant (BMT):** Long term survival 50-60% (20% relapse, 20-25% die from transplant-related complications). Higher survival if HLA-matched transplant from sib. Generally limited to age < 50.
  2) **Autologous BMT:** Long-term survival in 45-55%
  3) **Consolidative chemotherapy alone:**[190] High-dose cytarabine alone may induce long-term survival (50% at 4 yrs) although toxicity limits use
  4) **Differentiating agents:** All trans-retinoic acid (ATRA) produces complete remission in 80% of patient with M3 AML; continued therapy may induce long-term disease-free survival. Arsenic trioxide also effective.
  5) **Protein tyrosine kinase inhibitors:** Up to 30% of AML contains activating mutations in the FLT3 tyrosine kinase; FLT3 protein tyrosine inhibitors now in clinical trials
  6) **Re-induction for relapsed AML:** Repeat chemo may induce second remission in 25-40%; of these patients, additional treatment (e.g. BMT) may yield 30% long-term survival

# Hodgkin's Disease

**Cotswolds staging classification for Hodgkin's Disease**

| Stage | Involved lymph nodes or structures |
|---|---|
| I | Single lymph node region or lymphoid structure |
| II | Two or more lymph node regions or structures on the same side of the diaphragm. Hilar nodes are "lateralized" and are stage II if bilateral. Entire mediastinum is one region. Number of anatomic regions should be designated by subscript (e.g. II₃). |
| III₁ | Lymph node regions or lymphoid structures on both sides of diaphragm, including spleen, splenic hilum, celiac or portal nodes |
| III₂ | Lymph node regions or lymphoid structures on both sides of diaphragm, including paraortic, iliac, inguinal or mesenteric nodes |
| IV | Diffuse or disseminated involvement of one or more extranodal organs, with or without lymph node involvement |

**Subscript: A:** Asymptomatic  **B:** Associated fever, night sweats, weight loss > 10% body weight  **E:** Extranodal contiguous extension  **X:** Bulky disease (mediastinal mass > 10 cm or ≥ 1/3 of transverse diameter of thorax at T5-6)

---

[190] Cassileth PA *et al.* Chemotherapy compared with autologous or allogeneic BMT in the management of AML in first remission. *NEJM* 1998; 339(23):1649.

## Classification of Hodgkin's Disease

| Rye Classification | % Cases | 5-yr survival | WHO Classification |
|---|---|---|---|
| Lymphocyte predominance | 5-10 | 90 % | Lymphocyte predominance, nodular Lymphocyte rich classical HL |
| Nodular sclerosis | 40-80 | 70-80 % | Nodular sclerosis |
| Mixed cellularity | 20-40 | 50-60 % | Mixed cellularity Unclassifiable classical HL |
| Lymphocyte depletion | 2-15 | < 50 % | Lymphocyte depletion |

### Prognosis in advanced Hodgkin's disease[191]

Based on 5,141 patients treated 1983-1992 with combination chemotherapy for stage III-IV disease or stage I-II disease with "B" symptoms or bulky disease
**Risk factors: (1)** albumin < 4 g/dl **(2)** Hb < 10.5 g/dl **(3)** male gender **(4)** age ≥ 45 **(5)** stage IV disease **(6)** peripheral WBC > 15k **(7)** peripheral lymphocytes < 600/mm³ or < 8% of diff

| # Risk Factors | 0 | 1 | 2 | 3 | 4 | ≥ 5 |
|---|---|---|---|---|---|---|
| 5-yr remission | 84 % | 77 % | 67 % | 60 % | 51 % | 42 % |
| 5-yr survival | 89 % | 90 % | 81 % | 78 % | 61 % | 56 % |

# Non-Hodgkin's Lymphoma

## Ann Arbor Staging for Non-Hodgkin's Lymphoma

| Stage I | Single lymph node region (I) or single extralymphatic site (IE) |
|---|---|
| Stage II | Two or more lymph node regions or lymphatic structures on the same side of the diaphragm alone (II) or with involvement of limited, contiguous extralymphatic site (IIE) |
| Stage III | Lymph node regions or extralymphatic sites on both sides of diaphragm |
| Stage IV | Diffuse or disseminated foci of involvement of ≥ one extralymphatic organs, with or without lymph node involvement |

**Subscript: A:** Asymptomatic **B:** History of fever, sweats, weight loss > 10% body weight **E:** Extranodal extension **S:** spleen involved **X:** Bulky disease

### Prognosis in aggressive Non-Hodgkin's lymphoma [192]

Based on 2031 patients treated 1982-87 with combination chemotherapy containing doxorubicin. Subsequent studies suggest data applicable to indolent lymphoma.
**Risk factors: (1)** Age> 60 **(2)** LDH> normal **(3)** Low performance status (i.e. bed-ridden part of day) **(4)** Ann Arbor stage III or IV **(5)** Extra-nodal involvement > 1 site

| Age | Risk Factors | % of Cases | 5-yr Complete Remission (%) | 5-yr Overall Survival (%) |
|---|---|---|---|---|
| ≤ 60 | 0 | 22 | 92 | 83 |
| | 1 | 32 | 78 | 69 |
| | 2 | 32 | 57 | 46 |
| | 3 | 14 | 46 | 32 |
| > 60 | 0 | 18 | 91 | 56 |
| | 1 | 31 | 71 | 44 |
| | 2 | 35 | 56 | 37 |
| | 3 | 16 | 36 | 21 |

191 Hasenclever D et al. A prognostic score for advanced Hodgkin's disease. *NEJM* 1998; 339:1506-14.
192 Shipp M et al. A predictive model for aggressive non-Hodgkin's lymphoma. *NEJM* 1993; 329:987-94.

## Non-Hodgkin Lymphoma classification by aggressiveness [193]

| Classification | Types |
|---|---|
| **Highly aggressive**<br>5% of non-Hodgkin lymphomas<br>Survival measured in weeks if untreated or resistant to treatment<br>Often curable | • Burkitt's lymphoma<br>• Precursor B lymphoblastic leukemia/lymphoma<br>• Adult T-cell leukemia/lymphoma<br>• Precursor T lymphoblastic leukemia/lymphoma |
| **Aggressive**<br>50% of non-Hodgkin lymphomas<br>Survival measured in months if untreated or resistant to treatment<br>Often curable | • Follicular lymphoma (grade III)<br>• Diffuse large B-cell lymphoma<br>• Peripheral T-cell lymphoma<br>• Anaplastic large cell lymphoma, T/null cell<br>• Mantle cell lymphoma<br>• Extranodal NK-T-cell lymphoma, nasal type<br>• Natural killer cell large granular lymphocyte leukemia (aggressive) |
| **Indolent**<br>35-40% of non-Hodgkin lymphomas<br>Survival measured in years<br>Usually incurable | **B-cell**<br>• Small lymphocytic lymphoma (SLL)<br>• B-cell chronic lymphocytic lymphoma (CLL)<br>• Lymphoplasmacytic lymphoma<br>• Plasma cell myeloma or plasmacytoma<br>• Hairy cell leukemia<br>• Follicular lymphoma (grade I & II)<br>• Marginal zone B-cell lymphoma (extranodal; splenic +/- villous lymphocytes)<br><br>**T-cell**<br>• T-cell large granular lymphocyte leukemia (LGL)<br>• Mycosis fungoides<br>• T-cell prolymphocytic leukemia<br><br>**Natural killer cell**<br>• Natural killer cell large granular lymphocyte leukemia (indolent) |

193 Adapted from Freedman AS. Classification of the lymphomas. In: *UpToDate*. Rose BD (Ed). UpToDate, Wellesley, MA, 2002. Harris NL *et al.* World Health Organization classification of neoplastic diseases of the hematopoietic and lymphoid tissues. *J Clin Oncol* 1999; 17:3835-49.

# Staging Lung Cancer[194]

| T0 | No evidence of primary tumor | **Tis** | Carcinoma in situ |
|----|------------------------------|---------|-------------------|
| T1 | Tumor ≤ 3 cm surrounded by lung or visceral pleura, without evidence of invasion proximal to a lobar bronchus | | |
| T2 | (**1**) Tumor > 3 cm in greatest dimension (**2**) Involves main stem bronchus ≥ 2 cm distal to carina (**3**) Invades the visceral pleura (**4**) Atelectasis or obstructive pneumonitis that extends to hilum but does not involve entire lung | | |
| T3 | Tumor of any size with direct extension into the chest wall (including superior sulcus tumors), diaphragm, mediastinal pleura or pericardium; **or** a tumor in the main bronchus < 2 cm distal to the carina without involving the carina; **or** associated atelectasis or obstructive pneumonitis of the entire lung | | |
| T4 | Tumor any size that invades any of the following: mediastinum, heart, great vessels, trachea, esophagus, vertebral body, carina; **or** malignant pleural or pericardial effusion; **or** satellite tumor nodules within same lobe of lung | | |
| N0 | No demonstrable metastases to regional nodes | | |
| N1 | Metastases to peribronchial and/or ipsilateral hilar lymph nodes, or direct extension to intrapulmonary nodes | | |
| N2 | Metastases to ipsilateral mediastinal or subcarinal lymph nodes | | |
| N3 | Metastases to contralateral mediastinal, contralateral hilar, ipsilateral or contralateral scalene or supraclavicular lymph nodes | | |
| M0 | No (known) distant metastases | **M1** | Distant metastasis present |

## Prognosis and Survival by Stage

| Stage | TNM Classification | % of total | % Survival * | | Surgery |
|-------|--------------------|-----------|------|------|---------|
| | | | 1 year | 5 year | |
| IA | T1N0M0 | 13 | 94 | 67 | |
| IB | T2N0M0 | 23 | 87 | 57 | Resectable |
| IIA | T1N1M0 | 0.5 | 89 | 55 | |
| IIB | T2N1M0 or T3N0M0 | 7 | 73 | 39 | |
| IIIA | T3N1M0, T1-3N2M0 | 10 | 64 | 23 | N1 resectable |
| IIIB | TanyN3M0, T4NanyM0 | 20 | 37 | 7 | Unresectable |
| IV | TanyNanyM1 | 27 | 20 | 1 | |

* By pathological staging

## Reasons for classification as unresectable (inoperable)
• Distant metastasis • Involvement of trachea or contralateral mainstem bronchus
• Mediastinal lymph node involvement • SVC obstruction • Malignant pleural effusion
• Recurrent laryngeal nerve involvement • Small cell carcinoma

## Small cell carcinoma
15-25% of all lung cancer • Usually presents with large hilar mass and bulky mediastinal lymphadenopathy • 10% with occult brain mets at presentation

| Stage | TNM | % of cases | Survival | | | Treatment |
|-------|-----|-----------|--------|------|------|-----------|
| | | | Median | 1 yr | 5 yr | |
| Limited - confined to a hemithorax or XRT port | I-IIIB | 30 | 15-26 mo | 20-40% | 15-25% | XRT + Chemo |
| Extensive | IV | 70 | 7-11 mo | 5 % | 1 % | Chemo |

**Worse prognosis with:** • Mixed small/non-small cell pathology • Poor performance status (Karnofsky score) • Elevated LDH (limited stage) • Greater number of organs involved • Mets to CNS, bone marrow, liver • Male • Paraneoplastic syndromes

194 Mountain CJ et al. Revisions in the International System for staging lung cancer. *Chest* 1997; 111:1710-1717; Spira A, Ettinger DS. Multidisciplinary management of lung cancer. *NEJM* 2004; 350:379-392.

# Staging Colon Cancer [195]

| Tumor | | | |
|---|---|---|---|
| T0 | No evidence of primary tumor | **T3** | Invades subserosa or non-peritonealized pericolic or perirectal tissue |
| Tis | Carcinoma in situ; intraepithelial or invasion of lamina propria only | **T4** | Directly invades other organs structures, or perforates visceral peritoneum |
| T1 | Invades submucosa | | |
| T2 | Invades muscularis propria | | |

| Regional Lymph Nodes | | Distant Metastasis | |
|---|---|---|---|
| N0 | No regional lymph node metastasis | M0 | No distant metastasis |
| N1 | Mets in 1-3 regional lymph nodes | M1 | Distant metastasis |
| N2 | Mets in ≥ 4 regional lymph nodes | | |

## Stage Grouping

| T | N | M | AJCC * | MAC ** | Dukes # | 5-yr Survival |
|---|---|---|---|---|---|---|
| Tis | N0 | M0 | 0 | | | 100 % |
| T1 | N0 | M0 | I | A | A | 97 % |
| T2 | N0 | M0 | I | B1 | A | 90 % |
| T3 | N0 | M0 | II A | B2 | B | 78 % |
| T4 | N0 | M0 | II B | B3 | B | 63 % |
| T1,T2 | N1 | M0 | III A | C1 | C | 66 % |
| T3,T4 | N1 | M0 | III B | C2, C3 | C | |
| T any | N2 | M0 | III C | C1-3 | C | 37 % |
| T any | N any | M1 | Stage IV | | D | 4 % |

\* American Joint Committee on Cancer \*\* Modified Astler-Coller (MAC) staging system
# Gastrointestinal Tumor Study Group modification of Dukes staging system

## Factors associated with worse prognosis

• Poorly-differentiated histology • Invasive tumors • Lymphatic or perineural invasion • Male • Symptoms on presentation (including hemorrhage) • Obstruction or perforation • Young age at disease onset • Tumor arising at or below the peritoneal reflection • Tumor aneuploidy • Chromosome 18q allelic loss • p53 mutation

## Selected syndromes and median survival

• GI symptoms, stage C disease or direct extension to surrounding organs: 10-12 mo • Liver involvement or peritoneal seeding: 7-8 mo • Ascites or extra-abdominal mets: 4-5 mo

## Survival by Stage in 111,110 patients 1973-87

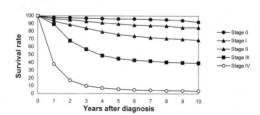

195 *AJCC Cancer Staging Manual*, 6th ed. Green FL, editor. New York: Springer-Verlag, 2002; Steele G *et al. Cancer of the Colon, Rectum and Anus.* In: *Cancer Manual*, 9th ed. Osteen RT (ed). Boston: American Cancer Society, 1996.

# *Staging Breast Cancer*[196]

## TNM Definitions

| Tumor | | | |
|---|---|---|---|
| **T0** | No evidence of primary tumor | **T1** | Tumor ≤ 2 cm in diameter |
| **Tis** | Carcinoma *in situ*: intraductal carcinoma, lobular carcinoma *in situ*, or Paget's disease of nipple | **T2** | Tumor 2 - 5 cm in diameter |
| | | **T3** | Tumor > 5cm in diameter |
| | | **T4** | Tumor of any size with direct extension to skin or chest wall |

| Regional Lymph Nodes | | Distant Metastasis | |
|---|---|---|---|
| **N0** | No regional nodes metastasis | **M0** | No distant metastasis |
| **N1** | Mets to moveable ipsilateral axillary LNs | | |
| **N2** | Mets to **(a)** fixed ipsilateral axillary LNs or **(b)** ipsilateral internal mammary LNs by exam or CT scan | **M1** | Distant metastasis |
| **N3** | Mets to **(a)** ipsilateral infraclavicular LNs ± axillary LNs **(b)** ipsilateral internal mammary LNs *and* axillary LNs or **(c)** ipsilateral supraclavicular LNs | | |

## Stage Grouping

| AJCC/UICC | T | N | M |
|---|---|---|---|
| Stage 0 | Tis | N0 | M0 |
| Stage I | T1 | N1 | M0 |
| Stage II A | T0,T1 | N1 | M0 |
| | T2 | N0 | M0 |
| Stage II B | T2 | N1 | M0 |
| | T3 | N0 | M0 |

| AJCC/UICC | T | N | M |
|---|---|---|---|
| Stage III A | T0-T3 | N2 | M0 |
| | T3 | N1 | M0 |
| Stage III B | T4 | N0-N2 | M0 |
| Stage III C | Any T | N3 | M0 |
| Stage IV | Any T | Any N | M1 |

## Factors associated with worse prognosis

- Larger primary tumor size
- Higher histologic grade
- Lymphatic invasion
- Greater number of lymph nodes involved
- Higher proliferative/mitotic/S-phase rate
- Higher expression of *Her-2/neu* (c-erbB-2) gene
- Reduced expression of estrogen and progesterone receptors

**Breast Cancer Survival (Disease-Specific) by Stage**

in 50,383 patients 1985-1989

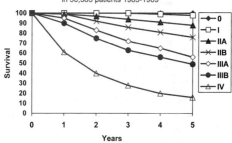

196 *AJCC Cancer Staging Manual*, 6th ed. Green FL, editor. New York: Springer-Verlag, 2002.

# Cancer of Unknown Primary Site [197]

## Pathological classification after biopsy

| Pathologic diagnosis after initial light microscopy (% of total) | Final diagnosis after special study or specific clinical features (% of total) |
|---|---|
| Moderate or well-differentiated adenocarcinoma (60%) | Specific subgroup (6%) No specific subgroup (54%) |
| Poorly differentiated carcinoma(PDC) or poorly differentiated adenocarcinoma (PDA) (30%) | Lymphoma, melanoma, sarcoma (3%) Specific carcinoma (1%) PDC, PDA (26%) |
| Poorly differentiated malignant neoplasm (PDMN) (5%) | Lymphoma (3%); PDC or PDA (1%) Melanoma, sarcoma, other (1%) |
| Squamous carcinoma (5%) | Specific subgroup (4%) No specific subgroup (1%) |

## Moderate or well-differentiated adenocarcinoma

- Clinical evaluation: abdominal CT; serum PSA in men; mammography in women
- Pathological studies: PSA stain in men; hormone receptor status in women

| Special Subgroups | Therapy | Prognosis* |
|---|---|---|
| Women with axillary-node involvement | Treat as primary breast cancer | Same as stage II breast cancer (70-80% at 5 yr) |
| Women with peritoneal carcinomatosis | Surgical cytoreduction and chemo for ovarian ca | 30-40% response rate |
| Men with blastic bone mets, high PSA or PSA tumor staining | Hormonal therapy for prostate cancer | Same as metastatic prostate cancer |
| Single peripheral nodal involvement | Lymph node dissection and XRT | Long-term survival reported |

\* If not in special sub-group, prognosis is poor (median survival of 4 months)

## Squamous carcinoma

| Location | Evaluation | Therapy | Prognosis |
|---|---|---|---|
| Cervical node | Pan-endoscopy | XRT ± neck dissection ± chemo | 30-50% 5-yr survival if high cervical node |
| Inguinal node | Pelvic & rectal exam, anoscopy | Lymph node dissection ± XRT | Potential long-term survivors |

## Poorly differentiated neoplasm, carcinoma or adenocarcinoma

- Clinical evaluation: chest and abdominal CT; serum hCG and AFP
- Pathological studies: immunoperox staining, electron microscopy, karyotype

| Special Sub-group | Therapy | Prognosis |
|---|---|---|
| Non-Hodgkin's Lymphoma (30-70% of PDN) | Chemo ± XRT | Same as lymphoma |
| Atypical germ cell tumors (young men w/ mid-line tumors, elevated AFP or hCG, abnormal chromosome 12 on karyotype) | Treat as germ cell tumor | Same as for extra-gonadal germ cell tumor |
| Neuroendocrine tumors | Cisplatin-based chemo | High response rate; 10-20% cured |
| Predominant tumor in retroperitoneum and peripheral nodes (esp. young, non-smoker) | Cisplatin-based chemo | High response rate |

---

197 Hainsworth JD, Greco FA. Drug Therapy: Treatment of patients with cancer of unknown primary site. *NEJM* 1993; 329(4): 259.

## Favorable prognostic factors[198]
- Single site of metastasis • Retroperitoneal or peripheral lymph node involvement
- Isolated axillary adenopathy (women = breast; rare in men)
- Blastic bone metastases or increased PSA in serum or tumor (men)
- Poorly differentiated malignant neoplasm (60% lymphomas)
- Extragonadal germ cell tumor • Squamous cell carcinomas
- Neuroendocrine carcinoma, high grade/poorly differentiated (small cell and others) or low- or well-differentiated (carcinoid and islet cell type)

# *Brain Mets from Primary Tumors*[199]

| Primary Tumor | Risk of Metastasis | % of total cases | | Symptom | % of cases |
|---|---|---|---|---|---|
| Lung | 34 % | 18-64 % | | Cognitive | 34 % |
| Breast | 21 % | 2-21 % | | Headache | 31 % |
| Melanoma | 49 % | 4-16 % | | Weakness | 24 % |
| Colon | 5 % | 2-11 % | | Seizure | 19 % |
| Renal/Bladder | 17 % | 2-8 % | | Ataxia | 11% |
| Leuk/lymphoma | - | 10% | | Visual change | 5 % |
| Other/unknown | - | 14 % | | None | 9 % |

- 5-10% with no identifiable primary
- 10-15 % with brain metastasis as initial manifestation

## Differential diagnosis
- Primary brain tumor • Abscess • HSV encephalitis • Granulomatous disease
- Demyelination • Infarction • Radiation necrosis
- Progressive multifocal leukoencephalopathy

## Treatment
- **Corticosteroids:** If symptomatic start IV or PO dexamethasone (Load 10 mg, then 4-6 mg q 6 hr) → improvement in 70% of patients and doubling of expected survival time. Relative contraindication: new lesions with no known history of malignancy (may confound diagnosis of CNS lymphoma or worsen infection)
- **Anticonvulsants:** Indicated if patient presents with seizures, but not prophylactic
- **Whole brain radiotherapy (XRT):** 80% of patients improve within 3 weeks • Median survival increased 4-5 months, with even likelihood of dying from systemic rather than brain disease
- **Surgery:** Indicated for **(1)** diagnosis in patient without known primary **(2)** solitary brain met **(3)** recurrent symptoms of life-threatening edema despite conservative management
- **Surgery followed by XRT:** Best outcome in patients with single brain metastasis, controlled systemic disease and good performance status (median survival: 1 yr)
- **Stereotactic radiosurgery:** Alternative to surgery in patients who are poor surgical candidates; if combined with whole brain XRT outcomes are similar to surgery plus XRT
- **Interstitial brachytherapy:** If tumor too large for radiosurgery
- **Chemotherapy:** For control of systemic disease, if appropriate

198 Greco FA, Hainsworth JD. Cancer of unknown primary site. In *Cancer: Principles and Practice of Oncology*, 6th ed. Devita VT et al, ed. Lippincott Williams and Wilkins, Philadelphia, 2001.
199 Chidel M et al. Brain metastases: presentation, evaluation and management. *Clev Clin J Med* 2000; 67(2):120-127; Lassman AB, DeAngelis LM. Brain metastases. *Neurol Clin* 2003; 21:1-23

# Pulmonary

## *Chest Anatomy - Radiographs* [200]

**Posteroanterior Chest View**

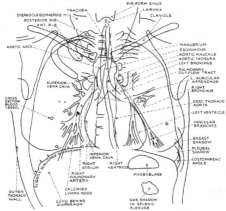

**Azygous Lobe**

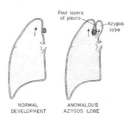

NORMAL DEVELOPMENT            ANOMALOUS AZYGOS LOBE

---

200  Meschan I. *Roentgen Signs in Diagnostic Imaging*, 2nd ed. Boston: Saunders; 1987. Pp. 4.72, 4.57, 4.82, 4.49. Reproduced with permission.

## Lateral Chest View

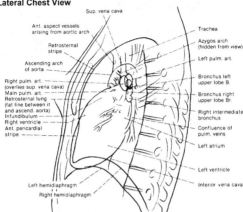

## Cardiac structures on PA chest radiograph

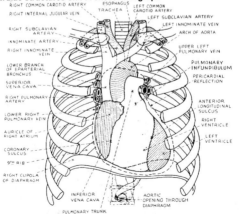

# *Chest Anatomy - CT* [201]

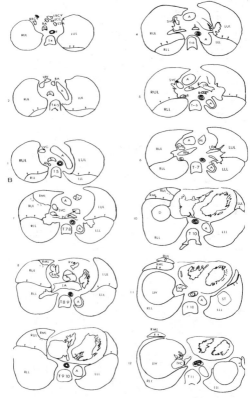

[201] Meschan I. *Roentgen Signs in Diagnostic Imaging*, 2nd ed. Boston: Saunders; 1987. P. 4.49. Reproduced with permission.

# Pulmonary Function Testing [202]

## Lung volumes in a healthy individual

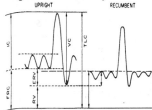

UPRIGHT          RECUMBENT

### Abbreviations

**ERV**= expiratory reserve vol.
**FEF$_{25-75\%}$**=forced expiratory flow from 25-75% VC
**FEV$_1$**= forced expiratory volume in 1 second
**FRC**= functional residual capacity
**FVC**= forced vital capacity
**IC**= inspiratory capacity
**RV**= residual volume
**TLC**= total lung capacity
**VC**= vital capacity

## Spirometry Patterns

- **Normal**: FVC, FEV$_1$, PEFR and FEF$_{25-75\%}$ > 80% predicted; FEV$_1$/FVC > 95% predicted ♦ Can be seen with intermittent disease (e.g. asthma), pulmonary emboli and pulmonary vascular disease

- **Obstructive**: Obstruction to airflow prolongs expiration ♦ FEV$_1$/FVC < 95% predicted and increased airway resistance ♦ Differential diagnosis: asthma, COPD, bronchiectasis, cystic fibrosis, bronchiolitis, proximal airway obstruction

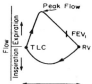

Flow-Volume Loop

- **Restrictive**: Reduced volumes without changes in airway resistance ♦ Decreased VC and TLC, FEV$_1$ and FVC decreased proportionately (FEV$_1$/FVC ratio > 95% pred) ♦ Must confirm lung volumes by helium dilution or plethysmography (reduced FVC on spirometry not specific for restrictive disease, although normal FVC predicts normal TLC) ♦ Differential diagnosis: interstitial disease, CHF, pleural disease, pneumonia, neuromuscular disease, chest wall abnormalities, obesity, lung resection

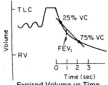

Expired Volume vs Time

- **Bronchodilator response**: Positive if FVC or FEV$_1$ increase 12% *and* ≥ 200 mL

- **Poor effort**: Most reliably diagnosed by technician performing test rather than spirometric values. Forced expiratory time (FET) < 6 seconds suggests inadequate expiration.

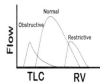

[202] American Thoracic Society. Lung function testing: Selection of reference values and interpretive strategies. Am Rev Resp Dis 1991; 144:1202-18.

## Grading of PFT abnormalities

| Obstruction | % Predicted FEV$_1$ | Restriction | % Predicted TLC# | % Predicted FVC |
|---|---|---|---|---|
| Mild | 70 - 100% | Mild | 70% - LLN* | 70% - LLN* |
| Moderate | 60 - 69% | Moderate | 50 - 69% | 60 - 69% |
| Mod-severe | 50 - 59% | Mod-severe | | 50 - 59% |
| Severe | 35 - 49% | Severe | < 50% | 35 - 49% |
| Very Severe | < 35% | Very Severe | | < 35% |

\# TLC superior to FVC in assessing restrictive disease
\* LLN= lower limits of normal

## Diffusion capacity (DL$_{CO}$)

- Expensive, imprecise and generally less helpful than widely believed. Measured value needs to be adjusted for hemoglobin and alveolar ventilation (V$_A$). Most useful for **(1)** evaluating pulmonary vascular disease **(2)** diagnosing pulmonary hemorrhage **(3)** assessing change in collagen-vascular or drug-related pulmonary disease.
- **Reduced:** emphysema, interstitial lung disease, pulmonary embolism, pulmonary vascular disease, lung resection, severe CHF
- **Increased:** pulmonary hemorrhage, mild CHF
- **Normal:** asthma, chronic bronchitis, chest wall and pleural abnormalities, neuromuscular disease

## Mechanical upper airway obstruction

- Most reliably diagnosed by contour of flow-volume loop and reproducibility (see below). If suspected, alert technician to emphasize performance of inspiratory limb of loop.
- **Variable extrathoracic:** Bilateral or unilateral vocal cord paralysis • Rheumatoid arthritis • Post-intubation vocal cord adhesions • Obstructive sleep apnea • Burns
- **Variable intrathoracic:** Non-circumferential tracheal tumors which make walls "floppy" • Relapsing polychondritis • Tracheomalacia following surgery • Mainstem bronchus tumors
- **Fixed upper airway obstruction:** Benign stricture after prolonged intubation • Tracheal tumor • Goiter • Small endotracheal or tracheostomy tube • Bilateral stenosis of mainstem bronchi (rare)

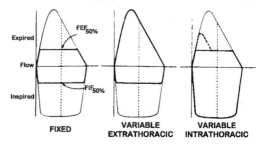

FIXED          VARIABLE EXTRATHORACIC          VARIABLE INTRATHORACIC

# Predicted Peak Flow (liters/min)[203]

| Age (yrs) | Women (height in inches) | | | | | Men (height in inches) | | | | |
|---|---|---|---|---|---|---|---|---|---|---|
| | 55 | 60 | 65 | 70 | 75 | 60 | 65 | 70 | 75 | 80 |
| 20 | 390 | 423 | 460 | 496 | 529 | 554 | 602 | 649 | 693 | 740 |
| 25 | 385 | 418 | 454 | 490 | 523 | 543 | 590 | 636 | 679 | 725 |
| 30 | 380 | 413 | 448 | 483 | 516 | 532 | 577 | 622 | 664 | 710 |
| 35 | 375 | 408 | 442 | 476 | 509 | 521 | 565 | 609 | 651 | 695 |
| 40 | 370 | 402 | 436 | 470 | 502 | 509 | 552 | 596 | 636 | 680 |
| 45 | 365 | 397 | 430 | 464 | 495 | 498 | 540 | 583 | 622 | 665 |
| 50 | 360 | 391 | 424 | 457 | 488 | 486 | 527 | 569 | 607 | 649 |
| 55 | 355 | 386 | 418 | 451 | 482 | 475 | 515 | 556 | 593 | 634 |
| 60 | 350 | 380 | 412 | 445 | 475 | 463 | 502 | 542 | 578 | 618 |
| 65 | 345 | 375 | 406 | 439 | 468 | 452 | 490 | 529 | 564 | 603 |
| 70 | 340 | 369 | 400 | 432 | 461 | 440 | 477 | 515 | 550 | 587 |

# Suspected Pulmonary Embolism [204]

## Criteria for quantifying clinical (pre-test) probability of PE [205]

| Criteria | Points |
|---|---|
| Suspected DVT | 3 |
| Alternative diagnosis less likely than PE | 3 |
| Heart rate > 100 bpm | 1.5 |
| Immobilization or surgery in past 4 weeks | 1.5 |
| Previous DVT or PE | 1.5 |
| Hemoptysis | 1 |
| Malignancy (active or treated within 6 months) | 1 |

| Category | Total Points | % of patients | Probability of PE |
|---|---|---|---|
| Low | 0-2 | 40 % | 3.6 % |
| Moderate | 3-6 | 53 % | 20.5 % |
| High | >6 | 7 % | 66.7 % |

## Accuracy of D-dimer assays

| Accuracy | Most | ←      → | Least |
|---|---|---|---|
| Assay | Quantitative ELISA | Qualitative whole blood Rapid ELISA Turbidimetric Immunofiltration | Latex agglutinin |
| Sensitivity | 97 % | 89-95 % | 70 % |

[203] Leiner GC *et al.* Expiratory peak flow rate. Standard values for normal subjects. Use as a clinical test of ventilatory function. *Am Rev Resp Dis* 1963; 88:644.

[204] Fedullo PF, Tapson VF. Clinical practice. The evaluation of suspected pulmonary embolism. *NEJM* 2003; 349:1247-56.; Clinical policy: Critical issues in the evaluation and management of adult patients presenting with suspected pulmonary embolism. *Ann Emerg Med* 2003; 41:257-70.

[205] Wells PS *et al.* Derivation of a simple clinical model to categorize patients probability of pulmonary embolism: Increasing the models utility with the SimpliRed d-dimer. *Thromb Haemost* 2000; 83:416-20.

| Clinical Probability | Strategies for ruling out pulmonary embolism [206] |
|---|---|
| Low | • Normal D-dimer assay *<br>*If D-dimer is positive:*<br>• Normal or low probability VQ scan<br>• Nondiagnostic V/Q# *plus* normal US<br>• Normal spiral CT scan *plus* normal US |
| Intermediate | • Normal V/Q scan<br>• Nondiagnostic V/Q# *plus* normal US *plus* normal D-dimer *<br>• Nondiagnostic V/Q# *plus* normal serial US ** *(if D-dimer abnormal)*<br>• Normal spiral CT scan *plus* normal US<br>• Normal pulmonary angiogram |
| High | • Normal V/Q scan<br>• Nondiagnostic V/Q# *plus* normal D-dimer* *plus* normal serial US **<br>• Normal pulmonary angiogram |
| **Clinical Probability** | **Strategies for ruling in pulmonary embolism** *(i.e. anticoagulation warranted)* |
| Low | • Elevated D-dimer *plus* high probability V/Q scan or abnormal US<br>• Abnormal pulmonary angiogram *(usually follows one or more abnormal tests: D-dimer, nondiagnostic V/Q#, spiral CT, US )* |
| Intermediate or High | • High probability V/Q<br>• Abnormal spiral CT<br>• Abnormal US *(1st test if suspected DVT; 2nd test after nondiagnostic V/Q# or normal spiral CT)*<br>• Abnormal pulmonary angiogram |

V/Q: ventilation-perfusion scan    US: Doppler ultrasonography of lower extremities
\*    Assumes use of highly sensitive assay
\#    Nondiagnostic VQ: neither normal nor high probability
\*\*   US repeated once, 3-7 days after initial negative results

## Pearls and nonsense
• Vital signs, EKG, chest x-ray, arterial blood gases all unreliable for confirming or ruling out diagnosis
• V/Q scanning of limited benefit in patients with severe underlying pulmonary disease
• Compression ultrasonography of femoral veins by itself is neither sensitive (50%) nor highly specific (68-75%) for PE.[207] However, may be appropriate initial test in patients with symptoms of both PE and deep vein thrombosis.
• Spiral CT scanning is emerging technology. Reported sensitivity for diagnosis of PE ranges from 57-100%. Newer scanners (helical, multi-detector) have improved accuracy.
• Spiral CT scanning requires significant contrast load and should be avoided in patients with underling severe renal insufficiency (especially in diabetes) or volume overload

[206] Wells PS *et al.* Excluding pulmonary embolism at the bedside without diagnostic imaging: Management of patients with suspected pulmonary embolism presenting to the emergency department by using a simple clinical model and d-dimer. *Ann Intern Med* 2001; 135:98-107; Kruip MJ *et al.* Diagnostic strategies for excluding pulmonary embolism in clinical outcome studies. A systematic review. *Ann Intern Med* 2003; 138:941-51.

[207] Kearon C *et al.* Noninvasive diagnosis of deep venous thrombosis. McMaster Diagnostic Imaging Practice Guidelines Initiative. *Ann Intern Med* 1998; 128:663-77.

# Pulmonary Embolism: PIOPED[208]

## Comparison of V/Q scan category with angiogram findings

| Scan category | PE present | PE absent | PE uncertain | No PAgram | Total |
|---|---|---|---|---|---|
| High probability | 102 (82%) | 14 (11%) | 1 (1%) | 7 (6%) | 124 (13%) |
| Intermediate | 105 (29%) | 217 (60%) | 9 (2%) | 33 (9%) | 364 (39%) |
| Low probability | 39 (13%) | 199 (64%) | 12 (4%) | 62 (20%) | 312 (34%) |
| Near-normal | 5 (4%) | 50 (38%) | 2 (2%) | 74 (56%) | 131 (14%) |
| **Total** | **251 (27%)** | **480 (52%)** | **24 (3%)** | **176 (19%)** | **931** |

## Probability of pulmonary embolism (PE) by V/Q scan result

| | Clinical (pre-test) probability | | | | | | |
|---|---|---|---|---|---|---|---|
| | "High" (80-100%) | | "Intermediate "(20-79%) | | "Low" (0-19%) | | All Probabilities |  |
| V/Q scan Category | Pts with PE | % | Pts with PE | % | Pts with PE | % | Pts with PE | % |
| High | 28/29 | 96 | 70/80 | 88 | 5/9 | 56 | 103/118 | 87 |
| Intermed | 27/41 | 66 | 66/236 | 28 | 11/68 | 16 | 104/345 | 30 |
| Low | 6/15 | 40 | 30/191 | 16 | 4/90 | 4 | 40/296 | 14 |
| Near Nml | 0/5 | 0 | 4/62 | 6 | 1/61 | 2 | 5/128 | 4 |
| **Total** | **61/90** | **68** | **170/569** | **30** | **21/228** | **9** | **252/887** | **28** |

V/Q: ventilation-perfusion scan

208 PIOPED Investigators. Value of the ventilation/perfusion scan in acute pulmonary embolism: Results of the Prospective Investigation of Pulmonary Embolism Diagnosis (PIOPED). *JAMA* 1990;263(20):2753-59.

# Pleural Fluid Analysis[209]

## Light's Criteria

- Any of following **excludes** transudates (98% sensitive, 83% specific for exudative effusion):
  (1) Pleural/serum LDH > 0.6
  (2) Pleural LDH > 2/3 upper limit for serum LDH
  (3) Pleural/serum Protein > 0.5
- Serum albumin - pleural albumin < 1.2 g/dL: more specific for exudate (92%) [210] but should not be used as only criteria

> **Always transudative**
> - CHF
> - Cirrhosis with ascites
> - Hypoalbuminemia
> - Nephrotic syndrome
>
> **Sometimes transudative**
> - Pulmonary embolism (35%)
> - Malignancy (10%)
> - Sarcoidosis
>
> **Sometimes exudative**
> - Diuretic-treated CHF

## Appearance

- Bloody: fluid hematocrit < 1% is non-significant; hematocrit 1-20 suggests cancer, PE, trauma; fluid hematocrit > 50% of serum hematocrit suggests hemothorax
- Turbid despite centrifugation suggests chylothorax or pseudochylothorax
- Putrid: suggests empyema • Viscid: mesothelioma
- "Anchovy paste" or "chocolate sauce": amebiasis

## Additional useful tests for exudative effusions

### Leukocytes
- Total WBC count rarely helpful
- Neutrophil predominance: **pneumonia, PE, pancreatitis**, abdominal abscess
- Lymphocyte predominance: **tumor, TB**, resolving acute process
- Eosinophilia (>10%): **blood or air in pleural space** • asbestos • drug reaction • paragonimiasis • uncommon in TB and malignancy

### Cytology (cell block and smears)
- 70% yield for metastatic adenocarcinoma, lower for other cancers
- Mesothelial cells nonspecific, but > 2-3% makes tuberculosis unlikely
- Send flow cytometry if lymphoma suspected

### Glucose
- Glucose < 60 mg/dL: **complicated parapneumonic effusion** (<40 mg/dL → chest tube) • **neoplasm** • TB • hemothorax • Churg-Strauss syndrome • rheumatoid arthritis or SLE • paragonimiasis

### Amylase
- Elevated in: esophageal perforation • pancreatic disease • malignancy

### Triglycerides
- Elevated in chylous effusions: > 110 mg/dl is 100% specific, <50 mg/dl excludes

### LDH
- Nonspecific indicator of inflammation

### pH
- < 7.0: complicated parapneumonic effusion (empyema)
- < 7.20: empyema, systemic acidosis, esophageal rupture, rheumatoid arthritis, TB, neoplasm, hemothorax, paragonimiasis

## Useful tests for tuberculous pleuritis
- Adenosine deaminase > 40 unit/L • Interferon $\gamma$ > 140 pg/mL • Positive PCR

## Useful tests for effusion of unknown cause
- Pulmonary embolism evaluation • Serial LDH measurement (reassuring if decreasing) • Thoracoscopy

---

209 Light RW. Pleural effusion. *NEJM* 2002; 346:1971-1977.
210 Roth BJ *et al.* The serum-effusion albumin gradient in the evaluation of pleural effusions. *Chest* 1990;98:546-49.

# Parapneumonic Effusions & Empyema[211]

| Class | Description | Features | Treatment |
|-------|-------------|----------|-----------|
| 1 | Insignificant parapneumonic effusion | • Small<br>• < 10mm thick on decubitus CXR | Antibiotics (thoracentesis not indicated) |
| 2 | Typical parapneumonic effusion | • ≥ 10mm thick<br>• Glucose > 40 mg/dl<br>• pH > 7.20<br>• Gram stain and culture negative | Antibiotics alone |
| 3 | Borderline complicated parapneumonic effusion | • pH 7.0-7.2 and/or LDH >1000<br>• Glucose > 40 mg/dl<br>• Gram stain and culture negative | Antibiotics plus serial thoracentesis If loculated, consider small (8-16F) chest tube +/- thrombolytics |
| 4 | Simple complicated parapneumonic effusion | • pH < 7.00 and/or glucose < 40 mg/dl and/or Gram stain or culture positive<br>• No loculations or frank pus | Small chest tube (8-16F) plus antibiotics |
| 5 | Complex complicated parapneumonic effusion | • Same as Class 4 but multi-loculated | Antibiotics plus thrombolytics via chest tube (rarely requires thoracoscopy or decortication) |
| 6 | Simple empyema | • Frank pus present<br>• Single locule or free flowing | Antibiotics and large (28F) chest tube +/- decortication |
| 7 | Complex empyema | • Frank pus present<br>• Multiple locules | Antibiotics plus thrombolytics via large (28F) chest tube; often requires thoracoscopy or decortication |

211 Light RW. A new classification of parapneumonic effusions and empyema. *Chest* 1995; 108:299-301.

# *Preoperative Pulmonary Evaluation*[212]

## Risk factors for perioperative pulmonary complications
- Smoking within 8 weeks of surgery
- COPD/significant airway obstruction
- Poor general health (ASA > 2)
- Elevated $P_aCO_2$
- Thoracic, AAA, or upper abdominal surgery
- Surgery lasting > 3 hours
- General anesthesia
- Long-acting neuromuscular blockade

## Pre-operative risk stratification
- Few patients have an absolute pulmonary contraindication to surgery
- Pre-operative spirometry should **not** be used to prevent surgery but rather as tool to optimize preoperative lung function. Appropriate if:
  - Asthma or COPD and unclear whether airflow has been optimized
  - Patients with unexplained dyspnea or pulmonary symptoms who are undergoing major surgery (intra-abdominal, thoracic, head/neck, vascular)
  - Patients undergoing lung resection
- **Respiratory Failure Index** [213]

| Factor | Score |
|---|---|
| Type of surgery | |
| AAA | 27 |
| Thoracic | 21 |
| Neuro, upper abdomen, peripheral vascular | 14 |
| Neck | 11 |
| Emergency surgery | 11 |

| Factor | Score |
|---|---|
| Albumin < 3 g/dL | 9 |
| BUN > 30 mg/dL | 8 |
| History of COPD | 6 |
| Functional status: partially or fully dependent | 7 |
| Age > 70 | 6 |
| Age 60-69 | 4 |

| Class | Points | Post-op respiratory failure |
|---|---|---|
| 1 | ≤ 10 | 0.5 % |
| 2 | 11-19 | 1.8 % |
| 3 | 20-27 | 4.2 % |
| 4 | 28-40 | 10.1 % |
| 5 | >40 | 26.6 % |

## Interventions to reduce perioperative risk
- Smoking cessation: beneficial if patient quits ≥ 8 weeks prior to surgery
- Inhaled ipratropium if clinically apparent COPD; β-agonists if wheezing
- Oral or inhaled steroids if COPD or asthma and pulmonary function not optimal (does not increase rate of infections or other postoperative complications, but potential adrenal suppression if ≥ 20 mg/day prednisone for ≥ 3 weeks)
- Defer elective surgery for acute exacerbations of pulmonary disease
- In high risk patients consider laparoscopic or shorter (< 3 hr) procedures, and spinal/epidural or regional rather than general anesthesia
- Avoid long-acting neuromuscular blockers (e.g. pancuronium)
- Post-op deep breathing exercises or incentive spirometry
- Epidural analgesia and nerve blocks for pain control

---

212 Smetana GW. Preoperative pulmonary evaluation. *NEJM* 1999;340(12):937-944; Arozullah AM et al. Preoperative evaluation for postoperative pulmonary complications. Med Clin North Am 2003; 87:153-73.

213 Arozullah AM et al. Multifactorial risk index for predicting postoperative respiratory failure in men after major noncardiac surgery. Ann Surg 2000; 232:242-53.

# Renal

## *Gaps and Deltas*

### Useful equations

Anion gap = $[Na^+] - [HCO_3^-] - [Cl^-]$
Calculated osmolarity = $([Na^+] \times 2) + ([glucose] \div 18) + ([BUN] \div 2.8) + ([ethanol] \div 4.6)$
Osmolar gap = Measured osmolality − calculated osmolarity
$\Delta$ gap ("delta-delta") = $\Delta$ Anion gap (measured − average normal) ÷ $\Delta HCO_3$ (average normal − measured)

### Causes of an elevated anion gap (> 11 mEq/L)

| *Acidosis present ("MUDPILES")* | *Acidosis absent* |
|---|---|
| • **M**ethanol<br>• **U**remia<br>• **D**iabetic ketoacidosis (also alcoholic and starvation ketoacidosis)<br>• **P**araldehyde<br>• **I**ron or isoniazid<br>• **L**actic acidosis (including metformin)<br>• **E**thylene glycol<br>• **S**alicylates<br>• Other: carbon monoxide, cyanide, hydrogen sulfide, sulfur, theophylline, toluene (glue-sniffing) | • Dehydration<br>• Alkalosis<br>• Sodium salts of unmeasured anions (citrate, lactate or acetate)<br>• Certain antibiotics (sodium penicillin, carbenicillin)<br>• Decrease in unmeasured cations (severe combined hypomagnesemia, hypocalcemia and hypokalemia) |

### Causes of a decreased anion gap (< 3 mEq/L)

| *Increase in unmeasured cations* | *Decrease in unmeasured anions* |
|---|---|
| • Hypercalcemia<br>• Hypermagnesemia<br>• Hyperkalemia<br>• Lithium intoxication<br>• Paraproteinemia | • Hypoalbuminemia<br>• Dilution |

### Causes of an elevated osmolar gap (> 10 mOsm/l)

| *With anion gap metabolic acidosis* | *No metabolic acidosis* |
|---|---|
| • Ethylene glycol<br>• Methanol<br>• Formaldehyde<br>• Uremia without dialysis<br>• Paraldehyde<br>• Alcoholic or diabetic ketoacidosis<br>• Lactic Acidosis | • Isopropyl alcohol<br>• Diethyl ether<br>• Mannitol<br>• Propylene glycol<br>• Severe hyperlipidemia or hyperproteinemia<br>• Sorbitol, glycerin or fructose<br>• IV contrast dye |

### Causes of a "delta-delta" gap

| *$\Delta$ Anion gap/$\Delta HCO_3$ < 1* | *$\Delta$ Anion gap/$\Delta HCO_3$ > 1.5* |
|---|---|
| • Non-anion gap acidosis or chronic respiratory alkalosis superimposed on anion gap acidosis, e.g. diarrhea and ESRD, salicylate intoxication<br>• DKA with urinary ketone losses<br>• Some cases of chronic renal failure | • Metabolic alkalosis superimposed on anion gap acidosis, e.g. vomiting and diabetic ketoacidosis<br>• Lactic acidosis (typical $\Delta/\Delta$ = 1.6) |

## Pearls and nonsense

- The absence of an anion gap does not exclude typical causes of anion gap acidosis, i.e. diabetic ketoacidosis may present without an anion gap [214]
- There is no identifiable cause of an elevated anion gap in 1/3 of patients [215]
- Large anion gaps (e.g. > 30 mEq/L) are most commonly diabetic ketoacidosis (DKA) or lactic acidosis; less commonly methanol or ethylene glycol. Higher anion gaps correlate with increased severity of illness.
- "Normal" anion gap is lab-dependent. The traditional value of 12 ± 4 mEq/L is high compared with results from newer instruments (normal range 7 ± 4 mEq/L). Time may be useful in individual patients.
- The Δanion gap/ΔHCO₃ oversimplifies complex acid-base relationships, and with minor deviations from unity (i.e. Δ/Δ = 0.7-1.5) the gap is as likely to misidentify a mixed acid-base disorder as to be correct [216]; however, with greater deviations (i.e. > 2) the presence of a mixed disorder is likely

# *Metabolic Acidosis*[217]

| Mechanism | Anion Gap? | Etiology |
|---|---|---|
| Increased acid production | Usually | • See table of anion gap acidoses (*page 141*) |
| Loss of HCO₃ | No | • Dilutional<br>• GI losses: diarrhea, ileal loop or tube/fistula drainage<br>• Renal losses: carbonic anhydrase inhibitors, topiramate, Type II RTA (proximal) |
| Decreased renal acid excretion | No | • Type I RTA (distal)<br>• Type IV RTA (hypoaldosteronism)<br>• Chronic renal failure (some cases) |
| Exogenous acid | No | • Toluene ingestion (hippuric acidosis)<br>• Ammonium chloride ingestion<br>• Hyperalimentation<br>• Lysine or arginine therapy |

## Urinary anion gap

$$\text{Urinary AG} = U_{Na} + U_K - U_{Cl} - U_{HCO3}$$

*Note: Calculated differently from serum anion gap; contribution of HCO₃ can be ignored if pH < 6.5*

Index of ammonium excretion: gap is **positive** if intrinsic renal disease (e.g. RTA), **negative** if normal or GI bicarbonate loss [218]

## Pathophysiologic consequences of severe acidemia

- Reduced cardiac contractility and output • Centralization of blood volume
- Increased pulmonary vascular resistance • Increased arrhythmias (re-entrant, VF)
- Reduced cardiovascular responsiveness to catecholamines • Insulin resistance
- Hyperkalemia • Obtundation and coma • Hyperventilation/dyspnea
- Decreased respiratory muscle strength and respiratory fatigue

214   Adrogue HJ *et al.* Plasma acid-base patterns in diabetic ketoacidosis. *NEJM* 1982; 307: 1603-10.
215   Gabow PA *et al.* Diagnostic importance of an increased serum anion gap. *NEJM* 1980; 303: 854-8.
216   Dinubile MJ. The increment in the anion gap: overextension of a concept? *Lancet* 1988; 2(8617): 951-3.
217   Adrogue HJ, Madias NE. Management of life-threatening acid-base disorders. *NEJM* 1998; 338: 26-34.
218   Battle DC *et al.* The use of the urinary anion gap in the diagnosis of hyperchloremic metabolic acidosis. *NEJM* 1988; 318:594-9.

## Bicarbonate therapy

- Should be limited to following scenarios:
  - Bicarbonate loss (e.g. diarrhea, Type I RTA) with moderate acidosis
  - Severe acidosis (e.g. pH < 7.15 or $HCO_3$ < 8 mEq/L) with metabolic consequences. Bicarbonate generally temporizes only until underlying cause is treated. Effectiveness in organic acidoses (e.g. diabetic ketoacidosis) unclear. Should **not** be used in hypercarbic respiratory acidosis.
  - Salicylate or tricyclic antidepressant toxicity (even if not acidemic)
- Bicarbonate should be administered as near-isotonic infusion (rather than bolus) to achieve pH > 7.20 or $HCO_3$ > 8-10 mEq/L (*See bicarbonate page 177*).
- Calculated $HCO_3$ deficit (in mEq) = $HCO_3$ deficit/liter × $V_D$ of $HCO_3$
  = (target $HCO_3$ – actual $HCO_3$) × (lean body wt × 0.5)
  **Note:** Calculation is approximate, and actual change in pH should be re-assessed 30 minutes after completing infusion
- Consequences of $NaHCO_3$ administration include hypernatremia, volume overload, "overshoot" alkalosis, and paradoxical worsening of intracellular acidosis.

# *Lactic Acidosis*[219]

## Diagnosis

- Exclude other causes of anion gap acidosis (see table on page 141)
- Lactic acidosis may alter tissue redox state and artifactually lower β-hydroxybutyrate level in co-existing ketoacidosis

## Type A: Clinically apparent hypoperfusion and tissue hypoxia

- Etiology: • Cardiogenic shock • Hypotension • Sepsis • Anemia/hemorrhage • CO poisoning
- Acidosis itself worsens cardiac, renal and hepatic dysfunction, which may in turn increase lactate production or reduce clearance
- High mortality related to underlying condition

## Type B: Clinically inapparent hypoperfusion

- Liver disease: Seen in fulminant hepatic failure or in acute decompensation of chronic liver disease (e.g. sepsis, GI bleeding). Correction of hypoglycemia may improve acidosis. Lactic acidosis in liver failure suggests very poor prognosis.
- Diabetic or alcoholic ketoacidosis: Etiology unclear; may be related to hypoglycemia in alcoholics
- Seizures: Usually transient unless underlying Type A mechanism
- Renal failure
- Malignant cell production: Usually acute leukemia or lymphoma
- Drugs: • metformin • nitroprusside (cyanide toxicity) • vasopressors • fructose and sorbitol (used as insulin-sparing sugars in TPN) • isoniazid • paraldehyde
- Toxins: • ethanol • methanol • salicylates • cyanide
- Hereditary enzyme deficiencies (gluconeogenesis, pyruvate oxidation, mitochondrial myopathies)
- Short gut syndrome: D-lactate absorbed but not metabolized

## Management

- Treat underlying condition
- Consider $NaHCO_3$ to keep pH > 7.15-7.20 (see bicarbonate therapy, above).
  **Note**: increased pH may cause increased lactate production.

---

219 Green R, Tannen R. Lactic acidosis. In: *Fluids and Electrolytes*, 3rd ed. Kokko JP, Tannen RL (eds). Philadelphia: Saunders, 1996.

# Renal Tubular Acidosis [220]

| | Distal (Type 1) | Proximal (Type 2) | Hypereninemic hypoaldosteronism (Type 4) |
|---|---|---|---|
| Defect | Inadequate distal acidification | Inadequate proximal $HCO_3$ reabsorption | Aldosterone deficiency or resistance |
| Etiology | • Autoimmune dis. (esp. Sjögren's) • Hypercalciuria • Cirrhosis • Obstruction • Sickle cell disease • 1° hyperPTH • Amphotericin B, lithium | • Myeloma • Heavy metals • Drugs: Ifos-famide, carbonic anhydrase inhibitors, topiramate • Cystinosis • Idiopathic | • Diabetic nephropathy • Chronic interstitial nephritis • Drugs: ACE inhibitors, NSAID, heparin, K+-sparing diuretics, cyclosporine |
| Urine pH | > 5.3 (exclude urease-splitting pathogen and extreme hypovolemia) | > 5.3 if above re-absorptive threshold; otherwise < 5.3 | Usually < 5.3 |
| Untreated plasma $[HCO_3]$ | May be < 10 mEq/L | > 12 mEq/L | > 15 mEq/L |
| Fractional $[HCO_3]$ excretion when plasma $[HCO_3] > 20$ mEq/L | < 3% | > 15-20% | < 3% |
| Plasma $[K^+]$ | Usually low-normal; ↑ in Na-reabsorption defect (sickle-cell, obstruction) | Normal or ↓ | ↑ |
| Urine anion gap (negative in GI loss) | Positive | Variable | Positive |
| Diagnosis | Response to $NaHCO_3$[a] or $NH_4Cl$[b] | Response to $NaHCO_3$[a] | ↓ Plasma aldo-sterone and plasma renin activity; TTKG < 5[c] suggestive in hyperkalemic pt |
| Amount $NaHCO_3$ to normalize plasma $[HCO_3]$ | 1-3 mEq/kg/d | 10-15 mEq/kg/d | 1-3 mEq/kg/day or correct hyper-kalemia |
| Other complications | • Nephrocalcinosis • Nephrolithiasis | • Rickets (children) • Osteomalacia • Osteopenia | • Hyperkalemia |

a: Response to **bicarbonate** (0.5-1.0 mEq/kg/hr infusion): Urine pH and fractional excretion of bicarbonate will remain constant in RTA type I, but will rise markedly in RTA type II

b: Response to **$NH_4Cl$** (0.1 g/kg): Urine pH in RTA type I should remain above 5.3 despite a 4-5 mEq/L fall in plasma $HCO_3$ within 4-6 hr

c: TTKG = trans-tubular K+ gradient = $(U_{K+} \times P_{Osm}) \div (P_{K+} \times U_{Osm})$, valid only if $U_{Osm} > P_{Osm}$

220 Rose BD, Post TW. *Clinical Physiology of Acid-Base and Electrolyte Disorders*, 5th ed. editor. New York: McGraw-Hill, Medical Pub. Division, 2001.

# Metabolic Alkalosis[221]

| Mechanism | Cause |
|---|---|
| Gastrointestinal H+ loss | • Vomiting or nasogastric suction<br>• Antacids (in uremia or milk-alkali syndrome) |
| Renal H+ loss | • 1° mineralocorticoid excess (including hyper-aldosteronism, Cushing's, licorice)<br>• Diuretics (loop or thiazide)<br>• Post-hypercapnia<br>• Hypercalcemia due to milk-alkali syndrome |
| Intracellular shift of H+ | • Hypokalemia |
| Alkali administration | • Citrate (transfusions), acetate (parenteral nutrition) |
| Volume contraction | • Massive diuresis<br>• Vomiting or NG suction in achlorhydria<br>• Sweat losses in cystic fibrosis<br>• Villous adenoma or laxative abuse |

## Urine chloride concentration in diagnostic evaluation

| < 25 mEq/L | > 40 mEq/L |
|---|---|
| Vomiting or NG suction<br>Diuretics (post-administration)<br>Laxative abuse<br>Post-hypercapnia<br>Cystic fibrosis<br>Low chloride intake | 1° mineralocorticoid excess<br>Diuretics (in effect)<br>Alkali load<br>Bartter's or Gitelman's syndrome<br>($U_{K+}$ > 30 mEq/L)<br>Severe hypokalemia (serum K+> 2.0 mEq/L) or hypomagnesemia |

## Consequences of severe alkalosis (pH >7.60 or $HCO_3$>45 mEq/L)
• Reduced cerebral blood flow • Tetany, seizures, lethargy, delirium and stupor
• Reduced coronary blood flow • Predisposition to refractory arrhythmias
• Reduced threshold for angina • Hypoventilation • ↓K, ↓Mg, ↓Ca, ↓PO₄

## Treatment[222]
• Treat underlying cause (i.e. suppress vomiting)
• Saline infusion if volume depleted
• KCI supplementation if hypokalemic or ongoing K+ losses (e.g. diuretics)
• H₂-blocker or proton pump inhibitor if ongoing nasogastric suction
• Addition of potassium-sparing diuretics to diuretic regimen; as second-line alternative consider addition of acetazolamide (250-375 mg PO qd-bid) with caution regarding "overshoot" acidosis and excessive K+-wasting
• Severe alkalosis (e.g. pH > 7.60 or $HCO_3$ > 45 mEq/L): Consider infusion of 0.1-0.2 N HCl (= 100-200 mEq H+ per liter) via central line at rate ≤ 0.2 mEq/kg/hr
• Calculated HCl deficit (in mEq) = $HCO_3$ excess/liter × $V_D(HCO_3)$
  = (actual $HCO_3$ - 40) × (lean body wt × 0.5)
**Note:** calculation is approximate, and actual change in pH should be re-assessed 30 minutes after completing infusion
• Consider hemodialysis for severe alkalosis in setting of cardiac or renal dysfunction

221 Rose BD, Post TW. Clinical Physiology of Acid-Base and Electrolyte Disorders, 5th ed. editor. New York: McGraw-Hill, Medical Pub. Division, 2001.
222 Adrogue HJ, Madias NE. Management of life-threatening acid-base disorders. NEJM 1998; 338: 107-111.

# Hyponatremia[223]

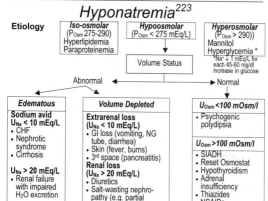

**Etiology**

| Iso-osmolar ($P_{Osm}$ 275-290) Hyperlipidemia Paraproteinemia | Hypoosmolar ($P_{Osm}$ < 275 mEq/L) | Hyperosmolar ($P_{Osm}$ > 290)) Mannitol Hyperglycemia * |
|---|---|---|

*$Na^+$ ↓ 1 mEq/L for each 45-60 mg/dl increase in glucose

**Volume Status**

**Abnormal** ← → **Normal**

**Edematous**

**Sodium avid**
$U_{Na}$ < 10 mEq/L
- CHF
- Nephrotic syndrome
- Cirrhosis

$U_{Na}$ > 20 mEq/L
- Renal failure with impaired $H_2O$ excretion

**Volume Depleted**

**Extrarenal loss**
($U_{Na}$ < 10 mEq/L)
- GI loss (vomiting, NG tube, diarrhea)
- Skin (fever, burns)
- 3rd space (pancreatitis)

**Renal loss**
($U_{Na}$ > 20 mEq/L)
- Diuretics
- Salt-wasting nephropathy (e.g. partial obstruction)
- ↓ Aldosterone

$U_{Osm}$ <100 mOsm/l
- Psychogenic polydipsia

$U_{Osm}$ >100 mOsm/l
- SIADH
- Reset Osmostat
- Hypothyroidism
- Adrenal insufficiency
- Thiazides
- NSAIDs
- Renal failure

## Differentiating causes of chronic hyponatremia

| Etiology | $U_{Osm}$ (mOsm/l) | $U_{Na}$ (mEq/l) | Response to $H_2O$ restriction | Response to $H_2O$ challenge |
|---|---|---|---|---|
| SIADH | > 100 | > 20 | $U_{Osm}$ remains high $P_{Osm}$ rises slowly | Water retained ($U_{Osm}$ remains high, $P_{Na}$ & $P_{Osm}$ fall) |
| Reset Osmostat | Variable (often > 100) | > 20 | $U_{Osm}$ rises or remains high $P_{Osm}$ rises slowly | Water load excreted ($U_{Osm}$ falls, $P_{Na}$ stays at "set point") |
| Psychogenic polydipsia | < 100 | Variable | $U_{Osm}$ stays low $P_{Osm}$ rises rapidly | No change |

## SIADH

**Diagnosis:** • Euvolemic • $P_{Na}$ and $P_{Osm}$ low • $U_{Osm}$ inappropriately high, despite adequate water intake (typically $U_{Osm}$ > $P_{Osm}$) • Absence of hypothyroidism, adrenal insufficiency, thiazides, etc • Uric acid typically low

**Etiology of SIADH**
- Neuropsychiatric disorders: infections (meningitis, encephalitis); cerebrovascular disease (stroke, intracranial bleeding, temporal arteritis); primary or metastatic tumors, psychiatric disease, Guillain-Barré syndrome, HIV
- Drugs: IV cyclophosphamide, carbamazepine, vincristine/vinblastine, antipsychotics, amitriptyline, MAOIs, bromocriptine
- Pulmonary disease: cancer, TB, pneumothorax, pneumonia, sarcoidosis

223 Rose BD, Post TW. *Clinical Physiology of Acid-Base and Electrolyte Disorders*, 5th ed. editor. New York: McGraw-Hill, Medical Pub. Division, 2001.; Adrogue HJ, Madias NE. Hyponatremia. *N Engl J Med* 2000;342(21):1581. Oster JR, Singer I. Hyponatremia, hyposmolality, and hypotonicity: Tables and fables. *Arch Intern Med* 1999; 159:333-6.

- Post-operative state
- Severe nausea
- Ectopic production of ADH: bronchogenic carcinoma (esp. small cell); also pancreas, duodenum, thymus
- Ectopic production of ADH-like compound: prolactinoma, Waldenström's
- Exogenous ADH: ddAVP, vasopressin, oxytocin
- Idiopathic

## Reset osmostat

- Patient will chronically regulate to lower-than-normal osmolarity/serum sodium (typically 125-130 mEq/L) but will respond appropriately to water load (i.e. within 4 hours will excrete 80% of 10-15 ml/kg $H_2O$ given IV or PO)
- Present in 1/3 of patients with SIADH
- Etiology: hypovolemia, quadriplegia, pregnancy, psychosis, TB, malnutrition
- Treatment: underlying condition only ($H_2O$ restriction unnecessary & ineffective)

## Manifestations of hyponatremia

- Symptoms proportional to rapidity of onset and severity of hyponatremia
- Early: nausea, malaise, lethargy
- Late: obtundation→ coma, seizures, respiratory arrest
- Pre-menopausal women at highest risk of neurologic deficits (may be irreversible)

**Management:**

- Sodium deficit (in mmol) = sodium deficit/liter × total body water
  = (120 − [Serum Na]) × wt (kg) × (0.5 in♀, 0.6 in♂)

**Symptomatic** hyponatremia ($Na^+$< 115 mEq/L or acute onset):

- Treat underlying conditions (e.g. Addison's) and stop offending drugs (e.g. HCTZ)
- If hypovolemic and no SIADH (i.e. dilute urine), replete deficit w/ normal or hypertonic saline (3% NaCl = 0.5 mEq $Na^+$/ml). If severe symptoms (e.g. seizures), use 3% NaCl. **If SIADH is present, normal saline may worsen hyponatremia.**
- If euvolemic (e.g. SIADH), use hypertonic (3%) saline
- Rate of correction: most symptoms reversed by rapid correction of only 3-7 mEq/l. Target should be 1.5-2.0 mEq/L per hour x 3-4 hours (or duration of symptoms), **but** total correction should be < 8-10 mEq/L in first 24 hr **and** < 18 mEq/L in first 48 hr. Monitor serum $Na^+$ frequently (e.g. every 4 hr initially)

**Asymptomatic** hyponatremia (typically $Na^+$ > 120 mEq/L and/or chronic):

- Treat underlying conditions (e.g. Addison's) and stop offending drugs (e.g. HCTZ)
- If volume depleted, correct deficit with normal saline
- If euvolemic (e.g. SIADH) should respond to **water restriction**
- Rate of correction: < 0.5 mEq/L per hour **and** < 8-10 mEq/L in first 24 hr **and** < 18 mEq/L in first 48 hr. Goal $Na^+$ is no higher than 125-130 mEq/L.

**Other treatment:**

- Loop diuretic impair the kidney's ability to retain free water and will augment effect of normal or hypertonic saline
- Potassium chloride supplementation if hypokalemic
- Demeclocycline or lithium indicated only in hyponatremia refractory to water restriction, salt loading (e.g. NaCl tablets) and loop diuretic

## Osmotic demyelination (pontine or extrapontine myelinolysis)

- Risk factors: **(1)** $Na^+$ correction of > 12-20 mEq/L in 24 hr **(2)** overcorrection of $Na^+$ to > 140 mEq/L **(3)** co-existing brain ischemia **(4)** pre-menopausal women
- Onset of symptoms typically delayed 2-6 days after correction of sodium
- MRI or CT may confirm suspected diagnosis (although findings may be delayed)
- If over-correction of hyponatremia occurs, hypotonic fluids and/or ddAVP may prevent or reverse neurological deficits
- Case reports suggest aggressive plasmapheresis may also improve outcomes [224]

---

224 Bibl D et al. Treatment of central pontine myelinolysis with therapeutic plasmapheresis. *Lancet* 1999;353(9159):1155.

# Hypernatremia[225]

## Etiology

| Mechanism | Cause |
|-----------|-------|
| Inadequate $H_2O$ intake | • Lack of thirst<br>• Poor intake or access to water |
| Renal losses of hypotonic fluid | • Central or nephrogenic diabetes insipidus (DI)<br>• Loop diuretics<br>• Osmotic diuresis (glucose, urea, mannitol)<br>• Post-obstructive diuresis<br>• Polyuric phase of ATN<br>• Intrinsic renal disease |
| Gastrointestinal losses of hypotonic fluid | • Vomiting<br>• Nasogastric drainage<br>• Enterocutaneous fistula<br>• Osmotic diarrhea (e.g. lactulose, malabsorption) |
| Other loss | • Insensible (skin, respiratory)<br>• Burns<br>• Excessive sweating |
| Hypertonic $Na^+$ gain ($U_{Na+} > 800$ mEq/L) | • Hypertonic saline or bicarbonate<br>• Hypertonic feedings (TPN, tube feeds)<br>• Ingestion of NaCl or sea water<br>• Hypertonic enemas or dialysis |

## Diabetes insipidus (DI)

- Most patients with DI have symptoms of polyuria (rather than hypernatremia) **unless** there is impaired thirst mechanism or access to free water
- Diagnosis: presence of low $U_{Osm}$ (< 300 mOsm/l) despite adequate stimulus to ADH secretion, i.e. elevated serum osmolality or sodium concentration after water deprivation
- After administration of ADH (10 mcg nasal ddAVP or 5 units vasopressin SC) patients with **central** DI will appropriately increase $U_{Osm}$ by ≥ 50%, while patients with **nephrogenic** DI will have little or no response
- Hypernatremia with mid-range urine osmolality (300-800mOsm/l) may be seen in:
  - Central DI with marked volume contraction
  - Partial DI (central or nephrogenic)
  - Osmotic diuresis, in which case daily solute excretion ($U_{Osm}$ x daily urine volume) is typically > 1000 mOsm

## Etiology of diabetes insipidus

| Central DI | Nephrogenic DI |
|------------|----------------|
| • Idiopathic<br>• Post-traumatic or post-surgical<br>• Space-occupying sellar lesions: cysts, tumors, histiocytosis, TB, sarcoid<br>• Inflammatory lesions: encephalitis, meningitis, Guillain-Barré, Lyme<br>• Vascular: aneurysms, infarction, Sheehan's | • Renal disease: medullary sponge kidney, amyloid, myeloma, Sjögren's<br>• Electrolytes: hypercalcemia, hypokalemia<br>• Drugs: lithium, foscarnet, ampho B, methoxyflurane<br>• Congenital |

---

225 Rose BD, Post TW. *Clinical Physiology of Acid-Base and Electrolyte Disorders*, 5th ed. editor. New York: McGraw-Hill, Medical Pub. Division, 2001; Adrogue HJ, Madias NE. *Hypernatremia. NEJM* 2000; 342: 1493-9.

**Clinical manifestations**

- Symptoms related to osmotic decrease in brain volume and include lethargy, confusion, and irritability. More advanced symptoms include seizures, coma, and intracerebral bleeding due to rupture of cerebral veins following brain shrinkage
- Symptoms are related to both rapidity of onset (acute >> chronic) and severity of hypernatremia (symptoms rare with [Na⁺] < 160 mEq/L)
- High mortality with [Na⁺] > 180 mEq/L, or [Na⁺] > 160 mEq/L for > than 48 hr

**Treatment**

- Free water deficit (in liters $H_2O$) = [($P_{Na+}$ ÷ 140) −1] × lean body weight (kg) x 0.4
- Actual fluid correction may need to account for ongoing losses
- Goal should be [Na⁺] ≤ 145 mEq/L
- If hypernatremia is chronic or of unclear duration, rate of correction should be ≤ 0.5 mEq/L per hour, or ≤ 10-12 mEq/L per day
- In acute hypernatremia e.g. accidental sodium loading occurring over several hours, [Na⁺] may be lowered at up to 1 mEq/L per hour
- Overly rapid correction may lead to cerebral edema producing seizures, irreversible neurologic damage or death
- May use D5W, ½ or ¼ normal saline as replacement fluid; normal saline generally ineffective unless profound volume depletion and should be **avoided**

# Hypokalemia[226]

## Etiology

| | |
|---|---|
| Trans-cellular shift | - Alkalosis<br>- Drugs: β-agonists (including pressors, bronchodilators, tocolytic agents and nasal decongestants), insulin overdose, methylxanthines, verapamil or chloroquine overdose<br>- Correction of megaloblastic anemia<br>- Periodic paralysis (familial or thyrotoxic)<br>- Delirium tremens |
| Renal loss (TTKG* > 3) | - Drugs: diuretics, fludrocortisone, high-dose steroids, high-dose penicillins, drugs causing hypomagnesemia (ampho B, aminoglycosides, cisplatin, foscarnet)<br>- Metabolic alkalosis<br>- Magnesium depletion<br>- Mineralocorticoid excess (1° aldosteronism, Cushing's, congenital adrenal hyperplasia, renovascular HTN, licorice)<br>- RTAs (type I > II)<br>- Bartter's, Gitelman's and Liddle's syndromes<br>- Acute myelogenous leukemia |
| Gastrointestinal loss | - Diarrhea (infectious or malabsorptive)<br>- Secretory tumors (villous adenoma, VIPoma, Zollinger-Ellison syndrome)<br>- Intestinal bypass or fistula |

\* TTKG = trans-tubular K⁺ gradient = ($U_{K+}$ × $P_{Osm}$) ÷ ($P_{K+}$ × $U_{Osm}$); valid only if $U_{osm}$>$P_{Osm}$

## Clinical manifestations

- Symptoms rare if [K⁺] > 3.0 mEq/L
- Early symptoms include weakness and constipation; as [K⁺] falls < 2.0 mEq/L may develop rhabdomyolysis or ascending paralysis with respiratory compromise
- Risk of lethal tachycardia, especially in setting of ischemia, CHF, LVH or digoxin
- ECG: U waves, T-wave flattening, and ST-segment changes

226 Gennari FJ. Hypokalemia. *NEJM* 1998; 339: 451-58.

## Treatment

*Note: Total body potassium deficit correlates poorly with serum levels (deficit is roughly 150-400 mEq per 1.0 mEq/L drop in serum [K+])*

- Correct underlying disorders, especially hypomagnesemia, alkalosis and volume contraction
- For [K+] < 2.0 mEq/L or [K+] < 3.0 mEq/L associated with symptoms or ECG abnormalities, give IV supplementation (maximum 20-40 mEq/hour via central IV line) with continuous cardiac monitoring
- Otherwise, give oral supplementation in form of KCl 20-40 mEq PO q4-24 hr. [1 inch banana or 1 oz orange juice contains ~ 1.6 mEq K+] [227]
- In patients with ongoing diuretic use daily K+ requirements are as high as 40-100 mEq; consider addition of K+-sparing diuretic such as amiloride, triamterene or spironolactone

# *Hyperkalemia*

## Etiology

| Mechanism | Cause |
|---|---|
| Spurious (plasma K+ normal) | • Hemolysis (during or after phlebotomy)<br>• Thrombocytosis or leukocytosis |
| Trans-cellular shift | • Metabolic acidosis<br>• Diabetic ketoacidosis<br>• Hyperosmolar states<br>• Drugs: β-blockers, succinylcholine, digitalis<br>• Hyperkalemic periodic paralysis<br>• Tissue destruction: rhabdomyolysis, crush injuries, tumor lysis, hemolysis<br>• Cardiac surgery |
| Increased intake | • Dietary (rare as isolated cause unless associated renal disease)<br>• Potassium salt drugs, e.g. penicillin G potassium |
| Decreased renal excretion | • Type IV RTA * (see table, page 143)<br>• Acute or chronic renal failure<br>• Decreased renal perfusion (CHF, sepsis)<br>• Adrenal insufficiency<br>• Congenital adrenal hyperplasia<br>• HIV<br>• Drugs: ACE inhibitors/receptor blockers, heparin, NSAIDs, cyclosporine, trimethoprim, pentamidine, K+-sparing diuretics |

* In absence of apparent cause, Type IV RTA (hyporeninemic hypoaldosteronism) accounts for 50-75% of cases. Trans-tubular K+ gradient (TTKG, see p. 149) is typically less than 5 when aldosterone is absent or inhibited.

## Clinical manifestations

- Cardiac arrhythmias, including idioventricular rhythm, sine-wave pattern VT, sinoventricular conduction and VF arrest
- ECG: peaked T waves, flattened P waves, prolonged P-R interval, widened QRS, and deepened S waves with merging into T waves
- Muscle weakness also seen with [K+] > 8 mEq/L

227 Somaia P. Effect of snack foods on cognitive processing in sleep-deprived monkeys. *JBIMA* 2003; Suite G; http://www.nal.usda.gov/fnic/foodcomp.

## Treatment

| Degree of hyperkalemia | Treatment |
| --- | --- |
| Mild<br>($K^+ < 6.0$ mEq/L) | **Decrease total body $K^+$ stores with**<br>• IV diuretic, e.g. furosemide 40-80 mg<br>• Kayexalate 30 g in 50 ml of 20% sorbitol, PO/PR<br>• Consider dialysis if renal failure |
| Moderate<br>($K^+$ 6.0-7.0 mEq/L) | **Shift $K^+$ into cells temporarily by adding**<br>• $NaHCO_3$ 50 mEq IV over 5 minutes (hypertonic; may exacerbate fluid overload or hypernatremia)<br>• D50 (50 g) plus insulin 10 units IV over 15 min<br>• Albuterol 10-20 mg nebulized over 15 minutes |
| Severe<br>($K^+ > 7.0$ mEq/L or ECG $\Delta$s) | **Protect myocardium by adding**<br>• $CaCl$ (central line) 5-10 ml 10% solution, or Ca gluconate (peripheral IV) 15-30 ml of 10% solution; either given IV over 2-5 minutes.<br>**Avoid** in suspected digitalis toxicity. |

# *Hypomagnesemia*

| Mechanism | Etiology |
| --- | --- |
| Gastrointestinal loss | • Malabsorption or small bowel bypass<br>• Acute or chronic diarrhea |
| Renal loss | • Diuretics (thiazide or loop)<br>• Alcohol<br>• Nephrotoxic drugs: aminoglycosides, amphotericin B, pentamidine, cyclosporine, cisplatin<br>• 1° aldosteronism<br>• Post-ATN or post-obstruction |
| Miscellaneous | • Poor intake/malnutrition<br>• Pancreatitis (sequestration)<br>• Diabetes (? mechanism)<br>• Post-operative or post-transfusion (citrate) |

## Clinical manifestations
- Secondary electrolyte disturbances: hypokalemia, hypocalcemia (↓PTH secretion/action, ↓ 1-hydroxylation of 25-OH vitamin D)
- Neuromuscular: weakness, anorexia, tetany, convulsions
- Cardiac: widened QRS, peaked or inverted T-waves, prolonged QT and PR intervals, S-T segment depression; polymorphic ventricular tachycardia (*torsades de pointes*); accentuation of digitalis toxicity

## Diagnosis
- Poor correlation between serum and tissue levels; if patient has evidence of hypomagnesemia (e.g. hypokalemia, *torsades*, etc.) consider empiric treatment for "normomagnesemic magnesium depletion"

- Fractional magnesium excretion:
  - In presence of Mg depletion, $FE_{Mg} < 1\%$ suggests extrarenal losses or "normomagnesemic" depletion
  - $FE_{Mg} > 4\%$ suggests renal losses
  - After supplementation, $FE_{Mg}$ increases substantially such that much of administered doses are renally wasted

$$FE_{Mg} (\%) = \frac{U_{Mg} \times P_{Cr}}{0.7 \times P_{Mg} \times U_{Cr}} \times 100$$

**Treatment**
- Symptomatic: Give $MgSO_4$, 1-2 grams IV slowly; may need daily replacement
- Asymptomatic or mild: Oral $Mg^{++}$ as gluconate, oxide, lactate or chloride. Typical dose 6-8 tabs PO daily in divided doses, or 2-4 tabs daily as maintenance in presence of ongoing losses (e.g. diuretics)

# $FENa^{228}$

- FENa = fractional excretion of sodium. A measure of sodium avidity of the renal tubule (represents % of filtered sodium that is excreted in the urine)

$$FE_{Na}(\%) = \frac{U_{Na}}{P_{Na}} \times \frac{P_{Cr}}{U_{Cr}} \times 100$$

- Normal value varies with $Na^+$ intake, GFR and volume status but is typically $\leq 1$ %
- Useful clinically in acute renal failure to differentiate between pre-renal azotemia (FENa < 1%) and acute tubular necrosis (FENa > 2%). FENa of 1-2% is indeterminate.

| FENa | Effective Intravascular Volume Status | |
|---|---|---|
| | **Hypovolemic** | **Normal or Volume Overloaded** |
| < 1% | • Pre-renal azotemia<br>• Cirrhosis or hepatorenal syndrome<br>• Congestive heart failure | • Non-oliguric ATN (10% of cases)<br>• ATN with underlying CHF or cirrhosis<br>• Drugs: ACE-I, NSAIDs<br>• Acute glomerulonephritis or vasculitis<br>• Acute interstitial nephritis *<br>• Acute renal allograft rejection<br>• Intratubular obstruction: myoglobin (rhabdomyolysis), contrast media<br>• Acute extrarenal obstruction * (FENa depends on duration/severity) |
| > 2 % | • Diuretics<br>• Chronic renal failure | • Oliguric ATN<br>• Non-oliguric ATN (90% of cases)<br>• Obstruction |

\* Seen in only some cases      ATN: acute tubular necrosis

**Pearls and nonsense**
- FENa more useful in oliguric than in non-oliguric renal failure
- Variability of FENa in non-oliguric patients without renal failure makes it a poor measure of volume status (unless **very** low, e.g. < 0.1-0.2 %)

228 Zarich S et al. Fractional excretion of sodium. Exceptions to its diagnostic value. *Arch Int Med* 1985; 145: 108-112.

# Diuretic Resistance [229]

## How diuretics work

- **Loop diuretics**: Inhibit Na-K-2Cl cotransporter at luminal surface of thick ascending limb. Effect mediated in part by $PGE_2$. No effect on distal tubule. Potent because distal Na delivery exceeds distal reabsorptive capacity.
- **Thiazides**: Act on distal convoluted tubule from luminal surface; inhibit NaCl cotransporter at luminal membrane. Synergistic when combined with loop diuretics.
- **Distal (potassium-sparing)**: Amiloride and triamterene block $Na^+$-channel uptake in collecting duct and decrease luminal negative voltage. Spironolactone and eplerenone antagonize aldosterone effect in collecting duct.
- **Carbonic anhydrase inhibitors**: Work proximally to decrease $H^+$ available for $Na^+$ exchange. Weak due to compensatory increase in distal $Na^+$ absorption.

## Pharmacodynamics

- Diuretics have typical sigmoid dose-response curve: No response unless threshold achieved (minimal effective dose), and no additional natriuresis once steep portion of curve exceeded (maximal inhibition of $Na^+$ reabsorption)
- Once effective dose established, higher rates of diuresis require increased **frequency** of dosing rather than escalating doses
- In normal individuals, the equivalent of 40 mg IV furosemide results in natriuresis of 200-250 mmol of $Na^+$ in 3-4 liters urine over 3-4 hours

## Renal adaptation to diuretics

- Increased distal sodium delivery causes compensatory distal reabsorption, which blunts effect of proximal tubule and loop diuretics
- Decreased effective circulating volume triggers intrarenal neurohumoral mechanisms, which cause compensatory "post-diuretic" NaCl retention

## Treatment of patients with diuretic "resistance"

| Cause of ineffective diuresis | Treatment Strategy |
|---|---|
| • Non-compliance | → Compliance |
| • High sodium intake (counteracts appropriate diuretic effect) | → 24-hr urine to assess $Na^+$ excretion (ideally < 100 mEq/day)<br>→ Low sodium diet |
| • NSAIDs (block cotransporters) | → Discontinue |
| • Inadequate diuretic dose<br>• Acute or chronic renal failure<br>• Blocked excretion: uremic toxins, probenecid, cirrhosis | → Increase loop diuretic dose |
| • ↓ Bioavailability due to gut edema | → Change PO to IV or increase dose<br>→ Use torsemide or bumetanide rather than furosemide |
| • ↓ Renal perfusion (CHF, cirrhosis) | → Low dose dopamine or ultrafiltration |
| • Hypoalbuminemia<br>• Intratubular binding to excreted albumin (nephrotic syndrome) | → Premix diuretic in albumin if serum albumin < 2.5 mg/dl |
| • Tubular $Na^+$ reabsorption (CHF, cirrhosis or chronic diuretic adaptation) | → Multiple daily doses or continuous IV infusion (see page 181)<br>→ Combine loop with thiazide diuretic |

[229] Brater DC. Diuretic therapy. *NEJM* 1998; 339: 387-395.

# Rheumatology

## *Autoantibodies[230]*

| Antibody | Disease Associations and Sensitivity | Comment |
|---|---|---|
| Antinuclear antibody (ANA) | SLE ≥ 95%<br>PSS 60-80%<br>Sjögren's 40-70%<br>PM/DM 30-80%<br>Raynaud's 20-60% | Serial negative ANA makes SLE less likely. Human lines (Hep2) more sensitive but less specific than rodent tissue. Titer not correlated with disease activity in SLE. In Raynaud's, positive ANA suggests worse prognosis. **Non-specific**; positive results in other connective tissue diseases (e.g. Sjögren's), drug reactions, pulmonary disease, hepatitis, cancer, chronic infections; also in healthy individuals (but titer ≥ 1:320 in only 3%). |
| α-dsDNA | SLE 30-70%<br>Chronic active hepatitis | Highly specific for SLE but less sensitive than ANA. Predicts renal disease. Rising titer accompanies and may precede disease flares. |
| α-ssDNA | | Non-specific and of little clinical utility |
| α-Sm | SLE ≤ 30% | Highly specific for SLE but insensitive. Not useful for monitoring disease activity. |
| α-nRNP | SLE 30-40%<br>MCTD 95%<br>Other CTDs | Neither specific nor sensitive for SLE. Diagnostic for mixed connective tissue disease (MCTD) if clinical features present. Presence in SLE with negative α-dsDNA correlates with "scleroderma-like" features and less nephritis. |
| α-Ro (SSA) | Sjögren's 60-90%<br>SLE 35-60% | Common in 1° or 2° Sjögren's; predicts extraglandular disease (e.g. vasculitis). In SLE correlates with photosensitivity, SCLE rash, thrombocytopenia, and neonatal heart block. May be positive in ANA-negative SLE. |
| α-La (SSB) | Sjögren's 40%<br>SLE 10% | Associated with α-Ro but less common. Suggests benign course of SLE if only positive antibody other than ANA. |
| α-histone | Drug-induced SLE<br>SLE 80% | Associated with drug-induced SLE but non-specific; absence does not rule out drug reaction if clinical features are typical |
| Rheumatoid factor (RF) | RA 80%<br>Sjögren's 50%<br>Other CTD | Non-specific (e.g. in fever & arthritis, more predictive of endocarditis than RA). Elevated titer in RA suggests aggressive course but not useful for following disease activity. |
| α-CCP | RA 80% | Slightly improved specificity compared with rheumatoid actor |

230 Moder KG. Use and interpretation of rheumatologic tests: a guide for clinicians. *Mayo Clin Proc* 1996; 71(4):391-6. Kavanaugh A et al. Guidelines for clinical use of the antinuclear antibody test and tests for specific autoantibodies to nuclear antigens. *Arch Pathol Lab Med* 2000;124:71-81. Hoffman GS, Specks U. Antineutrophil cytoplasmic antibodies. *Arthritis Rheum* 1998; 41:1521-8.

| Antibody | Disease Associations and Sensitivity | Comment |
|----------|-------------------------------------|---------|
| α-cardiolipin | Antiphospholipid antibody syndrome (APS) 80% | Associated with lupus anti-coagulant and false positive VDRL. Non-specific. Positive ANA suggests APS 2° to SLE. |
| α-centromere | CREST >60% Raynaud's 25% | Relatively sensitive and specific for CREST syndrome; in Raynaud's may predict progression to CREST. |
| α-Scl-70 | PSS 30-40% | Specific but insensitive for scleroderma (PSS). Predicts worse prognosis including pulmonary fibrosis. |
| α-Jo-1 | PM/DM 30-40% | Seen in idiopathic inflammatory myopathies. Predicts aggressive disease course including pulmonary involvement. |
| c-ANCA | WG 80-95% CSS | More specific than p-ANCA; 99% specific for vasculitis in patients with connective tissue disease, but utility in general population less clear (e.g. positive predictive value for WG < 20% if sinusitis alone) |
| p-ANCA | WG 10% | Nonspecific: WG, other vasculitides, glomerulo-nephritis, miscellaneous connective tissue disease, GI conditions, drug reactions, cystic fibrosis, chronic infections, etc. |

**Abbreviations**: α= anti; Ab= antibody; ANA= antinuclear antibody; ANCA= anti-neutrophil cytoplasmic antibody (c=anti-proteinase 3; p=anti-myeloperoxidase); APS= anti-phospholipid antibody syndrome; CREST= calcinosis, Raynaud's, esophageal dysmotility, sclerodactyly, telangiectasia; CCP = cyclic citrullinated peptide; CSS= Churg-Strauss syndrome; CTD= connective tissue disease; DM= dermatomyositis; dsDNA= double-stranded DNA; GN= glomerulonephritis; MCTD= mixed CTD; nRNP= ribonucleoprotein; PM= polymyositis; PSS= progressive systemic sclerosis; RF= rheumatoid factor; SCLE= subacute cutaneous lupus erythematosus; SLE= systemic lupus erythematosus; ssDNA= single stranded DNA; WG= Wegener's granulomatosis

**Comments**
- Post-test probability of disease related to prevalence and specific clinical scenario, e.g. positive rheumatoid factor of little value in medical inpatient without typical features of connective tissue disease [231]
- May be non-specific (e.g. positive p-ANCA in multiple diseases other than vasculitis) or may occur at low level in normal population or first-degree relatives of affected individuals
- Results may be assay and/or lab specific
- Data derived from referral patients, may be less predictive in general population
- Extractable nuclear antigens (ENA: dsDNA, Sm, nRNP, Ro/La, Scl-70, Jo-1) are virtually never positive if ANA is negative and should be ordered only following positive ANA

231 Shmerling RH, Delbanco TL. The rheumatoid factor: An analysis of clinical utility. *Am J Med* 1991; 91:528-34.

# Primary Vasculitis [232]

| | Vasculitis | Vessels affected | Diagnostic Features | Comments |
|---|---|---|---|---|
| **L A R G E** | Takayasu's arteritis | Aorta & 1° branches | Granulomas; arteriography | Age < 40 yrs, 80% female. Non-specific symptoms (fever, weight loss) followed by vascular disease |
| | Giant cell (temporal) arteritis (GCA) | Large and medium arteries | ↑ESR; granulomas | Mean age 70 yrs, 60% female. Headache, jaw claudication, visual loss, PMR common. |
| **M E D I U M** | Polyarteritis nodosa (PAN) | Med-small arteries | Hep B in 10%; arteriography | Mononeuritis multiplex, hypertension, abdominal pain |
| | Kawasaki disease | Lg-m-sm arteries | | Adult cases rare. Aneurysms of coronary arteries. |
| | Isolated CNS vasculitis | Med-small arteries | Arteriography | Diffuse vasculitis limited to CNS. Symptoms include confusion, headache, cranial nerve palsies. |
| **S M A L L** | Henoch-Schönlein purpura (HSP) | Capillaries, venules or arterioles | IgA deposits in vessels | Mean age < 20 yrs. Often follows URI. Symptoms: purpura, arthralgias, abdominal pain. Renal involvement common but renal failure rare (5%). |
| | Essential cryoglobulinemic vasculitis | | Cryoglobulins in serum and vessels; HCV Ab; ↓C4, nml C3 | 95% of cases caused by HCV. Symptoms: purpura, arthralgias, nephritis, neuropathy. Morbidity related to glomerulonephritis and chronic liver disease. |
| | Microscopic polyangiitis (MP) | | p-ANCA | Pathologically similar to PAN but affects smaller vessels; shares features with WG but lacks granulomas. Most common cause of pulmonary-renal syndrome. |
| | Wegener's granulomatosis (WG) | Capillaries, venules, arterioles and arteries | c-ANCA; necrotizing granulomas | Predilection for respiratory tract including sinuses, trachea and lungs. 80% will develop glomerulonephritis although only 20% at presentation. |
| | Churg-Strauss syndrome (CSS) | | ANCA (p> c); eosinophilia; necrotizing granulomas | Asthma initially, followed by eosinophilic tissue infiltration and vasculitis (typically within 3 yrs). Cardiac disease major cause of morbidity. |

**Abbreviations:** ANCA= anti-neutrophil cytoplasmic antibody; HCV= hepatitis C virus; PAN= polyarteritis nodosa; PMR= polymyalgia rheumatica; WG= Wegener granulomatosis

[232] Jennette JC, Falk RJ. Small vessel vasculitis. *NEJM* 1997; 337:1512-23. Hunder GG *et al.* The American College of Rheumatology 1990 criteria for the classification of vasculitis. *Arthritis Rheum* 1990;33:1065-7.

## Differential diagnosis of vasculitis
- Primary vasculitis (*see table*)
- Secondary vasculitis from connective tissue diseases: lupus, rheumatoid arthritis, Sjögren's, etc.
- Fibromuscular dysplasia (can mimic large vessel vasculitis)
- Cholesterol emboli
- Endocarditis or myxoma
- Mycotic aneurysm
- Thrombotic microangiopathy (thrombotic thrombocytopenic purpura, hemolytic-uremic syndrome, antiphospholipid antibody syndrome, eclampsia)

## Percent (%) organ system involvement in selected vasculitides

| Organ | Manifestations | HSP | Cryo | MP | WG | CSS |
|---|---|---|---|---|---|---|
| Skin | Purpura, livedo | 90 | 90 | 40 | 40 | 60 |
| Renal | GN, hematuria, ARF | 50 | 55 | 90 | 80 | 45 |
| Pulmonary | Infiltrates, hemoptysis | < 5 | < 5 | 50 | 90 | 70 |
| Upper airway | Sinusitis, ulcers | < 5 | < 5 | 35 | 90 | 50 |
| Musculoskeletal | Arthralgias, arthritis | 75 | 70 | 60 | 60 | 50 |
| Neurologic | Mononeuritis multiplex | 10 | 40 | 30 | 50 | 70 |
| GI | Abd pain, GI bleeding | 60 | 30 | 50 | 50 | 50 |

**Abbreviations:** ARF= acute renal failure; cryo= cryoglobulinemic; CSS= Churg-Strauss syndrome; GN= glomerulonephritis; HSP= Henoch-Schönlein purpura; MP= microscopic polyangiitis; WG= Wegener granulomatosis

# *ARA Criteria for SLE Classification*[233]

### Four or more of the following criteria
1) **Malar rash**: Fixed erythema, flat or raised, over malar eminences, tending to spare the nasolabial folds
2) **Discoid rash**: Erythematous raised patches with adherent keratotic scaling and follicular plugging; atrophic scarring may occur in older lesions
3) **Photosensitivity**: Skin rash as an unusual reaction to sunlight, by patient history or physician observation
4) **Oral ulcers**: Oral or nasopharyngeal ulcers, usually painless, seen by MD
5) **Arthritis**: Nonerosive arthritis involving two or more peripheral joints, characterized by tenderness, swelling, or effusion
6) **Serositis**:
   - Pleuritis: Convincing history of pleuritic pain or rub heard by a physician or evidence of pleural effusion, *or*
   - Pericarditis: By ECG or rub or evidence of pericardial effusion
7) **Renal disorder**:
   - Persistent proteinuria > 0.5 grams per day or greater than 3+, *or*
   - Cellular casts of any type
8) **Neurologic disorder**:
   - Seizures *or* psychosis (in absence of drugs or metabolic derangement, e.g. uremia, ketoacidosis, or electrolyte imbalance )
9) **Hematologic disorder**:
   - Hemolytic anemia with reticulocytosis, *or*
   - Leukopenia < 4000/mm$^3$ total on two or more occasions *or*
   - Lymphopenia < 1500/mm$^3$ on two or more occasions *or*
   - Thrombocytopenia < 100,000/mm$^3$ in absence of offending drugs

[233] Tan EM *et al.* The 1982 revised criteria for the classification of systemic lupus erythematosus (SLE). *Arthritis Rheum* 1992; 25:1271-7; Hochberg MC. Updating the ACR revised criteria for the classification of systemic lupus erythematosus. *Arthritis Rheum* 1997; 40(9)1725.

### 10) Immunologic disorder
- Anti-ds-DNA antibody in abnormal titer *or*
- Anti-Sm antibody *or*
- Antiphospholipid antibodies based on IgG/IgM anticardiolipin antibodies *or* a positive test for lupus anticoagulant *or* a false-positive serologic test for syphilis (> 6 months duration and confirmed by secondary testing)

### 11) Antinuclear antibody: Without drugs typical of "drug-induced" lupus syndrome

## Pearls and nonsense
- Criteria are intended for **classification** purposes rather than diagnosis. Criteria are non-specific, i.e. "false-positive" diagnosis of SLE possible with competing diagnoses such as endocarditis, drug reaction, etc.)
- Additional signs and symptoms suggestive of SLE but not included in classification criteria include: Raynaud's phenomenon, hair loss, unexplained fever, unexplained lymphadenopathy or splenomegaly, and unexplained thromboembolic phenomena.

# *Synovial Fluid Analysis*

- **Useful tests** [234]: total WBC • percent PMNs • crystal exam • gram stain • culture
- **Not useful:** glucose • LDH • protein
- **Gram stain/culture:** high yield in bacterial infections **except** gonorrhea and Lyme
- **Crystals:**
  - Uric acid (gout): thin, needle-like, negatively birefringent (yellow when ||, blue when ⊥ to polarized axis)
  - Calcium pyrophosphate (pseudogout): short rhomboid crystals, weakly positive birefringence (yellow when ⊥, blue when || to polarized axis)
  - Betamethasone (post-injection), calcium oxalate and lithium heparin (artifact from blood tube) can mimic uric acid

| Patterns * | Normal | Non-Inflammatory | Inflammatory | Purulent | Hemorrhagic |
|---|---|---|---|---|---|
| Appearance | Clear | Clear yellow | Cloudy yellow | Opaque | Opaque, red |
| Viscosity | High | High | Low | Low | Variable |
| WBC/mm³ | <200 | <2000 | 2000-50,000 | >50,000 | Variable |
| PMNs | <25% | <25% | >50% | > 75% | Variable |

\* non-specific with considerable overlap

**Non-inflammatory pattern:** • trauma • osteoarthritis • chronic or subsiding crystal synovitis (gout, pseudogout) • SLE • early rheumatoid arthritis (RA) • polyarteritis nodosa • osteonecrosis • scleroderma • amyloidosis • polymyalgia rheumatica • endocrine arthropathy • hypertrophic pulmonary osteoarthropathy • avascular necrosis • osteochondritis dessicans

**Inflammatory pattern:** • crystal synovitis (gout, pseudogout) • rheumatoid arthritis • reactive arthritis (Reiter's syndrome) • psoriatic arthritis • seronegative spondyloarthropathy (e.g. inflammatory bowel disease, ankylosing spondylitis, Behçet's) • juvenile chronic arthritis • sarcoidosis • some infectious arthritides (Lyme, gonococcal, viral, coagulase negative staph) • acute rheumatic fever

**Purulent pattern:** • infection: bacterial, fungal, TB • rarely RA, pseudogout

**Hemorrhagic pattern:** • trauma or fracture • Charcot joint • sickle-cell disease • coagulopathy (hemophilia, warfarin, thrombocytopenia, vWD) • tumor (especially pigmented villonodular synovitis)

[234] Shmerling RH *et al.* Synovial fluid tests: what should be ordered? *JAMA* 1990; 264:1009-1014.

# Arthritis & Fever [235]

| Causes | | Distinguishing features | |
|---|---|---|---|
| *Diagnosis* | *Confirmation* | *Symptom/Sign* | *Possible Diagnosis* |
| **Infectious arthritis** | | T > 40°C | Still's disease;  SLE |
|   Septic arthritis | Culture | | Bacterial arthritis |
|   Bacterial endocarditis | Blood cx | Antecedent fever | Viral; Lyme |
|   Lyme disease | Serology | | Reactive; Still's |
|   Mycobacteria/fungi | Culture, Bx | | Bacterial endocarditis |
|   Viral arthritis (parvo) | Serology | | |
| **Postinfectious or reactive** | | Migratory arthritis | Rheumatic fever |
|   Enteric infection | Cx/serology | | Gonococcal |
|   Reiter's syndrome | Genital cx | | Viral arthritis;   SLE |
|   Rheumatic fever | Clinical | | Acute leukemia |
|   Inflammatory bowel | Clinical | | Whipple's disease |
| **Systemic rheumatic disease** | | Effusion >> Pain | TB |
|   Systemic vasculitis | Biopsy/angio | | Bacterial endocarditis |
|   SLE | Serology | | Inflamm bowel disease |
|   Rheumatoid arthritis | Clinical | | Giant-cell arteritis |
|   Still's disease | Clinical | | Lyme disease |
| **Crystal-arthritis** | | Pain >> effusion | Rheumatic fever |
|   Gout / pseudogout | Microscopy | | Fam Mediterran. fever |
| **Other diseases** | | | Acute leukemia |
|   Familial Med. Fever | Clinical | | AIDS |
|   Malignancy | Biopsy | (+) Rheumatoid factor | Rheumatoid arthritis |
|   Sarcoidosis | Biopsy | | Viral arthritis |
| **Mucocutaneous syndromes** | | | Tuberculous arthritis |
|   Dermatomyositis | | | Bacterial endocarditis |
|   Behçet's disease | | | Sarcoidosis; SLE |
|   Henoch-Schönlein purpura | | | Systemic vasculitis |
|   Kawasaki disease | | Morning stiffness | Rheumatoid arthritis |
|   Erythema nodosum | | | Polymyalgia rheum. |
|   Erythema multiforme | | | Still's disease |
|   Pyoderma gangrenosum | | | Some viral/reactive |
|   Pustular psoriasis | | Symmetric small-joint synovitis | Rheumatoid arthritis |
| | | | SLE |
| | | | Viral arthritis (parvo) |
| | | WBC > 15k/mm³ | Bacterial arthritis |
| | | | Bacterial endocarditis |
| | | | Still's disease |
| | | | Systemic vasculitis |
| | | | Acute leukemia |
| | | Leukopenia | SLE; Viral arthritis |
| **Prompt arthrocentesis essential!** | | Episodic | Crystal-induced |
| • Gram stain 50-75% sensitive | | | Inflammatory bowel |
| • Culture >90% sensitive for | | | Lyme; Whipple |
|   diagnosis of septic arthritis | | | Familial Med. fever |
| | | | Still's disease; SLE |

235 RS Pinals. Polyarthritis and fever. *NEJM* 1994; 330(11):769-774. Adapted with permission of *The New England Journal of Medicine*, Copyright 1994, Massachusetts Medical Society.

# Toxicology

## *General Management* [236]

### Initial management
- **Treat the patient, not the poison!**
- **A**irway, **B**reathing, **C**irculation; consider co-existing trauma
- Cardiac and hemodynamic monitoring
- Consider empiric treatment with:
  - **Naloxone** 0.4 mg followed by 1-2 mg IM/IV (if suspected opiate ingestion)
  - **Thiamine** 100 mg IM/IV (alcoholism, malnutrition)
  - **Dextrose** 50% (if suspected hypoglycemia)
  - **Flumazenil** for isolated benzodiazepine ingestion; controversial in mixed overdose due to risk of seizure, although safe in one prospective trial [237]
- National Poison Control Center: 1-800-222-1222

### Laboratory analysis
- Electrolytes, BUN/creatinine, anion gap, ABG, osmolality; consider lactate, serum and urine toxicology screen including salicylate, acetaminophen, ethanol
- Osmolar gap (measured osmolality minus predicted osmolarity) – *see table page 141*
- Lactic acid – *see differential diagnosis on page 143*
- Pulse oximetry may **not** reveal methemoglobinemia or CO poisoning; use (blood) co-oximetry instead

### Decontamination
- Intubate trachea to protect airway if consciousness is depressed

| Charcoal ineffective for: |
| --- |
| • Alcohols (ethylene glycol, ethanol, methanol) |
| • Iron, lithium, potassium |
| • Acids and alkali |
| • Hydrocarbons |
| • Organophosphates, carbamates and DDT |

- Almost all oral poisonings are best managed with early **charcoal** (PO or NG).
  - Give single dose activated charcoal 0.5-1 g/kg. Repeat q 4 hr for massive or life-threatening ingestions. Charcoal is especially effective for large molecular weight compounds.
  - Follow first dose of charcoal with cathartic (e.g. **sorbitol** 0.5-1 g/kg)
  - If charcoal ineffective, consider bowel irrigation with **polyethylene glycol** 1.5-2 L/hr until clear.
  - Avoid charcoal and bowel irrigation if GI dysmotility
- Large bore orogastric lavage generally **not** indicated; reserve for comatose patients or those with known recent (i.e. < 1-2 hr) life-threatening ingestion. Specific contraindications: **(1)** corrosive or hydrocarbon ingestion **(2)** sharp object **(3)** coagulopathy **(4)** known or suspected varices.
- Decontaminate skin if warranted (e.g. radiation, insecticides, nerve agents)

---

236 Mokhlesi B *et al.* Adult toxicology in critical care: Part I: General approach to the intoxicated patient. *Chest* 2003; 123:577-92.

237 Weinbroum A *et al.* Use of flumazenil in the treatment of drug overdose: A double-blind and open clinical study in 110 patients. *Crit Care Med* 1996; 24:199-206.

## Drugs cleared by enhanced elimination [238]

| Alkaline diuresis | Hemodialysis | Hemoperfusion |
|---|---|---|
| Salicylates | Methanol | Theophylline |
| Barbiturates | Ethylene glycol | Phenobarbital |
| Fluoride | Salicylates | Phenytoin |
| Isoniazid | Lithium | Carbamazepine |
| Methotrexate | Barbiturates | Paraquat |
| Quinolones | Theophylline | Methotrexate |
| Uranium | | Dapsone |

## Specific antidotes

| Toxin or drug | Specific Antidote |
|---|---|
| Acetaminophen | N-acetylcysteine |
| Benzodiazepines | Flumazenil* |
| β-blockers | Atropine, glucagon |
| Calcium Ch blockers | Atropine, calcium, glucagon |
| Carbon monoxide | Hyperbaric oxygen |
| Cholinesterase inhibitors | Atropine, pralidoxime |
| Cyanide | Amyl nitrite/sodium nitrite/sodium thiosulfate |
| Digitalis | Digoxin Fab |
| Ethylene glycol | Fomepizole, ethanol, pyridoxine, thiamine |
| Heparin | Protamine sulfate |
| Iron | Deferoxamine |
| Isoniazid | Pyridoxine |
| Methanol | Fomepizole, ethanol, folinic acid, folate |
| Methotrexate/anti-folates | Folinic acid |
| Methemoglobinemia | Methylene blue |
| Opioids | Naloxone |
| Oral hypoglycemic agents | Dextrose, glucagon |
| Organophosphates | Atropine, pralidoxime |
| Sympathomimetics # | Phentolamine, benzodiazepines |
| Warfarin/rodenticides | Vitamin K, plasma |

* For reversal of benzodiazepine intoxication in non-dependent patient
# Including MAO inhibitor interactions, cocaine, epinephrine, ergotism

# *Common Toxic Syndromes* [239]

## Anticholinergic syndromes
- **Common signs:** . delirium with mumbling speech . tachycardia . dry flushed skin . dilated pupils . myoclonus . slightly elevated temperature . urinary retention . decreased bowel sounds . seizures and dysrhythmias may occur in severe cases
- **Common causes:** antihistamines . antiparkinsonian agents . atropine . scopolamine . amantadine . antipsychotics . antidepressants . antispasmodics . mydriatic agents . skeletal muscle relaxants . many plants (most notably jimson weed and *Amanita muscaria*)

---

238 Pond SM. Diuresis, dialysis and hemoperfusion. *Emerg Med Clin North Am* 1984; 2:29.
239 Kulig K. Initial management of ingestions of toxic substances. *NEJM* 1992;326(25):1677-81. Adapted with permission of *The New England Journal of Medicine*, Copyright 1992, Massachusetts Medical Society.

## Sympathomimetic syndromes

- **Common signs:** . delusions and paranoia . tachycardia (or bradycardia if the drug is a pure α-adrenergic agonist) . hypertension . hyperpyrexia . diaphoresis . piloerection . mydriasis . hyperreflexia . seizures, hypotension, and dysrhythmias may occur in severe cases
- **Common causes:** . cocaine . amphetamine, methamphetamine and derivatives (e.g. "ecstasy") . over the counter decongestants (ephedrine, pseudoephedrine) . herbal compounds including ephedra and ma huang . caffeine and theophylline may produce similar signs results from catecholamine release

## Opiate, sedative, or ethanol intoxication

- **Common signs:** . coma . respiratory depression . miosis . hypotension or bradycardia . hypothermia . pulmonary edema . decreased bowel sounds . hyporeflexia . needle marks . seizures may occur after overdoses of some narcotics, notably propoxyphene
- **Common causes:** . narcotics . barbiturates . benzodiazepines . ethanol . clonidine

## Cholinergic syndromes

- **Common signs:** . **Muscarinic:** SLUDGE (salivation, lacrimation, urination, defecation, GI cramps, emesis) . miosis . bradycardia . AV block . bronchoconstriction . rhinorrhea and bronchial secretions **Nicotinic:** . fasciculations . cramps . weakness . tachycardia . mydriasis
- **Common causes:** . organophosphate and carbamate insecticides . nerve agents . cholinesterase inhibitors (physostigmine, neostigmine, pyridostigmine, edrophonium) . some mushrooms

# Tricyclic Antidepressant Toxicity[240]

## Physiologic toxicity

- Class 1a antiarrhythmic effects (prolong QRS and QT) . Anticholinergic activity
- Induce catecholamine release and block reuptake; block α-adrenergic receptors

## Clinical manifestations

- Most lethal cases involve ingestions > 10 mg/kg, but life-threatening symptoms occur with doses as little as 500 mg. Co-ingestions in 70% of cases.
- Toxicity usually evident within 6 hr and rarely extends beyond 24 hr
- Symptoms may progress rapidly and unpredictably
- Plasma TCA levels have limited value in predicting toxicity
- Cardiovascular effects responsible for most morbidity and mortality:
  - Profound hypotension (most common cause of mortality)
  - Conduction delays with QRS widening (though 2° and 3° heart block unusual)
  - Ventricular arrhythmias including VT and VF (torsades is uncommon)
- Neurologic: Delirium, coma, seizures
- Anticholinergic effects: Altered mental status, hyperthermia, ileus

> **ECG signs of toxicity**
> - Sinus tachycardia at 120-160 bpm (common but rarely predicts serious toxicity)
> - Prolonged QRS duration -- toxicity rare when QRS < .10 sec; QRS ≥ 0.16 sec predicts seizures > ventricular arrhythmia
> - R in $_aV_R$ ≥ 3 mm (0.3 mV) or R/S ≥ 0.7 in $_aV_R$
> - Terminal 40 msec of QRS has rightward axis (120-170 °)
> - May have "Brugada" morphology (see page 31)

---

240 Liebelt EL, Francis PD. Cyclic Antidepressants. In: *Goldfrank's Toxicologic Emergencies*, 7th ed. Goldfrank LR, editor. New York: McGraw-Hill Medical Pub. Division, 2002; Glauser J. Tricyclic antidepressant poisoning. *Cleve Clin J Med* 2000; 67:704-6, 709-13, 717-9.

## Management
- GI decontamination with activated charcoal
- **Sodium bicarbonate** increases serum protein binding and counteracts Na-channel blockade. Indicated in any hemodynamic instability, seizure, or ECG alteration (other than isolated sinus tachycardia or prolonged QT interval)
  - Goal serum pH 7.50-7.55
  - Bolus 1-2 mEq/kg bicarbonate followed by "normal bicarbonate" (add 3 x 50mEq ampules to 0.85 L D5W) at 150-200 mL/hr infusion until ECG abnormalities and hypotension reverse
  - Recheck pH often to maintain > 7.50
- Hyperventilation for seizing or arresting patients (maintain pH > 7.50)
- Treat seizures aggressively with benzodiazepines (acidosis exacerbates toxicity)
- Hypotension usually responds to volume; give bicarbonate or vasopressors (norepinephrine preferred) if non-responsive
- Extracorporeal circulation (ECMO, cardiac bypass) for refractory hypotension
- Hemodialysis and hemoperfusion generally unhelpful

## Arrhythmias and cardiac arrest [241]
- **Pulseless electrical activity (PEA)**: Hyperventilation, bicarbonate to pH > 7.5 and saline infusion; if unresponsive, add epinephrine. Consider other causes.
- **Ventricular tachycardia (VT) or ectopy**: Lidocaine (1-1.5 mg/kg) – if responder, give continuous infusion. If non-responder, consider magnesium sulfate 25-50 mg/kg or phenytoin (25-50 mg/min). *Do not use procainamide;* avoid β- and Ca⁺⁺ channel blockers.
- **Ventricular fibrillation (VF)**: Treat per usual protocol (escalating shocks→ epinephrine 1 mg → shock) except:
  **(1)** Early use of bicarbonate and/or hyperventilation to raise pH > 7.5
  **(2)** Empiric magnesium if non-responsive to initial lidocaine bolus

## Triage
- All known/suspected ingestions warrant observation with serial ECGs & telemetry
- Disposition [242] (after GI decontamination and 6 or more hrs observation):

| Findings during observation | Disposition |
|---|---|
| • Asymptomatic | Psychiatric evaluation or discharge home |
| • Persistent, isolated sinus tachycardia<br>• Isolated prolonged QTc | Consider 24 hr observation |
| • Altered mental status<br>• Respiratory depression<br>• Cardiac conduction defects (QRS > 100 ms)<br>• Cardiac arrhythmias (other than sinus tach)<br>• Seizures<br>• Hypotension unresponsive to fluids | Inpatient admission and treatment. Continue monitoring for 24 hr beyond discontinuation of treatment. |

241 Cummins RO (ed). *Textbook of Advanced Cardiac Life Support.* Dallas: AHA, 1997
242 Foulke G. Identifying toxicity risk early after antidepressant overdose. *Am J Emerg Med* 1995; 13:123-6

# Ethylene Glycol & Methanol Toxicity [243]

## Physiologic toxicity
Liver metabolism leading to production of glycolic acid (ethylene glycol) and formic acid (methanol), resulting in anion-gap acidosis and multi-system effects

## Clinical manifestations
- **Ethylene glycol:** Onset 4-12 hr after ingestion • Intoxication → coma
  • Nausea/vomiting • Seizures or brain herniation • Cardiogenic or non-cardiogenic pulmonary edema • Oliguric renal failure with flank pain (oxaluria) • Hypocalcemia
- **Methanol:** Onset of symptoms may be delayed up to 30 hr • Headache → lethargy → coma and seizures • Visual changes or loss (sluggish or fixed/dilated pupils, papilledema) • Gastritis or pancreatitis • Bradycardia • Respiratory failure
- Presentation with either toxin may be delayed by ethanol co-ingestion

## Diagnostic evaluation
- Suspect if unexplained anion gap acidosis (see pages 141, 142)
- Osmolar gap (> 10) often present but absence does not exclude serious ingestion
- Serial urine microscopy for calcium oxalate crystalluria (ethylene glycol only)
- Ethylene glycol and methanol levels may be measured directly, but if ingestion is suspected therapy is warranted prior to confirmation
- Toxicity correlates best with degree of acidosis rather than EG or methanol level
- CT/MRI may show putamen or caudate lesions in severe methanol neurotoxicity

## Management goals - General
- Gastric suctioning if recent ingestion (use charcoal only for mixed ingestion)
- IV fluids to maintain urine output
- Sodium bicarbonate to correct acidosis. High doses may be required to reach goal pH 7.35-7.45. Correction of acidosis also limits tissue penetration of toxic metabolites and increases urinary excretion of acid metabolites.
- Calcium for *symptomatic* hypocalcemia
- Magnesium, thiamine and multivitamin in chronic alcohol abusers
- Lorazepam or diazepam for seizures. Hyperventilation, mannitol and intracranial pressure monitoring warranted if cerebral edema develops.
- Co-factors: glycolate clearance increased by pyridoxine (50 mg IM qid) and thiamine (100 mg IM qid); for methanol add leucovorin or folate (50 mg IV q4-6 hr)

## Antidote therapy
- **Indications**
  • Methanol or ethylene glycol level > 20 mg/dl (regardless of symptoms or acidosis)
  • Recent ingestion, serum levels not available and osmolar gap > 10 mOsm/l
  • Suspected ingestion and pH < 7.3, HCO3 < 20 mEq/L or Osm gap > 10 (2 of 3)
  • Anion gap acidosis with ocular signs or urinary oxalate crystals
- **Treatment**
  • Begin fomepizole (page 186) or **ethanol** (page 185) as soon as possible
  • Continue until ethylene glycol/methanol levels are undetectable (or < 20 mg/dl), pH is normal and patient is asymptomatic
  • If ethanol used, monitor levels frequently to assure therapeutic levels of 100-150 mg/dl

**Dialysis** indicated for
- Refractory acidosis (pH < 7.2)
- Deteriorating clinical status despite treatment
- Renal failure
- Visual symptoms or signs (methanol)
- Methanol or ethylene glycol levels > 50 mg/dl (relative indication if fomepizole used, pH is normal and patient is asymptomatic)

---
243 Barceloux DG *et al.* American Academy of Clinical Toxicology practice guidelines on the treatment of methanol poisoning. J Toxicol Clin Toxicol 2002; 40:415-46; Barceloux DG *et al.* American Academy of Clinical Toxicology Practice Guidelines on the Treatment of Ethylene Glycol Poisoning. Ad Hoc Committee. J Toxicol Clin Toxicol 1999; 37:537-60.

# *Acetaminophen (APAP) Toxicity* [244]

## Clinical manifestations

- Stage I (1-24 hr): anorexia, N/V; may be asymptomatic
- Stage II (24-72 hr): mild RUQ pain, asymptomatic increase in LFTs
- Stage III (72-96 hr): sequelae of hepatic necrosis including jaundice, renal failure, coagulopathy, encephalopathy, coma
- Patients with significant liver injury subsequently develop multi-system organ failure including hemorrhage, sepsis, ARDS, and cerebral edema. Death usually occurs 3-5 days after ingestion.

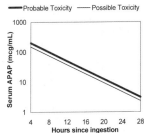

## Initial lab assessment

- Serum APAP level • AST
- PT/INR, lytes, glucose, renal function if patient is ill-appearing or AST is elevated

## Hepatic toxicity

- Toxicity increased by chronic ethanol, anticonvulsants, INH, malnourishment
- Rumack-Matthews nomogram [245] (inset) has high sensitivity but low specificity for toxicity. Initial level should be checked ≥ 4 hr after ingestion (although level < 50 mcg/ml between 1-4 hr suggests non-toxic dose).
  - **Probable** toxicity if log[level] ≥ 2.6 − (0.075 x hr since ingestion)
  - **Possible** toxicity (i.e. treatment indicated) if log[level] ≥ 2.48 − (0.075 x hr)
  - Use conservative time estimate since underestimation can result in lack of appropriate treatment [246]
- Toxic effects generally seen with ingestions ≥ 150 mg/kg; however, severe hepatitis or fulminant hepatic failure may occur after single doses of 7.5 g in normal adults or less than 4 g in alcoholics
- For extended release (Tylenol Arthritis formula®) ingestions, acetaminophen level should be re-checked in 4 hr if initial determination is below treatment line

## Treatment

- **Decontamination** with activated charcoal and/or bowel lavage
- **N-acetylcysteine** (p. 172) blocks production of toxic metabolites. Indicated for:
  - (1) APAP level on or above "possible toxicity" line on nomogram
  - (2) Suspected acute APAP ingestion and ↑ AST, regardless of serum [APAP]
  - (3) Serum level > 10 mcg/ml and time since acute ingestion completely unknown
  - (4) Chronic/repeated APAP ingestion at excessive doses *and*
    - AST > 2x normal, *or*
    - AST > normal and symptoms or APAP level > 10 mcg/ml, *or*
    - APAP level above expected for appropriate dose ( > 30 mcg/ml at 1 hr or > 10 mcg/ml at 4-6 hr after dose)
- Treatment should be initiated promptly for suspected ingestions ≥ 7.5 g (with completion of treatment pending serum APAP level). Acetylcysteine most effective if given within 8 hr of ingestion, but delayed administration (i.e. 24 hr post-ingestion) remains beneficial.

244 Bizovi K, Smilkstein M. Acetaminophen. In: Goldfrank LR, ed. *Goldfrank's Toxicologic Emergencies.* 7th edition. New York: McGraw-Hill Medical Pub. Division, 2002.

245 Rumack BH, Matthew H. Acetaminophen poisoning and toxicity. *Pediatrics* 1975:55(6):871-6.

246 Bridger S. Deaths from low-dose paracetamol poisoning. *BMJ* 1998; 316: 1724-5.

- **Standard dose:** 140 mg/kg PO load then 70 mg/kg q 4 hr x 17 doses
- Prolonged administration warranted in severe toxicity; continue drug until encephalopathy resolved and INR < 2
- **IV administration** warranted for **(1)** fulminant hepatic failure [247] **(2)** patient unable to take POs and high serum levels at or beyond 8 hr post-ingestion **(3)** pregnant patient (higher placental delivery prior to first pass metabolism)

### Prognosis
- Patients who survive through stage III (~ 5 days) generally recover completely
- Patients at high risk for death without liver transplant:
  - Persistent acidosis (pH < 7.30) after fluid and hemodynamic resuscitation
  - Combination of PT > 1.8 x control, creatinine > 3.3 mg/dl and grade III/IV encephalopathy
  - Abnormal INR that is rising on 4th day after overdose
  - Prothrombin time (sec) > hours since ingestion

# *Lithium Toxicity* [248]

### Epidemiology
- Most toxicity occurs in setting of chronic therapy or acute-on-chronic overdose
- Common triggers include: **(1)** worsening renal insufficiency, which can be caused by drug itself **(2)** pre-renal azotemia or volume depletion **(3)** drug interactions (diuretics, NSAIDs, ACE inhibitors, SSRIs) **(4)** advancing age **(5)** dosing errors

### Toxic manifestations

| Category | Lithium Level (mEq/L) | Neurological Effects |
|---|---|---|
| Therapeutic | 0.6 - 1.5 | Usually none |
| Mild | 1.5 - 2.5 | Weakness, lightheadedness, fine tremor |
| Moderate | 2.5 - 3.5 | Twitching, tinnitus, hyperreflexia, slurred speech, ataxia |
| Severe | > 3.5 | Confusion, clonus, coma , seizures 10% risk of permanent neurological deficits |

- Other findings: Dry mouth, nephrogenic diabetes insipidus, renal insufficiency, leukocytosis, hypothyroidism
- Acute ingestions can also produce GI symptoms (nausea, vomiting) and EKG abnormalities

### Treatment
- Aggressive volume repletion (with ½ NS to avoid hypernatremia in setting of diabetes insipidus) and electrolyte correction. Forced diuresis not helpful.
- Activated charcoal also not helpful. Limited evidence of benefit for whole bowel lavage with polyethylene glycol or multiple dose sodium polystyrene sulfonate (Kayexalate).
- **Dialysis** or **hemofiltration** (continuous arteriovenous or venovenous hemofiltration ± dialysis) highly effective. "Rebound" may require repeat treatment. Goal is [Li+] < 1 mEq/L at 6-8 hr post-dialysis. Indications:
  - [Li+] > 4 mEq/L, regardless of scenario
  - [Li+] > 2.5 mEq/L with moderate-severe neurological symptoms or renal insufficiency
  - Renal failure

---

[247] Keays R *et al.* Intravenous acetylcysteine in paracetamol induced fulminant hepatic failure: A prospective controlled trial. *BMJ* 1991; 303:1026-9.

Henry GC. Lithium. In: *Goldfrank's Toxicologic Emergencies,* 7th ed. Goldfrank LR, editor. New York: Graw-Hill Medical Pub. Division, 2002.

# Salicylate Toxicity [249]

## Epidemiology
- $2^{nd}$ most common cause of analgesic-related death, after acetaminophen
- Intentional overdose of ASA vs. accidental overdose of salicylate-containing compounds including ASA-narcotic combos, Pepto Bismol and oil of wintergreen

## Pharmacokinetics
- Rapidly absorbed from GI tract, though peak serum levels delayed 4-6 hr
- Normal $T_{1/2}$ of 2-4 hr increases to 20 hr at toxic levels
- Lethal dose 10-30 g (> 35 tablets ASA) or 150 mg/kg
- Therapeutic levels 15-30 mg/dl; toxicity usually at levels > 40 mg/dl, although severe poisoning may occur at lower levels, especially in elderly

## Pathophysiology
- Mixed respiratory alkalosis (central respiratory stimulation→hyperventilation) and metabolic acidosis (uncoupled oxidative phosphorylation→lactic acidosis)
- Hypoglycemia caused by hepatic damage, including low CSF glucose levels
- Acute lung injury (pulmonary edema) caused by unknown mechanism

## Presentation
- **Acute intoxication:** Nausea/vomiting, hyperventilation, tinnitus, lethargy or delirium
- **Severe toxicity:** Coma, seizures, hypoglycemia, fever, pulmonary edema. Signs may progress rapidly. Death occurs from cerebral edema and cardiovascular collapse due to acidosis.
- **Chronic intoxication:** More common in elderly (accidental or iatrogenic). Frequently unrecognized or misdiagnosed. Hearing loss, tinnitus, hyperventilation, non-specific confusion or agitation, dehydration, metabolic acidosis. Cerebral and pulmonary edema more common than in acute intoxication.

## Diagnosis
- Clinical diagnosis based on signs and symptoms, serum pH and salicylate levels (though serum levels correlate inexactly with toxicity). Patients with levels 30-40 mg/dl without symptoms or acidosis do not require treatment.
- Delayed absorption common; measure serial levels after acute ingestion
- Acidosis drives drug into tissues and thereby lowers serum levels; falling serum level reassuring **only** if pH stable or rising

## Treatment

- Multi-dose activated charcoal (acute ingestions only)
- Replace fluid deficits to promote renal clearance, but avoid overcorrection in light of risk of pulmonary edema. Forced diuresis not helpful.
- Bicarbonate (see page 177) to correct acidosis, enhance urinary elimination and prevent CSF penetration (serum pH goal 7.45-7.50, urinary pH ≥ 8)
- Correct hypokalemia to facilitate urinary alkalinization

| **Hemodialysis** indicated for: |
| --- |
| - Renal failure |
| - CHF or non-cardiogenic pulmonary edema |
| - Coma or seizures |
| - Progressive deterioration in vital signs |
| - Severe acidosis or electrolyte imbalance despite treatment |
| - Hepatic dysfunction with coagulopathy |
| - Salicylate level > 100mg/dl (or > 60 mg/dl in chronic ingestion) |

---

249 Flomenbaum NE. Salicylates. In: Goldfrank's Toxicologic Emergencies, 7th ed. Goldfrank LR, editor. New York: McGraw-Hill Medical Pub. Division, 2002. Mokhlesi B et al. Adult toxicology in critical care: Part II: Specific poisonings. Chest 2003; 123:897-922.

# Nerve Agents [250]

## Tabun (GA), Sarin (GB), Soman (GD), VX

- Highly toxic, irreversible acetylcholinesterases used as chemical warfare agents
- Chemically similar to organophosphate pesticides
- G agents are water-soluble, highly volatile, colorless, tasteless liquids that may have slight odor
- VX is an amber-colored, oily, odorless liquid that is less volatile (more persistent) and 10-fold more potent than G agents
- All are readily absorbed via inhalation, exposure to skin or eyes, or ingestion. Vapors are not toxic except via respiratory tract.

## Symptoms

- Usually start within 20-30 minutes of inhalation, but dermal exposure may cause insidious progression after delay of up to 18 hr
- Eye: Lacrimation, injection, miosis, pain, diminished vision
- Neurologic: CNS irritability, impaired judgment. Flaccid paralysis, coma, seizures, apnea at higher doses. Extensive muscarinic and nicotinic effects (see cholinergic syndrome, page 162)
- Respiratory: Major cause of mortality. Rhinorrhea, bronchial secretions, dyspnea, bronchoconstriction. Respiratory muscle paralysis, decreased central drive.
- Cardiac: Arrhythmias, bradycardia, hypertension
- GI: Abdominal pain, nausea/vomiting (early marker of severe toxicity)
- Other: Twitching, cramping, profuse sweating, drooling

> **Triage of exposed patients**
> - **Immediate treatment** for symptomatic patients. Conscious patients with full muscular control will need minimal care.
> - **Observation** for ≥ 18 h for those who may have had topical exposure to liquid. Carefully decontaminate hair and clothes.
> - **No treatment** if possible exposure to vapor only but no symptoms when presenting at medical facility -- patient unlikely to have been exposed and can be discharged safely

## Diagnosis

- RBC cholinesterase activity < 30% normal may aid in diagnosing unconfirmed cases. Do not withhold treatment awaiting results !

## Management

- Decontaminate patients by removing clothes and washing exposed skin with water or 0.5% hypochlorite (bleach). **Patients' skin and clothing can contaminate medical personnel by direct contact or vapor.** "Level A" biohazard gear preferred. Purifying respirators and latex gloves do not provide protection.
- Early airway management in patients with respiratory compromise or excessive secretions. Intubation and extensive suctioning may be needed. Avoid depolarizing paralytic agents (e.g. succinylcholine), which may cause prolonged neuromuscular blockade due to cholinesterase inhibition.
- Irrigate eyes with water or saline for 5 to 10 min

250 Holstege CP *et al*. Chemical warfare. Nerve agent poisoning. *Crit Care Clin* 1997; 13:923-42; Lee EC. Clinical manifestations of sarin nerve gas exposure. *JAMA* 2003; 290:659-62; Nerve agent fact sheet. Agency for Toxic Substances and Disease Registry. http://www.atsdr.cdc.gov

## Antidotes for Nerve Agents

| | Mild-mod symptoms<br>sweating fasciculations,<br>N/V, dyspnea | Severe symptoms<br>coma, seizures, apnea,<br>flaccid paralysis |
|---|---|---|
| Normal adult | Atropine 2 mg IV/IM<br>2-PAM* 15 mg/kg IV slowly | Atropine 6 mg IV/IM<br>2-PAM* 15 mg/kg IV slowly |
| Frail or elderly adult | Atropine 1 mg IV/IM<br>2-PAM* 5-10 mg/kg IV slowly | Atropine 2 mg IV/IM<br>2-PAM* 5-10 mg/kg IV slowly |

\* 2-PAM: pralidoxime HCl

- Repeat atropine 2 mg IV/IM q 2-5 min until symptoms resolved (**Note**: Atropine may not reverse miosis and nicotinic effects, including skeletal muscle weakness -- do not use as clinical endpoints). Typical total dose is 20 mg but some cases may require cumulative doses approaching 100 mg. Administer via endotracheal tube if needed.
- Diazepam or lorazepam for seizures
- Phentolamine 5 mg IV for pralidoxime-induced hypertension
- Topical atropine, tropicamide or homatropine for eye-related symptoms
- IM atropine (2mg) for severe rhinorrhea
- Activated charcoal for possible ingestion. **Do not induce emesis.**

Groovy Drugs

## Abciximab (ReoPro)
See Glycoprotein IIb/IIIa inhibitors, page 187

## Acetylcysteine[251] (Mucomyst)
<u>Action</u>: Prevents and treats acetaminophen overdose by repleting hepatic reducing capacity. Optimally given within 8 hr of ingestion, but beneficial up to 24 hr; also in patients with fulminant hepatic failure.[252]
<u>PO</u>: Load 140 mg/kg, then 70 mg/kg q4h x 17 doses. Dilute to 5% in cola or juice; serve chilled. Repeat dose if patient vomits within 1 hr of administration; use anti-emetic or nasogastric tube if recurrent vomiting.
<u>IV</u>: Not FDA-approved. Dilute 20% solution 1:3 in D5W. Give slowly over 1 hr (2 hr if intolerance). Load 140 mg/kg followed by 70 mg/kg q 4 hr x 12-17 doses.[253] Shorter 20 hr protocol (load 150 mg/kg, followed by 50 mg/kg over 4 hr, then 6.25 mg/kg/hr x 16 hr) used in U.K.[254]
<u>Side-effects</u>: N/V, diarrhea (PO); anaphylaxis, rash, bronchospasm, hypotension (IV).
<u>Interactions</u>: Charcoal prevents oral absorption; stagger other medications by 1-2 hr.
<u>Other uses</u>: Prophylactic use (600 mg PO bid x 2 days) in conjunction with saline loading may prevent contrast-induced worsening of azotemia.[255]

## Adenosine[256] (Adenocard)
<u>Action</u>: Slows AV node conduction. Locally acting coronary vasodilator. T½ <10 sec; metabolized by red blood cells. Use to interrupt reentrant tachycardias involving AV node. Efficacy comparable to verapamil with shorter T½. Also used as coronary vasodilator (e.g. perfusion imaging, rotational atherectomy).
<u>IV</u>: 6 mg IV **rapid push and flush** within 3 seconds, repeat 12 mg after one minute and may repeat 12mg again if needed. Give via central venous line if possible. **Myocardial perfusion imaging:** 140 mcg/kg/min × 6 min.
<u>Warnings</u>: Avoid in WPW or as diagnostic tool for irregular wide-complex rhythms (may cause anterograde bypass tract conduction in WPW with atrial fibrillation; ventricular fibrillation in 1%). Causes transient 1°-3° heart block or asystole. May cause bronchospasm. Prolonged effect in denervated (transplanted) hearts.
<u>Interactions</u>: Competitively antagonized by theophylline and caffeine (larger adenosine doses required); potentiated by dipyridamole (lower doses of adenosine required). Carbamazepine has additive effects when combined with adenosine and has been reported to cause high-grade AV block.
<u>Pregnancy</u>: Class C; no fetal effects anticipated.
<u>Side effects</u>: Transient flushing, lightheadedness, dyspnea, nausea, angina.

## Alteplase (tPA; Activase)
See Thrombolytic Agents, page 209

251 Smilkstein MJ. Efficacy of oral n-acetylcysteine in the treatment of acetaminophen overdose. *NEJM* 1988; 319:1557.
252 Harrison PM et al. Improvement by acetylcysteine of hemodynamics and oxygen transport in fulminant hepatic failure. *NEJM* 1991; 324:1852.
253 Smilkstein MJ et al. Acetaminophen overdose: a 48-hour intravenous N-acetylcysteine treatment protocol. Ann Emerg Med 1991; 20:23-28. Bizovi K, Smilkstein M. Acetaminophen. In: Goldfrank LR, ed. *Goldfrank's Toxicologic Emergencies*. New York: McGraw-Hill Medical Pub. Division, 2002.
254 Prescot LF et al. Intravenous N-acetylcysteine: the treatment of choice for paracetamol poisoning. *BMJ* 1997:1097-113.
255 Tepel M et al. Prevention of radiographic-contrast-agent-induced reductions in renal function by acetylcysteine. *NEJM* 2000; 343:180-4. Kay J et al. Acetylcysteine for prevention of acute deterioration of renal function following elective coronary angiography and intervention: A randomized controlled trial. *JAMA* 2003; 289:553-8.
256 DiMarco JP. Adenosine for paroxysmal supraventricular tachycardia: dose ranging and comparison with verapamil. *Ann Intern Med* 1990; 113(2):104-10.

# Aminoglycosides[257]

Divided dosing based on lean body weight:

| Drug | Load # | Total daily | Divided | Peak / Trough* (mcg/mL) |
|------|--------|-------------|---------|-------------------------|
| Gentamicin Tobramycin Netilmicin | 1.5-2 mg/kg | 3-5 mg/kg | q 8 h | 4-10 / < 1-2 |
| Amikacin Streptomycin | 7.5-15 mg/kg | 15 mg/kg | q 12 h | 15-35 / < 5-10 |

# Loading dose for critically ill only * High end of ranges in life-threatening infections only

Levels: Draw peak specimens 30 min after infusion and trough immediately prior to next dose. Adjust *dose* based on peak levels, *intervals* based on trough levels.

Anuric renal failure: Hemodialysis supplement: ½ normal dose after each hemodialysis. CAPD/CAVH supplement: 3-4 mg/L/d gent/netil/tobra; 15-20 mg/L/d amikacin; 20-40 mg/L/d streptomycin.

Renal insufficiency: Adjust dose to estimated creatinine clearance (*see page 8*). Give half of loading dose each half-life interval, or follow table: [258]

| Drug | CrCl 50-90 mL/min | CrCl 10-50 mL/min | CrCl <10 mL/min |
|------|-------------------|-------------------|-----------------|
| Gentamicin Tobramycin | 60-90% of normal dose Q8-12 | 30-70% of normal dose Q12 | 20-30% of normal dose q 24-48 |
| Netilmicin | 50-90% Q8-12 | 20-60% Q12 | 10-20% Q 24-48 |
| Amikacin | 60-90% Q12 | 30-70% Q12-18 | 20-30% q 24-48 |
| Streptomycin | 50% Q24 | Q24-72 | Q72-96 |

Once-daily dosing: Appears equally effective for most indications with reduced risk of nephrotoxicity. **Exceptions:** severe renal insufficiency (CrCl < 30 mL/min) or dialysis; use of other nephrotoxic agents; serious burns; ascites; endocarditis; mycobacterial disease; pregnant patients; children; patients with neutropenia (unless combined with β-lactam antibiotic); serious *Pseudomonas* infections. Monitor levels, e.g. twice weekly or if change in fluid status or renal function. Adjust dose as noted below in mild-moderate renal insufficiency.

**Adjustments in QD dose according to renal function w/ constant 24 h interval** [259]

| Estimated CrCl (mL/min) | Gentamicin or tobramycin (mg/kg) | Amikacin (mg/kg) | Dose interval (h) |
|-------------------------|----------------------------------|------------------|-------------------|
| >80 | 5.1 | 15.0 | 24 |
| 60-80 | 4.0 | 12.0 | 24 |
| 40-60 | 3.5 | 7.5 | 24 |
| 30-40 | 2.5 | 4.0 | 24 |
| <30 | Use conventional dosing | | |

Adverse Reactions: Nephrotoxicity, especially in volume-depletion, liver disease, prolonged therapy, elderly, or concurrent nephrotoxic drugs. Irreversible high-frequency ototoxicity (not assessable without special audiologic testing). Neuromuscular blockade especially with intraperitoneal or rapid IV infusion, or in myasthenia gravis; reverse with IV calcium. Endotoxin reactions reported with once-daily dosing.

# Aminophylline

Action: Phosphodiesterase inhibitor and nonspecific adenosine antagonist. Used as bronchodilator in acute and chronic bronchospasm; may also augment respiratory

---

257 Edson RS, Terrel C. The aminoglycosides. *Mayo Clin Proceedings* 1999; 74: 519-28.

258 Sarubbi FA, Hull JH. Amikacin serum concentrations: prediction of levels and dosage guidelines. *Ann Intern Med* 1978;89:612-8.

259 Gilbert DN *et al*. A randomized comparison of the safety and efficacy of once-daily gentamicin or thrice-daily gentamicin in combination with ticarcillin-clavulanate. *Am J Med* 1998; 105: 182-191.

muscle action. Therapeutic window is narrow and efficacy controversial.[260] Other uses include reversal of intravenous dipyridamole.

Kinetics: $T_{1/2}$ 3-15 hr in healthy nonsmokers; typically shorter in smokers. Hepatic metabolism.

IV: **Loading dose:** 6mg/kg IV over 20-30 min if not already using aminophylline. If already on methylxanthines, each 0.5mg/kg of aminophylline increases theophylline levels by 1 mcg/mL; if respiratory distress and levels unavailable, empirically load 2.5mg/kg. Maximum rate 25 mg/min IV.

| Maintenance Dose | 1st 12 hr | Followed by: |
|---|---|---|
| Smokers | 1mg/kg/h | 0.8mg/kg/h |
| Nonsmokers | 0.7mg/kg/h | 0.5mg/kg/h |
| Geriatric or cor pulmonale | 0.6mg/kg/h | 0.3mg/kg/h |
| CHF or liver disease | 0.5mg/kg/h | 0.1-0.2mg/kg/h |

Levels: Therapeutic: 5-15 mcg/dL; Toxic: > 20 mcg/dL (risk of seizure, arrhythmia). Measure levels 15-30 min after IV load; 4-8 h after maintenance infusion.

Renal failure: No adjustment. Supplement ½ dose after hemodialysis.

Interactions: $T_{1/2}$ shortened by phenytoin, barbiturates, tobacco, marijuana. $T_{1/2}$ lengthened by CHF or cirrhosis (20-30 hr), macrolide and quinolone antibiotics, cimetidine, propranolol, allopurinol, thyroid hormones

Pregnancy: Neonates sometimes have signs of theophylline toxicity. Nursing infants may receive up to 10% maternal dose.

# Amiodarone [261] *(Cordarone)*

Action: Complex antiarrhythmic with sodium, potassium, calcium, and beta-blocking activity. Unlike oral formulation, IV administration prolongs AV nodal refractoriness without short-term effect on SA node, intraventricular conduction, or QT interval.

Indications: **(1)** Antiarrhythmic of choice in VF/VT arrest **(2)** Treatment of hemodynamically stable VT, polymorphic VT or wide-complex tachycardia of unclear etiology **(3)** Control of ventricular rate in rapid atrial arrhythmias or accessory pathway conduction in pre-excitation syndromes **(4)** Pharmacological cardioversion of atrial fibrillation, or as an adjunct to electrical cardioversion in supraventricular tachycardias. Preferred to other antiarrhythmics particularly in patients with impaired LV function.

Kinetics: Rapid effect attributed to high peak serum concentration. Subsequent distribution results in fall of serum levels to 10% of peak concentration within 30-45 min of infusion. $T_{1/2}$ of parent compound is approximately 53 d, metabolite $T_{1/2}$ approximately 61 d.

IV: Best administered through central vein. **VF/VT arrest:** 300 mg rapid infusion in 20-30 mL NS or D5W (after epinephrine and defibrillation). **Stable arrhythmias:** Load 150 mg in (100mL D5W) over 10 min; then 900 mg mixed in 500mL D5W at 1 mg/min x 6 hr (360 mg) then 0.5 mg/min x 18 hr (540 mg). **Breakthrough events:** Bolus 150mg/100mL over 10 min. **Maintenance:** 0.5 mg/min. **Maximum daily dose:** 2.2 g.

Oral loading: 800-1600 mg PO qd (divide daily doses >1000 mg) x 1-3 weeks, reduce to 400-800 mg qd x1 month when arrhythmia controlled, then to 200-400 mg QD maintenance. Bioavailability approximately 50%.

Renal failure, liver failure: No dose-adjustment thought warranted.

Side effects (acute): Hypotension, CHF, *torsades* (rare), profound bradycardia, phlebitis, nausea, confusion, biochemical hepatitis, thrombocytopenia, fever.

Interactions: Precipitates with aminophylline, heparin, acetic acid or acetate, mezlocillin, cefazolin. Potentiates warfarin effect and increases digoxin levels (decrease usual doses by 50%).

---

260 Huang D et al. Does aminophylline benefit adults admitted to the hospital for an acute exacerbation of asthma? Ann Intern Med 1993;119(12):1155-60. Wrenn K et al. Aminophylline therapy for acute bronchospastic disease in the emergency room. Ann Intern Med 1991;115(4):241-7. Lam A, Newhouse MT. Management of asthma and chronic airflow limitation. Are methylxanthines obsolete? Chest 1990; 98(1):44-52.

261 Desai AD et al. The role of intravenous amiodarone in the management of cardiac arrhythmias. Ann Int Med 1997; 294-303.

## Amrinone *(Inocor)*
See inamrinone, page 192

# Anticholinesterases [262]
**Neostigmine, Physostigmine, Pyridostigmine.** *Also see edrophonium on page 183.*
Action: Reversible acetylcholinesterase inhibitors, increase acetylcholine concentration by blocking degradation. Restore muscle contraction. Decrease intraocular pressure. Action resembles organophosphates (which are irreversible anticholinesterases).
Indications: **(1)** Reversal of nondepolarizing neuromuscular blockade **(2)** myasthenia gravis **(3)** anticholinergic neurotoxicity (culprit drugs include atropine, belladonna alkaloids, tricyclics, phenothiazines, neuromuscular blockers, antihistamines) **(4)** colonic pseudo-obstruction **(5)** open-angle glaucoma **(6)** post-op urinary retention.
Warning: When reversing neuromuscular blockade co-administer atropine or glycopyrrolate to avoid muscarinic effects e.g. bradycardia/asystole, salivation, etc. Use cautiously in setting of asthma, diabetes, obstructed viscus.
Side effects: Cholinergic "crisis": bradycardia, seizures (esp. if given too rapidly); bronchospasm; excessive salivation, emesis, urination, defecation.
Interactions: Prolong effects of succinylcholine. Antagonized by Class 1a anti-arrhythmics, magnesium, corticosteroids. Cause severe hypotension when used with ganglionic blockers.

## Physostigmine
Indication: Anticholinergic drug toxicity. Tertiary amine crosses blood-brain barrier unlike neostigmine.
Kinetics: Onset 1-5 min. Duration 45-60 min.
IV: 2mg IV at rate ≤ 1mg/min. Repeat prn.

## Pyridostigmine
Indication: Reversal of nondepolarizing neuromuscular blockade; myasthenia gravis.
Kinetics: Onset 2-5 min IV, duration 2-4 hr. T½ 1.5-2h (ESRD 6h).
IV: 0.1-0.25 mg/kg (usual 10-20 mg) preceded by atropine 0.6-1.2 mg or glycopyrrolate 0.2 mg per each 5 mg pyridostigmine.
Renal failure: CrCl >50 mL/min: 50% usual dose; CrCl 10-50 mL/min: 35% usual dose; CrCl <10 mL/min: 20% usual dose.

## Neostigmine
Indication: Reversal of nondepolarizing neuromuscular blocker; myasthenia gravis; colonic pseudo-obstruction[263]; prevention of post-operative urinary retention.
Kinetics: Onset 4-8 min IV, duration 2-4 hr. T½ 1.3 hr (ESRD 3h)
IV: 0.5-2.0 mg (not to exceed 5 mg total dose) preceded by atropine 0.6-1.2 mg IV or with glycopyrrolate 0.2 mg per each 1 mg neostigmine. For colonic pseudo-obstruction: 2.0 mg IV.
Renal failure: CrCl 10-50 mL/min: 50% usual dose; CrCl <10 mL/min: 25% usual dose.

# Argatroban[264]
Indication: Prevention and treatment of thrombosis in heparin-induced thrombocytopenia (HIT), including those undergoing percutaneous coronary intervention (PCI).
Action: Direct thrombin inhibitor, synthetic derivative of L-arginine. Prolongs PT and aPTT, but does not alter vitamin K-dependent factor $X_a$ activity compared with warfarin alone.

---

262 Bevan DR *et al.* Reversal of neuromuscular blockade. *Anesthesiology* 1992;77(4):785-805.
263 Ponec RJ *et al.* Neostigmine for the treatment of acute colonic pseudo-obstruction. *NEJM* 1999; 341: 137-41.
264 Lewis BE *et al.* Argatroban anticoagulation in patients with heparin-induced thrombocytopenia. *Arch Intern Med* 2003;163:1849-1856.

Kinetics: Hepatic metabolism by CYP 3A4/5 enzyme; excreted into feces. $T_{1/2}$=30-51 min.

IV: Dilute to 1mg/mL in NS, D5W, or LR. **HIT treatment or prophylaxis:** Start 2 mcg/kg/min infusion. Check aPTT 2 hr after starting infusion. Adjust dose (up to 10 mcg/kg/min) until aPTT is 1.5-3 times baseline (but not >100 seconds). **PCI:** Bolus 350 mcg/kg IV over 3-5 minutes via large-bore IV and infuse 25 mcg/kg/min. Check activated clotting time (ACT) 5-10 min after bolus with goal 300-450 sec; use heparin-like ACT guidelines.

Overlap with warfarin: **Argatroban dose ≤ 2 mcg/kg/min:** Stop infusion when INR >4 on combined treatment and repeat INR in 4-6 hours. If INR is low, reinstitute infusion and repeat until desired INR is reached on warfarin alone. **Argatroban dose >2 mcg/kg/min:** Reduce dose to 2 mcg/kg/min and follow previous procedure.

Renal failure: No dosage adjustment necessary.

Hepatic dysfunction: 4-fold decrease in drug clearance. Reduce initial dose to 0.5 mcg/kg/min for moderate impairment

Interactions: Increased bleeding risk with antiplatelet drugs, thrombolytics, warfarin.

Adverse effects: Major bleeding, hypotension, fever, diarrhea.

Pregnancy: Class B

## Atracurium (*Tracrium*)

See Neuromuscular blockers, page 198

## Atropine

Action: Muscarinic acetylcholine receptor antagonist. Blocks vagal influence on SA and AV nodes reversing functional bradycardia and AV block. Inhaled bronchodilator in severe bronchospasm, significant systemic absorption (unlike ipratropium). Reduces oropharyngeal secretions for endotracheal intubation. Also used to counteract organophosphate and anticholinesterase drugs/toxicity.

Kinetics: Hepatic metabolism. Onset 1-2 min; $T_{1/2}$ 2 hr initially then 12h.

IV: **Asystole or "slow" pulseless electrical activity (PEA):** 1.0 mg IV, may be repeated in 3-5 min. May be administered via endotracheal tube at 2-3 times normal dose (diluted to 10 mL w/NS). **Bradycardia:** 0.5-1.0 mg q 3-5 min to max 0.04 mg/kg . **Anticholinesterase poisoning:** 2-3mg IV/IM q 20 min until muscarinic symptoms disappear, max 6 mg/hr.

Adverse effects: Paradoxical bradycardia for dose < 0.5 mg. Tachycardia may cause myocardial ischemia. Delirium, mydriasis, urinary retention. May exacerbate intestinal ileus or obstruction, myasthenia gravis.

## Beta-Adrenergic Blockers[265]

See individual entries for **esmolol** and **labetalol**

Action and indications: Antagonize circulating catecholamines. β-1-adrenergic activity: cardiac inotropy, chronotropy, dromotropy, lusitropy, vasoconstriction; β-2 effect: visceral smooth muscle relaxation including pulmonary bronchioles. Used to suppress angina, dysrhythmia, hypertension, anxiety, tremor, thyrotoxicosis, aortic dissection, pheochromocytoma crisis, reduce MI size, and postinfarction cardiac death. Role in compensated CHF. Significant interindividual variability in dose-response; titrate dose to target heart rate or blood pressure.

Adverse effects: Bronchospasm, bradycardia, AV block, hypotension, CHF, hypoglycemia in diabetes (especially in ESRD), depression, fatigue. May exacerbate peripheral vascular insufficiency.

Relative contraindications: Decompensated CHF, hypotension/shock, AV block or PR> 260ms, COPD or asthma, diabetes with severe or frequent hypoglycemia (masks symptoms), Raynaud's, peripheral vascular disease, allergic rhinitis.

---

265 Hoffman BB. β-adrenergic receptor antagonists. In: *Goodman and Gilman's Pharmacological Basis of Therapeutics*, 10th ed. Hardman JG (ed). New York: McGraw-Hill, 2002.

<u>Caution</u>: Additive AV block with diltiazem, verapamil, digoxin. Use cautiously in ischemic LV dysfunction, myasthenia gravis or if MAO inhibitors given within past 2 weeks. Treat β-blocker-induced CHF with beta-agonists, phosphodiesterase inhibitors, glucagon, atropine. Avoid agents with intrinsic sympathomimetic activity (ISA) in acute coronary syndromes and post-MI care. Sudden discontinuation can exacerbate angina or ischemia. Pre-treat with α-blocker in suspected sympathomimetic crises, e.g. pheochromocytoma or severe cocaine toxicity.

<u>Acute MI</u>: **Note:** All regimens should be modified as tolerated by hemodynamic status. **Metoprolol:** 5 mg IV q 5 min x 3 doses; after 15 min start 50 mg PO q12 hr x 24 hr, then increase to 100 mg PO bid. **Atenolol:** 5 mg IV over 5 min, repeat once after 10 min if tolerated; follow by 50 mg PO bid or 100 mg PO qd. **Propranolol:** 0.1 mg/kg by slow IV push divided into 3 equal doses at 2-3 min intervals (max 1 mg/min), may repeat after 2 hr if necessary; follow with 40 mg PO after 2 hr, then 40 mg PO q 4h x 7 doses; then start long-term therapy with 180-240 mg/d in divided doses.

**Comparative properties:**

| Name | T½ (h) (normal/ ESRD) | Typical Dose (mg) | Comments |
|---|---|---|---|
| Acebutolol | 7-9 / 7 | 200-600 bid | β1, ISA |
| Atenolol | 7 / 15-35 | 25-200 qd | β1, Low lipid solubility |
| Betaxolol | 14-22 / ? | 10-40 qd | β1, Low lipid solubility |
| Bisoprolol | 10-12/24 | 2.5-20 qd | β1, CHF, Low lipid solubility |
| Carvedilol | 6-10/ n/a | 3.125-25 bid | α1β1β2, CHF |
| Carteolol | 7 / 33 | 2.5-10 qd | β1β2, ISA, Low lipid solubility |
| Esmolol | 0.13 / 0.13 | IV only | β1 |
| Labetalol | 3-9 / 3-9 | 100-1200 bid | α1β1β2 |
| Metoprolol | 3.5/2.5-4.5 | 12.5-200 bid | β1, CHF |
| Nadolol | 19 / 45 | 20-240 qd | β1β2, Low lipid solubility |
| Penbutolol | 17-26/100 | 20-80 qd | β1β2, ISA |
| Pindolol | 3-4 / 3-4 | 5-30 bid | β1β2, ISA, Low lipid solubility |
| Propranolol | 2-6 / 1-6 | 10-160 qid | β1β |
| Timolol | 2.7 / 4 | 10-20 bid | β1β2 |

β1= β1 specificity β1β2= non-specific β-blocker α1β1β2= non-specific α and β-blocker CHF= studied in compensated CHF ISA= intrinsic sympathomimetic activity (partial β-1 agonism), may cause less bradycardia and negative inotropy, but **no** survival benefit in post-MI patients (unlike agents without ISA)

# Bicarbonate

<u>Action</u>: Systemic and urinary alkalinizing agent. Used in hyperkalemia (transiently shifts potassium intracellularly), severe metabolic acidosis (*see page 142*), intoxications (tricyclic antidepressants, ethylene glycol, methanol, phenobarbital, cocaine), diuresis of drugs (salicylates) and nephrotoxic agents (uric acid, myoglobin). Limited benefits. **Note:** Ventilation is the primary therapy of respiratory acidosis; restoring adequate perfusion the primary therapy of metabolic (lactic) acidosis from tissue hypoperfusion.

<u>Caution</u>: **Multiple adverse effects:** induces paradoxical intracellular acidosis by liberating $CO_2$ which crosses cell membrane more freely than $HCO_3$; shifts oxyhemoglobin saturation curve and reduces $O_2$ delivery; induces hypernatremia and hyperosmolarity; may precipitate exogenously-administered catecholamines.

<u>IV</u>: **Hyperkalemia or urgent intractable acidosis:** NaHCO₃ 1 mEq/kg bolus (1 amp = 50 mEq) then 0.5mEq/kg q 10 minutes as guided by arterial blood gas analysis. **Note:** Bicarbonate is distributed in total body water = 0.5-0.6 × body weight. Typical desired bicarbonate ≈ 8-10 mEq/L. Bicarbonate deficit (mEq) = (desired minus actual HCO₃ mEq/L) × 0.5 L/kg × body weight (kg). **Urinary alkalinization:** 2-5 mEq/kg IV over 4-8 hr (mix 3.5 amps [150 mEq] NaHCO₃ in 850 mL D5W = 150 mEq/L).

<u>Adverse effects</u>: (See "Caution") volume overload, hypercapnia, alkalemia, hyperosmolarity, hypocalcemia, hypokalemia.

## Bumetanide (*Bumex*)
*See Diuretics on page 181*

## Calcium
<u>Indications:</u> Hypocalcemia; reverse calcium channel blocker mediated hypotension; prophylax against hyperkalemic arrhythmias. No benefit in pulseless electrical activity.
<u>IV:</u> 20 mg elemental $Ca^{++}$= 1 mmol = 2 mEq. **Calcium chloride:** 1amp = 1g/10mL (10% solution) = 272mg or 13.6 mEq elemental $Ca^{++}$. Severe desiccant; should be given via central line. **Calcium gluconate:** 1 amp = 1g/10mL (10% solution) = 93 mg or 4.65 mEq elemental $Ca^{++}$. Gluconate form is less irritating (may be given via peripheral IV) but contains 1/3 elemental $Ca^{++}$ per unit volume compared to CaCl. **Hypocalcemia:** 10mL of 10% $CaCl_2$ (or 30 mL gluconate) in 500mL over 6 hr. **Acute hyperkalemia:** 5-10mL of 10% $CaCl_2$ (or 15-30 mL gluconate) IV over 1-5 min. **Tetany:** 10 mL of 10% CaCl (or 30mL gluconate) IV over 10 min.
<u>Caution:</u> Arrhythmogenic with digoxin. Causes bradycardia, paresthesias, hypercalcemia. Incompatible IV with phosphate, sulfate, carbonates. Correct hypokalemia before hypocalcemia. **Note:** Hypomagnesemia common in hypocalcemia.

## Chlorothiazide (*Diuril*)
<u>Action:</u> Parenteral thiazide diuretic. Used in combination with loop diuretic to prevent distal sodium reabsorption; effective in overcoming diuretic "resistance" in refractory edema or heart failure.
<u>Kinetics:</u> Onset 15 min, peak 30 min. $T_{1/2}$ 45-120 min, renal excretion.
<u>IV:</u> 500-1000 mg IV qd or bid. Ideally given 30 minutes prior to loop diuretic.
<u>Caution:</u> $K^+$ and $Mg^{++}$ wasting, monitor levels closely. May exacerbate hyponatremia or hypercalcemia.

## Cisatracurium (*Nimbex*)
*See Neuromuscular Blockers on page 198*

## Clonidine (*Catapres*)
<u>Action:</u> Central $\alpha$-2 adrenergic agonist reduces peripheral sympathetic activity, causes vasodilation and vagus-mediated bradycardia, decreased renin-angiotensin-aldosterone activity without reduction of renal blood flow. Used as antihypertensive; also in management of opiate and ethanol withdrawal.
<u>Kinetics:</u> $T_{1/2}$ 6-24 hr, 39-42 hr in ESRD. 50% liver metabolism, remainder excreted unchanged. Onset 30-60 min after PO dose, max effect 3-5 hr.
<u>PO:</u> **Urgent HTN:** 0.1-0.2 mg then 0.1 mg hourly (until max 0.8 mg or target BP). **Reduction of drug withdrawal symptoms:** 0.3-0.6 mg PO q 6h.
<u>Renal failure:</u> No adjustment.
<u>Caution:</u> Withdrawal syndrome (uncommon) 24-72 hr after stopping; usually sympathetic hyperactivity signs, rarely hypertension. Discontinue therapy by gradual dose reduction over 2-4 days. Use cautiously in angina or with β-blockers (withdraw β-blockers first).
<u>Side effects:</u> Dry mouth, sedation, postural hypotension, constipation, urinary retention.
<u>Interactions:</u> Decreased efficacy with tricyclics, prazosin, MAO inhibitors. β-blockers may reverse antihypertensive effects. Exacerbates sedation from other drugs.

# Corticosteroids [266]

| Drug | Approximate equivalent dose (mg) | Relative anti-inflammatory potency | Relative mineralocorticoid potency | Biological half-life [†] |
|---|---|---|---|---|
| Betamethasone | 0.6-0.75 | 25 | 0 | Long |
| Cortisone | 25 | 0.8 | 0.8 | Short |
| Dexamethasone | 0.75 | 25 | 0 | Long |
| Fludrocortisone * | n/a | 10 | 125 | Intermed |
| Hydrocortisone | 20 | 1 | 1 | Short |
| Methylprednisolone | 4 | 5 | 0.5 | Intermed |
| Prednisolone | 5 | 4 | 0.8 | Intermed |
| Prednisone | 5 | 4 | 0.8 | Intermed |
| Triamcinolone | 4 | 5 | 0 | Intermed |

* Not used for glucocorticoid effects
[†] Short = 8-12 hr, Intermediate = 12-36 hr, Long = 36-72 hr

## Dalteparin *(Fragmin)*
See Heparin, Low Molecular Weight on page 191

## Dantrolene [267]
Action: Selective skeletal muscle relaxation; interferes with calcium release from sarcoplasmic reticulum. Used to treat malignant hyperthermia, along with oxygen, cooling, and correction of acidosis. Possible role in neuroleptic malignant syndrome.
Kinetics: Onset rapid. Half-life 4-8 hr after IV.
Dose: 1 mg/kg rapid IV. Repeat rapidly as necessary until reversal of process (usually 2.5mg/kg) or maximum dose of 10 mg/kg. Follow with 1-2 mg/kg PO qid x 3 days.
Interactions: Causes marked cardiac depression when combined with verapamil. Potentiates non-depolarizing neuromuscular blockers.

## Desmopressin (ddAVP, *Stimate*) [268]
See also Vasopressin on page 212
Action: Synthetic vasopressin analog. Induces release of endothelial von Willebrand factor and hepatic factor VIII. Used to replace ADH; also to control hemorrhage in uremia, hemophilia A (when factor VIII activity > 5%) and von Willebrand disease.
Kinetics: Bleeding time minimized in 1-2 hr.
Dosage: Hemorrhage: 0.3 mcg/kg SC or IV (mixed in 50-100mL NS) over 15-60 min. Nasal spray: Use 150 mcg/0.1mL formulation only, one spray per nostril. Administer 30 min before surgery. Central diabetes insipidus: 2 mcg IV qd-bid, or 10-40 mcg nasal spray (1-4 sprays of 10 mcg/0.1 mL formulation) qd-bid; titrate to urine output, serum sodium and osmolality.
Caution: Restrict free water access 12-24h after each dose. Tachyphylaxis may occur after prolonged use. After 2-3 doses for hemorrhage, must wait 3-4 d to rebuild von Willebrand factor stores.
Side effects: IV: Water intoxication, platelet-aggregation and thrombosis, myocardial ischemia, hypotension with rapid infusion, abdominal distress. Nasal: Water intoxication, flushing, headache, congestion.

266  Schimmer BP, Parker KL. Adrenocortical Steroids. In: *Goodman and Gilman's Pharmacological Basis of Therapeutics*, 10th ed. Hardman JG (ed). New York: McGraw-Hill, 2002.
267  Wedel DJ *et al.* Clinical effects of intravenously administered dantrolene. *Mayo Clin Proc* 1995;70(3):241-6; Guze BH, Baxter LR Jr. Current concepts: Neuroleptic malignant syndrome. *NEJM* 1985;313(3):163-6.
268  Manucci PM *et al.* Deamino-8-d-arginine vasopressin shortens the bleeding time in uremia. *NEJM* 1983;308:8-12.

# Digoxin

**Action & Kinetics:** Reduces ventricular rate in atrial arrhythmias and prevents re-entrant arrhythmias by enhancing vagal tone and suppressing A-V conduction; weak inotropy by inhibiting Na-K-ATPase and increasing cytosolic $Ca^{++}$. Reduces CHF hospital admissions without overall mortality benefit [269]; but may increase mortality in women.[270]

**Kinetics:** $T\frac{1}{2}$ 36-44 hr, ESRD 80-120 hr. Cleared primarily by kidneys, 18-28% cleared via stool, liver. Loading dose saturates skeletal muscle receptors; without a loading dose, therapeutic effect delayed for 1-3 weeks, depending on renal function. Onset 20-30 min IV; 2 hr PO (once steady state is reached). Oral bioavailability 60-80%.

**Dosing:** "**Digitalization:**" Usually PO. Give total load of 8-12 mcg/kg, 50% initially then 25% q 6-8 hr thereafter. **Maintenance:** Typically 0.125-0.25mg qd.

**Renal failure:** Halve load. CrCl > 50 mL/min: 100% q 24h; CrCl 10-50 mL/min: 25-75% q 36h; CrCl < 10 mL/min: 10-25% dose q 48h. CAVH supplement 24-75% Q36 hr.

**Contraindications:** Hypertrophic cardiomyopathy; significant AV block; Wolff-Parkinson-White with possible antegrade conduction. *Relative contraindications:* cardioversion; risk of toxicity including cor pulmonale; diastolic LV dysfunction; amyloidosis.

**Levels:** Therapeutic 0.5-0.8 ng/mL for CHF [271], higher ($\geq 2$ ng/mL) for SVTs. Toxicity may occur at "therapeutic" levels, especially acutely. Levels generally unhelpful in atrial fibrillation (endpoints: heart rate and toxicity). Measure column-separated digoxin levels in ESRD.

**Toxicity:** Arrhythmias ($\uparrow$ automaticity, $\uparrow$ A-V block; many arrhythmias possible but most common serious include high-grade A-V block $\pm$ junctional escape and VT/VF); hyperkalemia; anorexia, nausea, vomiting, malaise, fatigue, confusion, insomnia, depression, vertigo, green/yellow halo around lights. Increased risk for toxicity with renal insufficiency, underlying cardiac disease, electrolyte abnormalities (esp. $\downarrow K^+$, $\downarrow Mg^{++}$, $\uparrow Ca^{++}$), hypothyroidism, advanced pulmonary disease, drug interactions, concomitant use with sympathomimetics.

**Interactions: Drugs that increase digoxin level:** Quinidine, verapamil, diltiazem, amiodarone, propafenone, flecainide ($\downarrow$ clearance), broad-spectrum antibiotics ($\downarrow$ enteric bacterial breakdown), $\downarrow$ renal blood flow (beta-blockers, CHF), anticholinergics, omeprazole ($\uparrow$ absorption) **Drugs that lower digoxin level:** $\downarrow$ absorption (GI edema, antacids, cholestyramine, metoclopramide, sulfasalazine, neomycin); $\uparrow$clearance (ACE inhibitors, nitroprusside, hydralazine, phenytoin, rifampin; St. John's wort).

# Digoxin Immune Fab [272] *(Digibind)*

**Indication: Life-threatening** digoxin toxicity, typically arrhythmia or hyperkalemia or digoxin level >10 ng/mL.

**Action:** Affinity of digoxin for Digibind is greater than for Na,K-ATPase. Fab has large volume of distribution.

**IV:** Loading dose (# vials) = (serum digoxin level in ng/mL) $\times$ (weight in kg) $\div$100. Dispensed in 0.5 mg/vial, 0.5 mg will bind 0.5 mg digoxin. Give IV over 30 minutes or bolus if necessary through a 22 micron filter.

**Caution:** $K^+$ levels may drop precipitously after administration. May precipitate acute CHF. Digoxin toxicity may also require potassium, lidocaine, phenytoin, procainamide, propranolol, atropine, pacemaker. Renal failure may cause spuriously elevated digoxin levels by certain assays.

**Contraindications:** History of sensitivity to sheep products, previous Fab.

---

269 Digitalis Investigation Group. The effect of digoxin on mortality and morbidity in patients with heart failure. NEJM 1997; 336:525-33.

270 Rathore SS et al. Sex-based differences in the effect of digoxin for the treatment of heart failure. NEJM 2002; 347:1403-11.

271 Rathore SS, et al. Association of serum digoxin concentration and outcomes in patients with heart failure. JAMA 2003;289:871-8.

     ey AR et al. Digoxin Immune Fab therapy in the management of digitalis intoxication: Safety and
     y results of an observational surveillance study. J Am Coll Cardiol 1991;17(3):590-8.

# Diltiazem IV [273] *(Cardizem)*

<u>Action:</u> Slow calcium-channel antagonist. Prolongs AV nodal refractoriness. Used IV to slow ventricular response to atrial fibrillation or flutter, to interrupt SVTs involving AV node, and to control rest angina. Lowers BP by relaxing vascular smooth muscle without significant reflex tachycardia. Negative inotrope.

<u>Kinetics</u>[274]: IV response time 5 min, peak 11 min. Plasma elimination half-life 3.4 hr. Extensive hepatic metabolism via cytochrome P450 degradation.

<u>IV:</u> **Tachycardias:** 0.25 mg/kg (avg 20 mg) given over 2 min. If unsatisfactory response after 15 min give additional 0.35 mg/kg. **Continuous infusion:** mix 250 mg (50 mL) diltiazem + 250 mL fluid = 0.833 mg/mL and infuse 5-15 mg/hr. Change to oral after 3h.

<u>Renal failure:</u> No adjustment.

<u>Contraindications:</u> Undiagnosed wide-complex tachycardia, WPW, 2° AV block or higher, sick-sinus syndrome, hypotension, concurrent β-blockers.

<u>Side-effects:</u> Hepatitis, edema, blurred vision, flushing, injection site reaction.

<u>Pregnancy:</u> Class C.

# Diuretics, Loop [275]

<u>Action:</u> Cause natriuresis and obligate diuresis via inhibition of renal Na-K-2Cl cotransporter at luminal surface of thick ascending limb of loop of Henle.

| Kinetics and dosing | Furosemide (Lasix) | Bumetanide (Bumex) | Torsemide (Demadex) |
|---|---|---|---|
| Oral bioavailability | 10-80 % (typically 50%) | 70-100 % | 80-100 % |
| T ½ (normal) | 1.5 – 2 hr | 1 hr | 3-4 hr |
| T ½ (ESRD, cirrhosis, CHF) | 2.5 - 2.8 hr | 1.3 – 2.3 hr | 4 – 8 hr |
| **Bolus dosing** | | | |
| Starting dose (IV) | 20 - 40 mg | 0.5 – 1 mg | 10 – 20 mg |
| Maximum dose * | 500 mg | 10 mg | 200 mg |
| **Continuous infusion** | | | |
| Loading dose | 40 mg | 1 mg | 20 mg |
| Infusion rate | | | |
| Normal renal function | 10 – 20 mg/h | 0.5 – 1 mg/h | 5 – 10 mg/h |
| Renal insufficiency | 20 – 40 mg/h | 1 –2 mg/h | 10 – 20 mg/h |

* "Typical" maximum effective dose in renal insufficiency, lower doses usually needed with normal renal function. Doses of up to 2000 mg furosemide per day have been administered without major adverse effects.

<u>Adverse effects:</u> Hearing loss (reversible or permanent), electrolyte wasting (Mg++, K+, Cl), rash, interstitial nephritis.

# Dobutamine [276]

<u>Uses:</u> Inotrope for circulatory failure from decreased myocardial contractility, e.g. MI, decompensated CHF, cardiac surgery. Also increases CO in right ventricular infarct unresponsive to volume.

<u>Action:</u> Racemic mixture: L-isomer is α-1 agonist, D-isomer is nonspecific β-agonist. Reduces SVR as it increases inotropy. No dopaminergic activity. Hemodynamic effect comparable to dopamine + nitroprusside. Less chronotropy than isoproterenol. Onset 1-2 min, peak effect 5-10min, half-life 2.4 minutes

<u>Renal failure:</u> No dose adjustment.

273 Goldenberg IF *et al.* Intravenous diltiazem for the treatment of patients with atrial fibrillation or flutter and moderate to severe congestive heart failure. *Am J Cardiol* 1994;74(9):884-9.

274 Dias VC *et al.* Pharmacokinetics and pharmacodynamics of intravenous diltiazem in patients with atrial fibrillation or atrial flutter. *Circulation* 1992; 86(5):1421-8.

275 Brater DC. Diuretic therapy. *NEJM* 1998; 339: 387-395.

276 Chatterjee K *et al.* Dobutamine in heart failure. *Eur Heart J* 1982; 3(Suppl D): 107-14; Leier CV, Unverferth DV. Drugs five years later. Dobutamine. *Ann Intern Med* 1983;99(4):490-6.

IV: Mix 250mg in 250mL NS or D5W = 1 mg/mL. Begin at 0.5 mcg/kg/min (2.1 mL/hr for 70 kg patient). Usual range 2– 20 mcg/kg/min, maximum 40 mcg/min.
Caution: Enhances AV conduction especially in atrial fibrillation. May precipitate or exacerbate ventricular arrhythmias.
Contraindications: Hypertrophic cardiomyopathy. Incompatible IV with alkali (theophylline, bicarbonate).

# Dopamine

Indications: **(1)** First-line vasopressor for hypotension refractory to fluids **(2)** Increases cardiac contractility (inotropy) in circulatory failure (often used in conjunction with nitroprusside) **(3)** First–line catecholamine for bradycardia refractory to atropine (preferred over isoproterenol) **(4)** May improve renal blood flow, especially at low doses along with a vasopressor (as in septic shock).
Action: At low doses (1-5 mcg/kg/min) produces renal, mesenteric, cerebral vasodilatation via dopaminergic receptors without cardiac effects. At intermediate range (5-10 mcg/kg/min) stimulates β-1 and α-adrenergic receptors, acting as inotrope and vasopressor. At high doses (>10 mcg/kg/min) acts predominantly as α-agonist vasopressor. Significant interindividual variability in dosage ranges and overlap of hemodynamic effects (i.e. must titrate dose to achieve desired effect). Onset of effect < 5 min, duration < 10 min.
IV: Mix 400 mg in 250 mL D5W or NS = 1.6 mg/mL. Begin at 1 mcg/kg/min (2.6 mL/hr for 70 kg patient). If "renal dose" desired, titrate to vital signs at each dose; ↑ HR and ↑ BP imply "renal dose" is exceeded. Vasopressor effect maximized at doses > 40 mcg/kg/min; consider switching to norepinephrine.
Caution: Start with 10% of dose in patients with circulating MAO inhibitors. Avoid cyclopropane or halogenated hydrocarbon anesthetics. Enhances AV conduction especially in atrial fibrillation. May exacerbate psychoses. Treat extravasation aggressively (see phentolamine, page 204). Spuriously elevates LV filling pressures (via constriction of pulmonary veins).
Incompatibility: Alkali (bicarbonate, theophylline) inactivate dopamine. Interaction is slow enough that drugs may co-infuse in a single catheter.
Pregnancy: Class C.

# Doxacurium (Nuromax)
See Neuromuscular blockers, page 198

# Drotrecogin Alfa (Activated Protein C, Xigris)[277]
Action: Recombinant human activated protein C with profibrinolytic, antithrombotic, and antiinflammatory properties (inhibits clotting factors $V_a$ and $VIII_a$, as well as PAI-1).

| Indications [278] | Contraindications |
|---|---|
| Reduction of mortality in patients with *severe sepsis* who meet **all** of following criteria: <br> **1)** Evidence of life-threatening infection, as manifested by abnormalities of temperature, HR, BP and WBC count <br> **2)** Acute organ failure, present for less than 24 hours, involving one or more major organ systems <br> **3)** High risk of death, i.e. APACHE II score ≥ 25 (see page 46) <br> **4)** Commitment to aggressive treatment | • Active internal bleeding <br> • Hemorrhagic stroke (within 3 months) <br> • Intracranial or intraspinal surgery, or severe head trauma (within 2 months) <br> • Trauma with an increased risk of life-threatening bleeding <br> • Existing epidural catheter <br> • Intracranial neoplasm or mass lesion or evidence of cerebral herniation |

277 Bernard GR *et al.* Efficacy and safety of recombinant human activated protein C for severe sepsis. *NEJM* 2001; 344:699-709.

278 Siegel JP. Assessing the use of activated protein C in the treatment of severe sepsis. *NEJM* 2002; 347:1030-1034.

Kinetics: Inactivated by endogenous plasma protease inhibitors. Biphasic elimination, $T_{\frac{1}{2}}$= 13 - 90 min.

IV: 24 mcg/kg/hr IV infusion x 96 hours, no dosage adjustment necessary in hepatic/renal dysfunction. Administration of drug needs to be completed within 12 hours of solution preparation. Administer via dedicated line.

Adverse effects: Bleeding, including major risk of intracranial and GI hemorrhage.

Drug Interactions: Carefully weigh risk of bleeding with potential benefit when using the following medications concomitantly or recently: heparin, thrombolytics (within 3 d), oral anticoagulants or glycoprotein IIb/IIIa inhibitors (within 7 d), aspirin > 650mg/d or other platelet inhibitors (within 7 d).

Suggestions: Stop 2 hr before surgery, epidural catheter, or percutaneous procedure. Restart 1 hr after percutaneous procedure & 12 hours after surgery or epidural catheter. Discontinue if full-dose heparin therapy required for thrombosis. Consider using as sole anticoagulant during hemodialysis. Consider prophylactic gastroprotective agent.

Caution: Use with caution if platelets < 30K, INR > 3, GI bleeding within 6 weeks, ischemic stroke within 3 months, intracranial arteriovenous malformation or aneurysm, severe hepatic disease, and any other condition where bleeding would be a significant danger or would be difficult to manage due to location. Costs ≥ $ 5000 for each 4 day course.

Pregnancy: Category C.

## Edrophonium *(Tensilon)*

Action: Rapid-acting anticholinesterase used to diagnose myasthenia gravis (MG) or to increase vagal tone. Onset of effect in 30-60 sec; duration 10 min.

Positive Test: Increase in muscle strength (ptosis, diplopia, respiration, dysphonia/phagia/arthria, limb strength) but when adverse reactions like fasciculations (orbicularis oculi, facial muscles, limb muscles) and side effects.

Adverse Reactions: *Eye:* lacrimation, diplopia, spasm of accommodation, pupillary constriction. *CNS:* seizure, dysarthria, dysphonia, dysphagia. *Resp:* secretions, bronchoconstriction, hypoventilation. *Cardiac:* bradycardia, vagal hypotension. *GI:* salivation, gastric and intestinal secretions and peristalsis, N/V/D. *Other:* skeletal weakness and fasciculations, urinary incontinence.

Dosage: 10mg (1mL) in tuberculin syringe. Use cardiac monitor and keep atropine available. Give 2 mg (0.2mL) IV. If no adverse reaction in 45 seconds may give remainder of dose; otherwise give atropine 0.5mg IV. To test for adequacy of MG drugs give 1-2 mg one hour after PO drugs.

Overdose: Atropine or pralidoxime; cardiac monitoring, anti-seizure measures.

## Enalaprilat *(Vasotec IV)*

Action: Parenteral angiotensin converting enzyme inhibitor. Active metabolite of orally-administered prodrug enalapril. Used as antihypertensive. Not generally used as afterload-reducer in absence of hypertension.

IV: 1.25 mg over 5 min, then 1.25-5.0 mg q 6 hr, response in 15 min; may repeat 0.625 mg in 1 hr if response inadequate. Decrease dose in patients on diuretics. Max 5 mg q 6 hr. Manufacturer suggests this protocol regardless of oral enalapril dose (1.25 mg IV ≈ 5 mg PO enalapril).

Renal failure: Dose 0.625 mg IV q 6 hr for CrCl< 30 mL/min.

Side-effects: Hypotension especially in intravascular volume depletion; lowers GFR and can cause renal failure (reversible) in renal insufficiency or renovascular disease; hyperkalemia; angioedema; agranulocytosis; cough. Trend towards excess mortality when used in acute MI.[279]

Pregnancy: Contraindicated; fetal morbidity and mortality in 3rd trimester.

---

279 CONSENSUS II. *NEJM* 1992; 327: 678-684.

## Enoxaparin (Lovenox)
*See Heparin, Low Molecular Weight on page 190*

## Epinephrine (Adrenalin)
Action: Nonspecific adrenergic agonist; has $\beta$-2 activity unlike norepinephrine (NE). Twice as potent inotrope and chronotrope compared to NE, but equipotent vasopressor. At low doses (< 4 mcg/kg/min) $\alpha$ effects less prominent; $\beta$-2 mediated vasodilation with compensatory increase in cardiac output. Potent bronchodilator.
Indications: Cardiac arrest, anaphylaxis, severe bronchospasm and laryngospasm, cardiogenic shock especially post cardiac surgery.
IV: **Cardiac arrest:** Bolus 1 mg (10mL of 1:10,000) q 3-5 min IV followed by 20 mL flush; or infusion (mix 30 mg in 250 mL fluid) beginning at 100 mL/h; or endotracheal 2.5 mg diluted to 10 mL with NS q 3-5 min. Limited data support bolus doses of 3-5 mg IV q 3-5 min. May be useful after vasopressor. 280 **High dose for asystole:** 0.1 mg/kg IV q 3-5 min. **Shock:** Mix 4 mg in 250mL D5W = 16 mcg/mL. Start 2 mcg/min, titrate to effect up to ~20 mcg/min. **Note:** $\alpha$-effects predominate > 4 mcg/min.
Subcutaneous: **Bronchospasm and anaphylaxis:** 0.1 mg SC, equivalent to 20 mcg/min IV. Local vasoconstriction reduces absorption.
Adverse effects: Increased myocardial oxygen demand, tachyarrhythmias, decreased splanchnic perfusion, hypertension, hyperglycemia, hypokalemia, CNS activation
Interactions: MAO inhibitors and tricyclics dramatically potentiate activity. Halothane anesthetics sensitize myocardium to arrhythmias.

## Epoprostenol 281 (Flolan, Prostacyclin, PGI₂)
Action: Short-acting vasodilator with diverse effects including inhibition of platelet aggregation. Prolongs survival in primary pulmonary hypertension; also used in secondary pulmonary hypertension
Kinetics: Rapid hydrolysis in blood, $T_{1/2}$ 6 minutes.
IV: Initial infusion may be administered peripherally, chronic infusion administered through central venous catheter via ambulatory infusion pump. Maximal tolerated dose determined by initiating infusion at 2 ng/kg/min, then increasing dose by increments of 2 ng/kg/min q $\geq$ 15 min until dose-limiting clinical effects or patient intolerance (hypotension, n/v, headache, abdominal pain). Subsequently reduce dose by 2-4 ng/kg/min to establish chronic infusion rate. (Mean initial dose in one trial was 5.3 ng/kg/min, mean dose after 12 weeks was 9.2 ng/kg). Chronic infusion rate should be adjusted based on symptoms or adverse effects. Increase chronic infusion by increments of 1-2 ng/kg/min q $\geq$ 15 min. Decreases should be made at decrements of 2 ng/kg/min q 15 min or longer.
Side-effects: Hypotension, nausea, vomiting, headache, flushing, lightheadedness, restlessness, anxiety, abdominal pain, dyspnea, tachycardia, bradycardia.
Caution: Exacerbates R → L shunting (hypoxemia) across patent foramen ovale.

## Eptifibatide (Integrilin)
*See Glycoprotein IIb/IIIa inhibitors on page 187*

## Esmolol (Brevibloc)
Action: Intravenous $\beta$-blocker. Slows AV node conduction in atrial fibrillation and flutter.282 Combine with nitroprusside for aortic dissection; combine with phentolamine

---

280  Wenzel V et al. A comparison of vasopressin and epinephrine for out-of-hospital cardiopulmonary resuscitation. *NEJM* 2004; 350:105-13.  McIntyre KM. Vasopressin in asystolic cardiac arrest [Editorial]. *NEJM* 2004; 350:179-181.

281  RJ Barst et al. A comparison of continuous intravenous epoprostenol (prostacyclin) with conventional therapy for primary pulmonary hypertension. *NEJM* 1996; 334(5):296-301; *Med Lett Drugs Ther* 1996; 38(968):14-15.

282  Byrd RC et al. Safety and efficacy of esmolol (an ultrashort-acting beta-adrenergic blocking agent) for control of ventricular rate in supraventricular tachycardias. *JACC* 1984;3(2 Pt 1):394-9.

for pheochromocytoma crisis. Reduces myocardial ischemia [283] but more hypotensive than other β-blockers. [284] May be used to test tolerability of β-blockers in patients with strong relative contraindications.

Kinetics: β1-selective, T½ 9 min, distribution time 2 min. Steady-state 5 min with load, 30 min without. β-blockade remits 10-20 min after stopping. Esterified in RBCs.

IV: Mix 5g in 500mL D5W = 10mg/mL. Load 500 mcg/kg over one minute then 50 mcg/kg/min. Titrate q 4 minutes by increasing infusion 50 mcg/kg/min and re-loading each time (skip load as target effect approaches). Maximum 300 mcg/kg/min.

Renal failure: No dose adjustment.

Transition to alternative agent: Decrease infusion by 50% 30 minutes after 1st dose of oral agent (digoxin, Ca⁺⁺ or β-blocker). Discontinue infusion 60min after 2nd dose of oral agent if response is satisfactory.

Caution: Bronchospasm, A-V block. IV irritant; avoid extravasation, and use concentration ≤10mg/mL. NaHCO₃ incompatible.

Side effects: Pallor, nausea, flushing, bradycardia or asystole, pulmonary edema.

# Ethanol [285]

Action: Second line treatment (after fomepizole) for ethylene glycol and methanol poisoning. Prevents build-up of toxic metabolites by competitively binding to alcohol dehydrogenase. Target levels 100-150 mg/dL, must be checked frequently (q 1-2 hr initially) along with glucose. **Conversions**: Specific gravity of absolute ethanol is 0.79 mg/mL = 79 g/100 mL. 10% ethanol in D5W = 7.9 g/100 mL.

IV: Load 600-800 mg/kg ethanol over 1 hr, followed by initial infusion at 66 mg/kg/h in non-drinkers or 154 mg/kg/h in chronic alcoholics.

PO: For severe poisoning in which medical care will be delayed several hours, give 4 x 1 oz doses of 80 proof alcohol (whiskey).

Hemodialysis: Double infusion rate or supplement dialysis bath with 200 mg/dL ethanol.

Caution: Hypoglycemia and folate depletion may occur during prolonged infusion. 10% solution is hyperosmolar, may cause local phlebitis unless administered through central line.

# Fenoldopam [286] *(Corlopam)*

Indications: Parenteral treatment of severe hypertension.

Action: Arterial vasodilator. Activity mainly through stimulation of $DA_1$ receptors. Increases renal/splanchnic blood flow despite decrease in arterial BP. Also has direct natriuretic and diuretic effects. Dose-dependent hypotension for 24-48 hr; possible tachyphylaxis. May improve renal perfusion and increase urine output in acute hypertension. Does not appear to protect against contrast-induced nephropathy. [287]

IV: Mix 10 mg in 250mL D5W or NS (40 mcg/mL). Begin 0.1 mcg/kg/min, titrate in 0.05-0.1 mcg/kg/min increments q 15 min. Usual dose range 0.1-1.6 mcg/kg/min. Overlap with oral antihypertensive agents once BP is stable.

Pharmacokinetics: Onset 5 minutes, steady state 20 minutes. Rapidly metabolized by liver. Unaffected by renal failure. Infusion may be tapered or stopped abruptly.

Adverse effects: Flushing, dizziness, headache, reflex tachycardia, nausea, hypokalemia, elevated intraocular pressure.

Contraindications: None

Caution: Hypovolemia, cerebrovascular disease, ß-blockers (hypotension), glaucoma.

Pregnancy: Class B.

---

283 Kirshenbaum JM *et al.* Use of an ultrashort-acting beta-receptor blocker (esmolol) in patients with acute myocardial ischemia and relative contraindications to beta-blockade therapy. *JACC* 1988;12(3):773-80.

284 Deegan R. Beta-receptor antagonism does not fully explain esmolol-induced hypotension. *Clin Pharm Ther* 1994;56(2):223-8.

285 Barceloux DG *et al.* American Academy of Clinical Toxicology practice guidelines on the treatment of methanol poisoning. J Toxicol Clin Toxicol 2002; 40:415-46.

286 Post JB 4th, Frishman WH. Fenoldopam: a new dopamine agonist for the treatment of hypertensive urgencies and emergencies. *J Clin Pharmacol* 1998; 38(1):2-13; Med Lett Drugs Ther 1998; 40:57-8.

287 Stone GW *et al.* Fenoldopam mesylate for the prevention of contrast-induced nephropathy: A randomized controlled trial. *JAMA* 2003; 290:2284-2291.

# Flumazenil [288] *(Romazicon)*

Action: Competitive antagonist of benzodiazepines (BDZ) at the GABA$_A$/benzo receptor. Used to reverse sedation and respiratory depression from benzodiazepines.

IV: **Known isolated benzodiazepine overdose:** 0.2 mg over 30 sec. If still lethargic give 0.3 mg over 30 sec. May repeat 0.5 mg over 30 sec q min to maximum cumulative dose of 3 mg. May re-bolus 0.5 mg/h to maintain wakefulness. BDZ intoxication unlikely if no response after 5 mg. **Reversal of procedural sedation:** 0.2 mg over 15 sec, if sedated after 45 sec give 0.2 mg IV. Repeat q1 min up to total 1 mg.

Kinetics: Metabolized by liver. Elimination half-time ~50-60 min if liver normal.

Caution: May provoke withdrawal syndrome including seizures in chronic BDZ users and in concurrent tricyclic antidepressant overdose. Half-life of BDZ may exceed that of flumazenil. Sedation may be reversed earlier than is respiratory depression.

Side-effects: Agitation, myoclonus, nausea, vomiting, dizziness.

# Fomepizole [289] *(4-methylpyrazole, Antizol)*

*Orphan Medical 1-888-8ORPHAN; www.antizol.info*

Indications: Treatment of ethylene glycol and methanol poisoning. Preferred over ethanol because **(1)** does not cause inebriation and **(2)** no need to monitor levels. However, much more expensive ($1200 per 1.5 g vial). Possible (unproven) benefit in isopropanol and diethylene glycol ingestions, and alcohol-disulfiram reactions.

Action: Competitive inhibitor of alcohol dehydrogenase with stronger binding affinity than ethanol.

IV: Load 15 mg/kg (in 100 mL NS or D5W), then 10 mg/kg q 12 hr x 4 doses, then 15 mg/kg q 12 hr. Infuse slowly over 30 minutes. Continue infusion until pH normalizes and ethylene glycol or methanol levels < 20 mg/dL. During hemodialysis, increase frequency to q 4 hr or infuse 1-1.5 mg/kg/h (see product information for specific instructions).

PO: Load 15 mg/kg, then 5 mg/kg 12 hr later, then 10 mg/kg q 12 hr.

Pharmacokinetics: Acidosis resolution begins within 4 hr of initial dose. Typical duration of treatment 30-60 hr (Goal: normal pH and ethylene glycol or methanol levels < 20 mg/dL). Hepatic metabolism. Significant clearance during hemodialysis.

Toxicity: Generally well-tolerated. Hypertriglyceridemia, nausea, dizziness, headache.

Contraindications: None

Pregnancy: Class C.

# Fondaparinux *(Arixtra)*

Action: Pentasaccharide sequence of heparin that binds with antithrombin III to inactivate factor Xa. Inhibits thrombin formation. Does not inactivate thrombin and has no effect on platelets.

Kinetics: Primarily eliminated via kidney; $T_{1/2}$ 17-21 hr.

SC: **Pulmonary embolism:** 7.5 mg qd for ≥ 5 days [290] (use 10 mg if weight > 100 kg). **DVT prophylaxis:** 2.5 mg qd starting 6-8 hr post-op (giving earlier increases risk of bleeding) for up to 11 days.

Renal dysfunction: Use with caution if CrCl 30-50 mL/min, contraindicated if CrCl <30 mL/minute.

Contraindications: Severe renal impairment, weight < 50 kg, active bleeding.

Interactions: Increased bleeding risk when used with ASA, NSAIDs, antiplatelet agents, warfarin and other anticoagulants.

---

[288] Med Lett Drugs Ther 1992; 34(874):66-8; Hoffman RS, Goldfrank LR. The poisoned patient with altered consciousness. Controversies in the use of a 'coma cocktail.' *JAMA* 1995;274(7):562-9; Shapiro BA *et al.* Practice parameters for intravenous analgesia and sedation for adult patients in the intensive care unit: An executive summary. *Crit Care Med* 1995;23(9):1596-1600.

[289] Brent J *et al.* Fomepizole for the treatment of ethylene glycol poisoning. *NEJM* 1999;340:832-8; Brent J *et al.* Fomepizole for the treatment of methanol poisoning. N Engl J Med 2001; 344:424-9.

[290] The MATISSE Investigators. Subcutaneous fondaparinux versus intravenous unfractionated heparin in the initial treatment of pulmonary embolism. *NEJM* 2003; 349:1695-1702.

Adverse Effects: Major bleeding (especially in elderly, low body weight, or renal dysfunction) and thrombocytopenia (rare). Spinal/epidural hematomas associated with neuraxial anesthesia or spinal punctures before and during treatment. Protamine ineffective for reversing anticoagulant effect
Pregnancy: Class B.

## Fosphenytoin *(Cerebyx IV)*
See Phenytoin on page 205

## Furosemide *(Lasix)*
See Loop diuretics on page 181

## Glucagon[291]
Action: Peptide hormone. Part of insulin counterregulatory system and therefore useful in hypoglycemia. Transiently decreases GI motility via relaxation of smooth muscle. Positive inotrope in supraphysiologic doses (activates cAMP independently of adrenergic receptors); used in hypotension or bradycardia unresponsive to catecholamines, especially after $Ca^{++}$channel or β-blockers. Inotrope > chronotrope.
Kinetics: $T_{1/2}$ 8-18minutes. Onset 1 min, comparable to insulin.
IV: **Hypoglycemia**: Reserve for patients who cannot receive immediate glucose. Give 1mg IV/IM/SC, may repeat q 15 min 1-2 times. **Bradycardia due to calcium channel or β-blocker toxicity**: 1-5 mg bolus over 2-5 minutes.
Caution: Hepatic glucose stores are rapidly depleted in fasting/starved patients or those with liver disease; use glucose instead. Promotes insulin release in insulinoma with resultant hypoglycemia. Elicits catecholamine release by pheochromocytoma.

## Glycoprotein IIb/IIIa Inhibitors [292]
Indications: Treatment of acute coronary syndromes (MI, unstable angina) and as adjunct to percutaneous coronary interventions (PCI) - see specific agents below. Routinely used along with ASA and heparin.
Action: Inhibit platelet cross-linking and aggregation by blocking of fibrinogen and vWF. Prolong bleeding time but do not directly affect PT or aPTT in absence of concurrent heparin treatment.
Contraindications: Active bleeding with 30 days, or GI/GU bleeding within 6 weeks; history of thrombotic stroke within 3 mo; history of any hemorrhagic stroke; bleeding diathesis; warfarin with INR > 1.5; platelet count < 100-150 K; major surgery or trauma within 4-6 weeks; intracranial neoplasm; severe, uncontrolled hypertension; suspected aortic dissection; acute pericarditis.
Caution: Weight < 50 kg and recent use of thrombolytics all increase risk of bleeding. Minimal data on use in renal insufficiency.
Toxicity: Major bleeding, thrombocytopenia (0.5-1 %).
Overdose: Platelet transfusion for serious bleeding (may be more effective for abciximab than for tirofiban).

## Abciximab [293] *(ReoPro)*
Monoclonal antibody to GP IIb/IIIa receptor
FDA Approved indications: During percutaneous coronary interventions (PCI) or for unstable angina, if PCI planned within 24 hr. Intended for use in conjunction with heparin and ASA.

---

291  Hall-Boyer K *et al*. Glucagon: hormone or therapeutic agent? *Crit Care Med* 1984;12:584.

292  Bhat DI, Topol EJ. Current role of platelet glycoprotein inhibitors in acute coronary syndromes. *JAMA* 2000;12(12):1549-1558.

293  EPIC, *NEJM* 1994; 330:956-961. EPILOG, *NEJM* 1997; 336:1689-96. EPISTENT, *Lancet* 1998; 352:87-92.

<u>Pharmacokinetics:</u> > 90% platelet inhibition within 2 hr of bolus. $T_{1/2}$ 25 minutes. Irreversibly binds platelets, platelet recovery seen in 48 hr.
<u>IV:</u> **PCI:** Bolus 0.25 mg/kg 10-60 min prior to intervention, then infuse 0.125 mcg/kg/min (10 mcg/min max) x 12 hr. **Acute coronary syndromes with planned PCI:** Bolus 0.25 mg/kg, then infuse 10 mcg/min x 18-24 hr before PCI and 1 hr post-PCI.
<u>Caution:</u> Renal insufficiency.
<u>Pregnancy:</u> Category C

## Eptifibatide [294] (*Integrilin*)

Peptide inhibitor of GP IIb/IIIa receptor
<u>FDA approved indications:</u> Percutaneous coronary interventions (PCI); acute coronary syndromes with or without planned PCI.
<u>Pharmacokinetics:</u> Platelet function inhibited within 1 hr. Bleeding time normalizes within 15 minutes of discontinuation; platelet function recovers by 4 hr. Clearance is primarily renal.
<u>PCI:</u> Bolus 180 mcg/kg, with second bolus 180 mcg/kg ten minutes later; then infuse 2.0 mcg/kg/min for 18-24 hr (minimum 12 hr recommended).
<u>Acute coronary syndromes:</u> Bolus 180 mcg/kg, then infuse 2.0 mcg/kg/min for up to 72 hr.
<u>Renal insufficiency:</u> Avoid if Cr > 4 mg/dL, or consider tirofiban. If serum Cr 2-4 mg/dL use same bolus but decrease infusion rate to 1 mcg/kg/min. Max dosages when creatinine 2-4 mg/dL are 22.6 mg (bolus) and 7.5 mg/hr (infusion rate).
<u>Incompatibility:</u> Do not give in same IV line as furosemide.
<u>Pregnancy:</u> Category B

## Tirofiban [295] (*Aggrastat*)

Non-peptide inhibitor of GP IIb/IIIa receptor
<u>FDA approved indications:</u> Acute coronary syndromes including percutaneous coronary interventions, in conjunction with ASA and heparin.
<u>Pharmacokinetics:</u> Platelet function inhibited within 5 minutes. Platelet function recovers within 4-8 hr of discontinuation. Clearance is primarily renal.
<u>Dose:</u> Bolus 0.4 mcg/kg/min x 30 minutes, then infuse 0.1 mcg/kg/min for 48-108 hr.
<u>Renal insufficiency:</u> Reduce infusion rate by 50% if CrCl < 30 mL/min.
<u>Incompatibility:</u> Do not give in same IV line as diazepam.
<u>Pregnancy:</u> Category B

## Haloperidol [296] (*Haldol*)

<u>Action:</u> Antipsychotic and sedative via dopaminergic blockade. Does not depress respiratory drive.
<u>Kinetics:</u> Half-life 10-38 hr (average 20 hr). Liver metabolism.
<u>IV/IM:</u> **Acute psychosis and severe agitation:** 2-10 mg q 15-20 min until symptoms abate, then 25% of initial dose q 6 hr. Total dose usually < 10-15 mg/d. May give IV over 2-3 min [297]; has also been given as IV infusion at 3-25 mg/hr in delirious ICU patients. Start with 0.5 mg in elderly or debilitated. Oral agents such as risperidone, olanzapine or quetiapine have more favorable side effect profiles and may be preferable in elderly.
<u>Renal failure:</u> Half-life unknown. No dosage adjustment. Not dialyzed.
<u>Caution:</u> Reduce dose in liver (extreme care) and renal failure. Thyrotoxicosis exacerbates extrapyramidal effects. High doses may cause $QT_c$ prolongation and polymorphic ventricular tachycardia.

---

294 PURSUIT *NEJM* 1998; 339:436-443.
295 PRISM *NEJM* 1998; 338:1498-1505. PRISM-Plus *NEJM* 1998;338:1488-1497.
296 Riker RR *et al.* Continuous infusion of haloperidol controls agitation in critically ill patients. *Crit Care Med* 1994;22(3):433-40. Jacobi J *et al.* Clinical practice guidelines for the sustained use of sedatives and analgesics in the critically ill adult. *Crit Care Med* 2002; 30:119-41.
297 Not FDA approved for IV administration.

Side-effects: Anticholinergic, extrapyramidal, orthostatic hypotension. Neuroleptic malignant syndrome, tardive dyskinesia (risk greater in elderly with prolonged higher-dose therapy), leukopenia, rash, hyperprolactinemia.
Pregnancy: Suspected teratogen in 1st trimester.

# Heparin [298] (Unfractionated)

Action: Accelerates antithrombin III inhibition of factors II (thrombin), IXa, and Xa, thereby inhibiting thrombin-induced activation of factors V and VIII. Anticoagulant in treatment/prophylaxis of thrombosis and thromboembolism, coronary syndromes; also used during cardiovascular procedures.
Kinetics: Anticoagulation increases disproportionately with increasing dose. Biological $T\frac{1}{2}$ 30 min after 25 unit/kg bolus, but $T\frac{1}{2}$ 60 min after 75 unit/kg. No important difference among bovine, porcine, sodium or calcium heparins.
IV: **Treatment of venous thromboembolism:** 80 units/kg IV then 18 units/kg/h *or* 5000 units IV then 1333 unit/h. Adjust 6 hr afterwards for aPTT 1.5-2.5 × control. **Prevention of venous thromboembolism:** 5000 units SC q 8-12h. High-risk patients should have dose adjusted to increase aPTT to upper-normal limits. **Unstable angina:** 80 units/kg IV then 18 units/kg/h, or 5000 unit bolus then 1333 units/h. Adjust 6 hr afterwards for aPTT 1.5-2.5 × control. **Myocardial infarction with thrombolytics:** [299] 60 units/kg IV bolus then 12 units/kg/h (max 4000 unit bolus and 1000 units/h for patients > 70 kg) or 5000 IV bolus then 1000 units/h. Adjust dose per nomogram below. Monitor aPTT q6h during first 24h of therapy and 6h after each heparin dosage adjustment. Frequency of aPTT monitoring can be reduced to daily when aPTT is stable within therapeutic range. Check platelet count between days 3 to 5.
Renal failure: Half-life unchanged. No dosage adjustment.
Dosage adjustment:[300]

| aPTT (sec) | Rebolus | Stop | Δ infusion | Next aPTT |
|---|---|---|---|---|
| < 35s (<1.2×control) | 80 units/kg | - | ↑ 4 units/kg/h | 6 h |
| 35-45s (1.2-1.5×control) | 40 units/kg | - | ↑ 2 units/kg/h | 6 h |
| 46-70s (1.5-2.3×control) | - | - | - | Next AM |
| 71-90s (2.3-3×control) | - | - | ↓ 2 units/kg/h | Next AM |
| > 90s (>3×control) | - | 60 min | ↓ 3 units/kg/h | 6 h |

Adverse effects: Hemorrhage, especially in seriously ill, alcohol abusers, use with other anticoagulants or antiplatelet agents. Thrombocytopenia and thromboembolic complications (see Heparin-induced Thrombocytopenia, page 81). Osteoporosis after chronic use. Hyperkalemia (Type IV RTA) especially in renal insufficiency and diabetes.
Interactions: Increased bleeding with ASA, GP IIb/IIIa inhibitors, NSAIDs, other antiplatelet agents, warfarin, dipyridamole.
Caution: Rebound thrombosis may occur when discontinuing heparin in acute coronary syndromes without revascularization; consider tapering over 4-8 hr.
Overdose: see Protamine, page 208.
Pregnancy: Class C. Does not cross placenta; anticoagulant of choice though has been reported to cause premature/still births.

298 Hirsh J et al. Heparin and low-molecular-weight heparin: mechanisms of action, pharmacokinetics, dosing, monitoring, efficacy, and safety. Chest 2001; 119:64S-94S; Hirsh J et al. Guide to anticoagulant therapy: Heparin: A statement for healthcare professionals from the American Heart Association. Circulation 2001; 103:2994-3018.
299 Ryan TJ et al. 1999 Update: ACC/AHA guidelines for the management of patients with acute myocardial infarction. Executive summary and recommendations. Circulation 1999; 100:1016-30.
300 Raschke RA et al . The weight-based heparin dosing nomogram compared with a "standard care" nomogram. A randomized controlled trial. Ann Intern Med 1993; 119:874-81.

# Heparin, Low Molecular Weight (LMWH) [301]

*Also see alternative antithrombins including Argatroban (page 175), Fondaparinux (page 186), and Lepirudin (page 194).*

General Indications: **(1)** Prevention and treatment of DVT (tinzaparin) **(2)** Pulmonary embolism **(3)** Acute coronary syndromes [302] and percutaneous coronary interventions [303] (enoxaparin, dalteparin) **(4)** Acute stroke (enoxaparin)

Action: See unfractionated heparin (UH). Have more targeted effects on factor Xa and less anti-thrombin activity compared to UH. Better subcutaneous bioavailability and more predictable dose-response curves compared to UH, allowing fixed dosages without monitoring or dose adjustment in most patients.

Monitoring: Usually unnecessary. Minimal effect on aPTT or thrombin time. Consider monitoring plasma anti-factor Xa concentration ("heparin level") in patients with renal insufficiency or weight <50 kg or > 80 kg. Draw anti-Xa level 3-6 hr after dose; target 0.4-1.0 units/mL for active thrombosis and 0.1-0.2 units/mL for prophylaxis.

Adverse effects: Hemorrhage, especially if used in combination with anti-platelet drugs or NSAIDs. **Particular risk for epidural hematoma after spinal/epidural anesthesia or lumbar puncture.** May cause less heparin-induced thrombocytopenia and osteopenia than unfractionated heparin.

Interactions: Increased bleeding with ASA, antiplatelet drugs, NSAIDs, warfarin, dipyridamole.

Overdose: Protamine (page 208) may be used but relatively ineffective.

Pregnancy: Enoxaparin – class B, safe in breastfeeding. All others – class C.

## Enoxaparin (Lovenox)

Indications: **(1)** Prevention & treatment of DVT [304] **(2)** Unstable angina and non-Q wave MI (better outcomes compared with UH) [305] and percutaneous coronary interventions **(3)** Acute ischemic stroke. [306]

Kinetics: Peak effect 3-5 hr after SC administration. $T_{1/2} = 3$- 4.5 hr SC. Excreted renally, with doubling of $T_{1/2}$ in renal failure.

Dose: **Treatment of venous thromboembolism:** 1 mg/kg SC q12h or 1.5 mg/kg SC q 24h. **Prevention of venous thromboembolism:** Medical patients at risk: 40 mg/kg qd; orthopedic surgery: 30 mg SC bid; abdominal surgery: 40 mg SC qd, start 2 hr prior to surgery if no epidural. **Acute coronary syndromes/non-ST-elevation MI:** 1 mg/kg bid x 2-8 days, combine with ASA. **Acute coronary syndromes/ST-elevation MI:** 30 mg IV bolus followed immediately by 1 mg/kg SC q12 hr. **Percutaneous coronary intervention:** (1) If initial 30 mg IV load given or if ≥ 2 SC doses already given and if procedure within 8 hr of last dose, no additional enoxaparin needed. If procedure within 8-12 hr of last dose, give 0.3 mg/kg IV. (2) If only one SC dose given without IV load, give 0.3 mg/kg IV. (3) If no prior enoxaparin, give 1 mg/kg IV without IV load or give 0.75 mg/kg IV in combination with GP IIb/IIIa inhibitor. **Arterial Sheath Removal:** 6-8 hours after last SC dose, 4 hours after IV PCI dose if > 8-12 hr since last SC dose. **Acute ischemic stroke:** 1 mg/kg SC q 12 hr in patient

301 Hirsh J et al. Heparin and low-molecular-weight heparin: mechanisms of action, pharmacokinetics, dosing, monitoring, efficacy, and safety. Chest 2001; 119:64S-94S; Aguilar D, Goldhaber SZ. Clinical uses of low-molecular weight heparins. Chest 1999; 115:1418-1423.

302 Wong GC et al. Use of low-molecular-weight heparins in the management of acute coronary artery syndromes and percutaneous coronary intervention. JAMA 2003; 289:331-42.

303 Kereiakes DJ et al. Low-molecular-weight heparin therapy for non-st-elevation acute coronary syndromes and during percutaneous coronary intervention: An expert consensus. Am Heart J 2002; 144:615-24.

304 Levine M et al. A comparison of low-molecular-weight heparin administered primarily at home with unfractionated heparin administered in the hospital for proximal deep vein thrombosis. NEJM 1996; 334(11): 677-81.

305 Cohen M et al. A comparison of low-molecular weight heparin with unfractionated heparin for unstable coronary artery disease. ESSENCE Study Group. NEJM 1997; 337:447-452; Antman EA et al. Enoxaparin prevents death and cardiac ischemic events in unstable angina/non–Q-wave myocardial infarction (TIMI 11B trial). Circulation 1999; 100: 1593-1601.

306 Kay R et al. Low-molecular heparin for the treatment of acute ischemic stroke. NEJM 1995; 333: 1588-93.

started on warfarin while awaiting therapeutic INR, then discontinue.
FDA Warning: Not recommended for anticoagulation of prosthetic heart valves, especially during pregnancy, due to reports of valve thrombosis (including deaths).[307] Controversial. [308]

## Tinzaparin (Innohep)
Indications: (1) Treatment of DVT and PE (2) Thromboembolism prevention.
Kinetics: Peak 3.7 hr after administration, T1/2 3-4h, renal elimination
Dose: **Treatment of DVT or PE:** 175 units/kg SC qd for ≥ 6 days and until adequate anticoagulation with warfarin. **Post-op prevention of DVT:** General surgery: 3,500 units SC given 2 hr pre-op and qd post-op; orthopedic surgery: 75 units/kg SC qd starting 12-24h post-op or 4,500 units SC given 12h pre-op and qd post-op.

## Dalteparin *(Fragmin)*
Indications: (1) Prevention of DVT (2) Acute coronary syndromes [309]
Kinetics: Peak effect 4 hr after administration. $T_{1/2}$ = 3-5 hr SC. Excreted renally, with approximate doubling of $T_{1/2}$ in renal failure.
Dose: **Prevention of venous thromboembolism:** 2500 units SC qd (normal risk) or 5000 units SC qd (high risk, e.g. malignancy); begin 1-2 hr pre-op and continue 5-10 days post-op. **Prevention of DVT after hip replacement:** 2500 units 2 hr pre-op and 4-8 post-op, then give 5000 units qd starting >6 after 1st dose x 14 days . **Acute coronary syndromes:** 120 units/kg (max 10,000) SC q 12 hr until clinically stable, usually 5-8 days; combine with ASA 75-165 mg PO qd. **Percutaneous coronary intervention:**[310] May proceed without further dosing if within 8 hr of ACS dose; otherwise supplement 60 units/kg IV.

# Hydralazine *(Apresoline)*
Action: Predominantly arteriolar vasodilator. Reflex tachycardia in healthy subjects, blunted tachycardia in patients with CHF.
Indication: CHF in combination with nitrates; hypertension in combination with diuretic or β-blocker; hypertensive emergencies (especially in pregnancy).
Kinetics: Biological exceeds biochemical T1/2 of 3-7 hr. Liver metabolism; fast-acetylators need 25% more; slow-acetylators more susceptible to lupus-like syndrome.
IV: 5-10 mg q 20 min up to max 40 mg (20 mg in pregnancy) repeated prn to target BP. Transfer to oral in 24-48 hr.
PO: Begin 10 mg qid, titrate up to 300 mg/day in divided doses bid-qid.
Renal failure: T1/2 7-16 hr. Give q 8-16h for CrCl <10 mL/min. Not dialyzed.
Caution: Slow-acetylators should probably not receive > 200 mg/d.
Side-effects: Lupus syndrome rare < 200 mg/day. Fluid retention from renin release. Reflex tachycardia (contraindicated in angina). Polyneuropathy, drug fever rare.
Pregnancy: Animal (not human) teratogen. Emergency agent of choice.

# Ibutilide [311] *(Corvert)*
Action: Short-acting class III antiarrhythmic used to convert atrial fibrillation (AF) or flutter to sinus rhythm. Dose-related QT prolongation associated with antiarrhythmic activity. Ibutilide treatment prior to electrical cardioversion reduces energy threshold and

307 http://www.fda.gov/medwatch/SAFETY/2002/lovenox.htm
308 Ginsberg JS et al. Anticoagulation of pregnant women with mechanical heart valves. Arch Intern Med 2003; 163:694-8.
309 Long-term low molecular weight heparin in unstable coronary-artery disease: FRISC II prospective randomised multicentre study. Lancet 1999; 354: 701-7.
310 Invasive compared with non-invasive treatment in unstable coronary-artery disease: FRISC II prospective randomised multicentre study. Lancet 1999; 354:708-15.; Kereiakes DJ et al. Dalteparin in combination with abciximab during percutaneous coronary intervention. Am Heart J 2001;141:348-52.
311 Stambler BS et al. Efficacy and safety of repeated intravenous doses of ibutilide for rapid conversion of atrial flutter or fibrillation. Circulation 1996;94(7):1613-1621.

increases success rate.[312]

Kinetics: Rapid redistribution terminates drug effect. Elimination $T\frac{1}{2}$ ~6 hr (variable).

IV: **AF or flutter < 48 hr duration:** 1 mg infused over 10 min (0.01 mg/kg if < 60kg). Repeat once if arrhythmia persists 20 min after start of infusion. Continue ECG monitoring ≥ 4-6 hr post-infusion (longer if hepatic dysfunction). Consider initiation of long-term oral anti-arrhythmic if cardioversion successful. Start IV heparin prior to infusion and continue anticoagulation for 4 weeks afterward. **AF of unclear duration or lasting > 48h:** Anticoagulate > 3 wks before cardioversion and 4 wks afterwards.

Renal failure: No apparent dosage adjustment warranted. Not studied in liver disease.

Caution: Avoid other antiarrhythmics (especially class I or III agents) before and within 4 hr of administering drug. Do not give if decompensated CHF, EF < 30% or recent MI. Avoid in hypokalemia, hypomagnesemia, $QT_c$ > 440ms or hemodynamic instability.

Warning: Can cause lethal polymorphic ventricular tachycardia (torsades de pointes). In one study 15/180 patients developed polymorphic VT; in 12/15 it resolved spontaneously or with cessation of ibutilide, but 3/15 required emergency cardioversion. VT generally begins during or shortly after infusion, and is more common in women, CHF, reduced EF and those with slower heart rates. Low incidence (<2%) of self-limited high-grade AV block and bundle-branch block.

Interactions: Excess risk of torsades if co-administered with drugs that prolong QT (antiarrhythmics, tricyclic antidepressants, phenothiazines, $H_1$-antagonists).

# Inamrinone *(Inocor)*

Action: Inotrope-vasodilator. Additive to digoxin and catecholamines; potent direct systemic, pulmonary, coronary vasodilator. Reportedly causes little change in myocardial oxygen demand. Resembles dobutamine hemodynamically with less tachyphylaxis. Increases infarct size in dogs. Used acutely in CHF refractory to diuretics and afterload reduction. **Note:** Studies of similar phosphodiesterase inhibitors used orally for treatment of CHF suggest increased mortality.

Kinetics: Hepatic/renal clearance. $T\frac{1}{2}$ extended in CHF, range 3-15 hr.

IV: Bolus 0.75 mg/kg over 10-15 min then 5-15 mcg/kg/min titrated to clinical effect (max 10 mg/kg/day). May re-bolus 0.75 mg/kg 30 min after starting therapy.

Mix: Add 300mg (60mL) to 60mL NS (not D5) for 2.5 mg/mL. Renal failure: Give 50-75% dose for CRCL <10 mL/min.

Side Effects: Dose-related vasodilation/hypotension, especially if hypovolemic; thrombocytopenia (1-2%, dose-related); increased AV conduction with increased ventricular response in atrial fibrillation; idiosyncratic hepatotoxicity, nausea/vomiting/abdominal discomfort.

Caution: Atrial fibrillation, hypotension, hypertrophic cardiomyopathy.

# Insulin

Action & kinetics: Anabolic hormone maintains glucose homeostasis via glucose translocation, inhibition of glycogenolysis and gluconeogenesis, and stimulation of glycogen synthesis; also suppression of lipolysis and ketogenesis. Drives potassium into cells. Used in hyperglycemia, diabetic ketoacidosis, acute hyperkalemia. Intensive therapy improves morbidity and mortality in critically ill patients.[313]

Kinetics: Renal excretion. Plasma half-life 5-15 min.

IV (regular only): Mix 100 units in 100 mL NS or D5W; flush first 10 mL through tubing and waste. **Ketoacidosis:** Bolus 0.1 units/kg, then start 0.1 units/kg/h. Rebolus and increase infusion rate if glucose does not fall 50-70 mg/dL/hour. Halve rate when glucose is < 250 mg/dL. **Severe hyperkalemia:** Onset 15-30 min. Give 10 units along with 50 g dextrose 50% during first hour. May re-bolus or infuse 20 units insulin in 1 liter 10% dextrose at 50 mL/h.

Renal failure: $T\frac{1}{2}$ increased. Give 75% dose if CrCl 10-50 mL/min; 50% if CrCL <10 mL/min.

---

312 Oral H *et al.* Facilitating transthoracic cardioversion of atrial fibrillation with ibutilide pretreatment. *NEJM* 1999; 340(24):1849-1854.

313 Van den Berghe G *et al.* Intensive insulin therapy in critically ill patients. *NEJM* 2001; 345:1359-1367.

**Subcutaneous** insulin preparations:

| Insulin | Onset | Peak | Duration |
|---|---|---|---|
| Aspart (Novolog®) | 15 min | 45 min | 3-5 h |
| Lispro (Humalog®) | 15 min | 0.5-1.5 h | 6-8 h |
| Regular | 30-60 min | 2-4 h | 8-12 h |
| NPH | 1- 1.5 h | 4-12 h | 24 h |
| Lente | 1-2.5 3 h | 7-15 h | 24 h |
| Ultralente | 4-8 h | 10-30 h | >36 h |
| Glargine (Lantus®) | Slow | - | 24 h |

**An intensive insulin protocol for critically ill hyperglycemic patients:** [314]

1) Check bedside blood glucose (BBG) and begin insulin infusion:

| | | Insulin Infusion (units/h) | |
|---|---|---|---|
| Glucose (mg/dL) | IV insulin bolus | Type 1 | Type 2 |
| 80 -119 | 0 | 1.0 | 0.5 |
| 120-179 | 0 | 2.0 | 1.0 |
| 180-239 | 0 | 3.5 | 2.0 |
| 240-299 | 4 units | 5.0 | 3.5 |
| 300-359 | 8 units | 6.5 | 5.0 |
| ≥ 360 | 12 units | 8.0 | 6.5 |

2) Check bedside glucose every hour (by fingerstick or arterial line sample) and titrate insulin as below. Glucose can be checked every 2 hours when glucose is 100-150 mg/dL with < 15 mg/dL change from last test *and* insulin rate is unchanged for 4 hr. Check glucose and titrate drip every 30 min if: • Glucose > 200 or < 75 mg/dL • Insulin drip is > 10 units/h • Adjusting dose of catecholamines vasopressors • Patient is receiving mannitol or a large dose of IV steroids

3) Titrate insulin (1 unit regular insulin/1 mL NS, piggybacked on maintenance IV):

| Glucose | Action |
|---|---|
| < 50 | • Stop insulin and give 25 mL D50W<br>• Recheck glucose in 30 min<br>• When glucose > 75 mg/dL, restart insulin at 50% of previous rate<br>• If insulin drip is stopped for > 6 hours, restart as if initiating drip |
| 50-75 | • Stop insulin and give 25 mL D50W if previous glucose >100 mg/dL<br>• Recheck glucose in 30 min<br>• When glucose > 75 mg/dL, restart insulin at 50% of previous rate<br>• If insulin drip is stopped for > 6 hours, restart as if initiating drip |
| 75-100 | • If < last test and change > 10 mg/dL, decrease rate by 50%<br>• If < last test and change ≤ 10 mg/dL, decrease rate by 0.5 unit/h<br>• If ≥ last test, continue current rate |
| 101-150 | • Continue current rate |
| 151-200 | • If < last test and change > 20 mg/dL, continue same rate<br>• If ≤ last test and change ≤ 20 mg/dL, increase rate by 0.5 unit/h<br>• If > last test, increase rate by 0.5 unit/h |
| > 200 | • If < last test and change > 30 mg/dL, continue same rate<br>• If ≤ last test and change ≤ 30 mg/dL, increase rate by 1 unit/h<br>• If > last test, increase rate by 1 unit/hr<br>• If glucose > 240 mg/dL, bolus as per step 1 above and increase rate by 1 unit/hr<br>• Recheck glucose in 30 min<br>• If glucose > 200 and has not decreased after 3 insulin rate increases, then bolus as per step 1 above and double insulin rate<br>• If insulin rate doubled at last adjustment, increase by 1 unit/hr increments 3 times before doubling again |

---

[314] Adapted with permission from Furnary AP *et al.* Continuous insulin infusion reduces mortality in patients with diabetes undergoing coronary artery bypass grafting. *J Thorac Cardiovasc Surg* 2003; 125:1007-21.

# Isoproterenol *(Isuprel)*

Indications:  2nd line agent (after dopamine) for bradycardia unresponsive to atropine if transcutaneous or transvenous spacing is unavailable; temporizing measure prior to overdrive pacing for *torsades de pointes*

Action & kinetics:  Nonspecific β-adrenergic agonist.  Potent inotrope and chronotrope.  Hepatic metabolism.  Plasma T½ < 5 min.  Onset < 5 min, duration <1 hr.

IV:  Mix 1 mg in 500ml D5W = 2 mcg/mL.  Start at 2 mcg/min ( 60 mL/h), titrate up to 10 mcg/min (300 mL/h).

SC/IM:  Undiluted solution 1mL (0.2mg).

Contraindication:  Digitalis induced bradycardia, angina

Side effects:  Hypotension from vasodilatation; tachycardia; ischemia and increased infarct size during MI; malignant ventricular arrhythmias.

# Kayexalate

*See sodium polystyrene sulfonate, page 208*

# Labetalol

Action:  Selective α-1 antagonist, nonselective β-antagonist.  α:β 1:3 oral, 1:7 IV.  No β-1 agonism (ISA) but may be partial β-2 agonist.  Dose-related antihypertensive effect without reflex brady/tachycardia.  Tachyphylaxis uncommon.  Predominant β-effect makes it a 2nd line agent for sympathomimetic crises [315] (e.g. cocaine overdose, pheochromocytoma); pure α-antagonists preferred, e.g. phentolamine

Kinetics:  T½ 5-8h.  IV onset 3-5 min.  Liver clearance with extensive first-pass metabolism; reduce dose in liver disease.

Renal failure:  T½ unchanged.  No dosage adjustment.  Not dialyzed.

IV:  Mix 200mg in 160 mL NS (1 mg/mL) or 200 mg in 250 mL NS(2 mg/3 mL).  Give 20 mg over 2 minutes then 40-80 mg q 10 min to max 300 mg for rapid BP control.  Push IV slowly over 2 minutes, **while supine**, then infuse 2 mg/min to maximum of 2400 mg/day.  Stop infusion after satisfactory BP.  Change to PO by abruptly stopping infusion and waiting for BP to rise.

PO:  1:1 PO-IV conversion (total daily dose).  Usual dose 200-400 mg bid, max 1200 mg bid.  Titrate on **standing** BP.

Caution:  Postural hypotension.  Abrupt discontinuation may precipitate angina, hypertension, myocardial ischemia like all β-blockers.  β-predominance may precipitate paradoxical hypertension in sympathomimetic crisis.

Side effects:  Bradycardia, 3° AVB (all less than in pure β-blockers).  Postural hypotension, paresthesias, hepatocellular damage, tremor, low-titer insignificant (+) antinuclear antibody, halothane hypotension.

Pregnancy:  Category C.  Some increase in fetal adverse effects reported, but drug of choice for severe maternal hypertension.

# Lepirudin [316] (recombinant hirudin, *Refludan*)

Action:  Direct thrombin inhibitor.  Indicated for anticoagulation in heparin-induced thrombocytopenia or treatment of HIT thromboembolic complications.  Acts on free and clot-bound thrombin, resistant to platelet factor-4.  Prolongs aPTT.  Possible role in acute coronary syndromes.[317]

IV:  Bolus 0.4 mg/kg (max 44 mg), then infuse 0.15 mg/kg/h (max 16.5 mg/h).  Monitor

---

315  Hollander JE. Management of cocaine-associated myocardial ischemia. *NEJM* 1995; 333: 1270-6.

316  Greinacher A *et al.* Recombinant hirudin (lepirudin) provides safe and effective anticoagulation in patients with heparin-induced thrombocytopenia: a prospective study. *Circulation.* 1999; 99:73-80. Greinacher A *et al.* Lepirudin (recombinant hirudin) for parenteral anticoagulation in patients with heparin-induced thrombocytopenia *Circulation.* 1999; 100:587-93.

317  OASIS-2 Investigators. Effects of recombinant hirudin (lepirudin) compared with heparin on death, myocardial infarction, refractory angina, and revascularisation procedures in patients with acute myocardial ischaemia without ST elevation: A randomised trial. *Lancet* 1999; 353:429-38.

aPTT after 4 hr, target aPTT 1.5-2.5 × normal. Low aPTT: Increase infusion by 20%; high aPTT: hold 2 hr and decrease infusion by 50%. Do not exceed an infusion rate of 0.21 mg/kg/h without ruling out coagulation abnormalities preventing appropriate aPTT response. **Combined with thrombolytic therapy:** Bolus 0.1 mg/kg, then infuse 0.15 mg/kg/h.

Pharmacokinetics: Elimination $T_{1/2}$ 1.3 hr. Prolonged in renal insufficiency and elderly.

Renal insufficiency: Reduce bolus in all cases by 50%, then adjust infusion as follows: for CrCl 45-60 mL/min or Scr 1.6-2.0 mg/dL give 50% infusion rate; for CrCl 30-44 mL/min or Scr 2.1-3.0 mg/dL give 30% infusion rate; for CrCl 15-29 mL/min or Scr 3.1-6.0 mg/dL give 15% infusion rate. Avoid in all patients with further reductions in renal function.

Toxicity: Major bleeding, allergic reactions including stridor.

Caution: ↑ bleeding risk with renal insufficiency, liver disease, recent surgery or stroke.

Pregnancy: Class B.

# Levothyroxine (T4)

Action: Thyroid hormone. Must undergo peripheral conversion to T3 for biological activity. Conversion blocked by severe non-thyroid illness.

Kinetics: Onset of action 6-12 hr. Half-life one week.

IV: **Myxedema coma:** [318] Bolus 300-600 mcg IV as a 100 mcg/mL solution (higher end of range for more severe symptoms). If lower range dose given and no response by 6-12 hr, re-bolus with 100-300 mcg (or more) after first 24 hr. If combined with liothyronine (T3) therapy, bolus initially with 4 mcg/kg.

PO: Oral bioavailability 50-80%. **Maintenance:** Average dose 1.6 mcg/kg. Start at 12.5-50 mcg in elderly or cardiac disease and titrate upwards every 2-3 weeks. **Non-compliant patients:** Long half-life allows "directly observed therapy" in form of weekly dosing (7 x usual daily dose).

Caution: Cardiovascular effects (ischemia, arrhythmia especially atrial fibrillation, high output CHF).

Drug interactions: Estrogens bind T4, higher doses may be needed. Decreased oral absorption with iron, antacids, bile resins, calcium. Thyroid replacement increases clotting factor metabolism, thereby increasing warfarin effect and potential for bleeding.

# Lidocaine

Action: Class IB antiarrhythmic depresses automaticity. Used to suppress ventricular arrhythmias, especially in association with acute ischemia. Not warranted as routine prophylaxis in acute MI.

Kinetics: $T_{1/2}$ 1.5-2 hr initially lengthens to 3h with infusions >1day. $T_{1/2}$ increases with CHF, age, liver disease. Extensive hepatic metabolism; metabolites accumulate in renal failure and may cause CNS toxicity. Rapid redistribution of initial load ($T_{1/2}$ ~4-8min) requires re-bolus.

IV: Mix 1 gram in 125 mL D5W (8 mg/mL) for fluid restricted or 1 gram in 1 L for (1 mg/mL). **Ventricular tachycardia or fibrillation:** Load 1-1.5 mg/kg over 1-2 min then 0.5-0.75 mg/kg q 5-10 min to max 3 mg/kg. May give initial bolus via ETT at 2-4 mg/kg. **Maintenance:** 30-50 mcg/kg/min (1-4mg/min). Re-bolus 0.5 mg/kg and increase infusion for breakthrough arrhythmias. Reduce infusion after 1 day. No need to taper before discontinuing.

Renal failure: Minimal $T_{1/2}$ change: no dose change, not dialyzed. However, active metabolite accumulates in renal failure and may contribute to neurological side effects.

Side-effects: Neurologic, including drowsiness, slurred speech, paresthesias, confusion (seen almost universally > 7mcg/mL). Severe: seizures.

Interactions: Half-life prolonged by beta-blockers (which decrease hepatic blood flow) and by cimetidine (reduces hepatic metabolism). Lidocaine potentiates action of neuromuscular blocking agents.

Levels: Therapeutic: 1.5-5.0 mcg/mL. Seizures seen at levels > 5 mcg/mL.

---

[318] Wartowsky L. Myxedema coma. In: *Werner and Ingbar's Thyroid: a Fundamental and Clinical Text*, 8th ed. Braverman LE, Utiger RD (eds). Philadelphia : Lippincott, 2000.

# Liothyronine (T3; *Cytomel, Triostat IV*)

<u>Action:</u>  Biologically active form of thyroid hormone (converted from T4 in periphery).

<u>Kinetics:</u>  Onset of activity within 2-4 hr. Biologic half-life ~ 2.5 days, compared to ~ 7 days for T4.

<u>Indication:</u>  T3 is generally avoided except in severe hypothyroidism (myxedema coma) in which **(1)** T4 monotherapy would pose unacceptably delay in recovery or **(2)** concurrent severe non-thyroid illness inhibits peripheral conversion from T4 to T3.

<u>Dose:</u>  No prospective studies and lack of expert consensus on optimal dosing. Load 10-20 mcg PO/IV, check patient response after 4 hr and give additional doses accordingly. Mortality benefit noted with at least 65 mcg/day during initial treatment. Alternatively,[319] load 12.5 mcg PO/IV, then 12.5 mcg q 6h x 48 hr. If no response (HR, BP or T°) in 15-21 hr, increase dose to 25 mcg x 2 doses; reduce dose if evidence of myocardial ischemia (especially falling BP in face of rising T°). Doses as low as 2.5 mcg appear to reverse metabolic abnormalities. Usually given in combination with levothyroxine (T4).

<u>Adverse effects:</u>  Cardiovascular (ischemia, hypertension, CHF, cardiac arrest).

# Magnesium

<u>Action:</u>  Hypomagnesemia common with diuretics, alcohol, nephrotoxic agents (aminoglycosides, amphotericin). Shortens QT interval and may suppress polymorphic VT associated with hypomagnesemia. Correction of deficit facilitates correction of hypocalcemia, hypokalemia. Anticonvulsant in eclampsia. No benefit to supplementation in acute MI.[320] Anecdotal evidence for use in a variety of other medical conditions.[321]  **Note:** In severe hypo-magnesemia deficit is 1-2 mEq/kg; half of administered Mg is excreted renally. Replace half in first day and remainder in 2-3 days. Serum levels correlate poorly with body stores.

<u>IV:</u>  1-2 g IV as 10% solution in 50-100 mL D5W or NS over > 20-30 minutes. 1 g MgSO$_4$ = 8.12 mEq. ***Torsades de Pointes*** 1-2 g IV over 5 min. **Eclampsia:** 2-4 g IV push over 2-4 min then 1-4 g/h titrated to respiratory drive, loss of patellar reflexes, levels. Levels of 4-7 mg/dL therapeutic in eclampsia and seizures. Levels > 7 mg/dL toxic.

<u>IM:</u>  IV dose given as 1g of 25% solution q 4-6h.

<u>Side effects:</u>  Hypotension, hypothermia, CNS depression, respiratory paralysis. Atropine-responsive bradycardia. Extreme caution in renal failure.

# Metaraminol *(Aramine)*

<u>Action:</u>  Sympathomimetic amine that acts directly and indirectly on α > β-adrenergic receptors to cause vasopressor effect. Positive inotrope. Similar to norepinephrine but less potent, slower onset and longer duration of action.

<u>Indication:</u>  Hypotension refractory to fluids. Bolus may be used in hypotension associated with MI or coronary intervention prior to availability of other catecholamine infusions.

<u>Kinetics:</u>  Onset 1-2 min IV, 10 min IM. Duration 20-60 minutes. Excreted renally.

<u>IV:</u>  Mix 100 mg in 500 mL NS or D5W. Administer dose according to a rate of infusion that maintains desired BP. In elderly, a bolus of 0.01 mg/kg and infusion rate of 0.05 mg/kg/h should provide reliable BP control. Wait 10 min prior to additional doses. No maximum dose.

<u>IM/SC:</u>  2-10 mg (IV route preferred; may cause local reactions including skin sloughing).

<u>Renal/liver disease:</u>  No adjustment; avoid in cirrhosis.

<u>Caution:</u>  Drug interactions with MAO inhibitor (increased pressor effects), tricyclics (decreased pressor effects) and halothanes (arrhythmias). May cause arrhythmias (β-

319  Emerson CH. Myxedema Coma. In: *Intensive Care Medicine*, 5th ed. Irwin RS, Rippe JM, editors. Philadelphia: Lippincott Williams & Wilkins, 2003.

320  Antman E. Early administration of intravenous magnesium to high-risk patients with acute myocardial infarction in the Magnesium in Coronaries (MAGIC) trial. *Lancet* 2002; 360:1189-96.

321  Wolf MA. Personal communication.

effect) or volume contraction (α-effect).

## Methylene Blue [322]

Action: Reduces methemoglobin from ferric to ferrous state via NADPH-dehydrogenase. Requires NADPH generated by pentose phosphate pathway, itself requiring G6PD.

Indication: Symptomatic methemoglobinemia > 40%. Note: remove toxins as warranted with charcoal, catharsis, hemodialysis. Exchange transfusion or hemodialysis indicated if > 70% MetHb.

IV: 1-2 mg/kg of 1% solution, repeat in 1 hr if cyanosis persists.

Contraindication: G6PD deficiency (causes hemolysis). Consider alternative treatment with ascorbic acid.

Adverse reactions: Colors urine bright blue-green. Irritates bladder. Cumulative doses > 7mg/kg can cause dyspnea, chest pain, tremor, cyanosis, hemolysis.

## Midazolam [323] *(Versed)*

Action: Benzodiazepine used for sedation and as anticonvulsant. Also has amnestic, anxiolytic, and muscle relaxant properties. **Note:** High risk for respiratory depression. Dose must be individualized and titrated to desired effect. Hemodynamic and oximetric monitoring is **essential**.

Kinetics: Liver metabolism, renal excretion. Onset 2-5 min, T½ 3 -11h.

IV: **Procedural sedation:** 0.01-0.05 mg/kg IV over 2 min repeated prn Q10-15 min or 0.07- 0.1 mg/kg IM. Observe for 2 min before re-bolusing; > 5 mg usually unnecessary. Use 0.25-0.5 mg as initial IV dose in elderly. Reduce dose by 30% if pre-treatment with narcotic. **Continuous infusion for ventilated patient:** Bolus 0.02 - 0.08 mg/kg, then infuse 0.04 - 0.2 mg/kg.hr. **Status epilepticus:** Bolus 0.2 mg/kg IV, then infuse 0.75- 10 mcg/kg/min (adjusted to EEG monitoring). Therapeutic levels may require intubation and blood pressure support.

Renal failure: T½ unchanged, distribution different. Use 50% for CrCl <10.

Contraindications: Narrow-angle glaucoma.

Adverse reactions: Respiratory depression, hypotension.

Pregnancy: Teratogenic.

## Milrinone *(Primacor)*

Action: Phosphodiesterase-III inhibitor used as inotrope-vasodilator in CHF. Also see inamrinone (page 192).

IV: Add 80 mL NS or D5W to 20mg/20mL vial to make 200 mcg/mL. Load 50 mcg/kg over 10 min, then infuse 0.375 (minimum), 0.50 (standard), or 0.75 mcg/kg/min. Duration typically less than 72 hr.

Kinetics: Onset 5-15 min. Terminal elimination T½ 2.4 hr. 70% protein-bound, 80% urine elimination, remainder glucuronide.

Renal Failure: Adjustments in bolus may be necessary. Infusion adjusted based on CrCl (mL/min): for 50 mL/min give 0.43 mcg/kg/min, decrease infusion by 0.05 mcg/kg/min for every additional 10 mL/min decrease in CrCl (to 10ml/min). For CrCl 5ml/min, rate is 0.2 mcg/kg/min.

Incompatibility: Precipitates IV furosemide.

Caution: Studies of long-term oral milrinone for treatment of CHF suggest ↑ mortality.

Side Effects: Hypotension, tachycardia, aggravates ventricular arrhythmia, accelerates ventricular response to atrial fibrillation. Headache. Contains bisulfite.

## Mivacurium (Mivacron)

*See Neuromuscular Blockers on page 198*

[322] Jaffe ER. Methaemoglobinemia. *Clin Haematol* 1981;10(1):99; Mansouri A. Review: methemoglobinemia. *Am J Med Sci* 1985;289(5):200.

[323] Jacobi J *et al.* Clinical practice guidelines for the sustained use of sedatives and analgesics in the critically ill adult. *Crit Care Med* 2002; 30:119-41.

# Naloxone *(Narcan)*
<u>Action</u>: Direct opiate competitive antagonist, no agonist properties. Indicated in opiate overdose, reversal of opiate sedation/hypotension.
<u>Kinetics</u>: T½30-80 minutes in adults. IM more prolonged than IV. Liver metabolism.
<u>IV/IM/SC</u>: **Opiate intoxication**: 0.4-2 mg (1-5 mL) IV q2-3 min to total 10mg, then question opiate intoxication. **Postop**: 0.1- 0.2 mg IV q2-3min. **Infusion**: mix 2mg/250mL= 0.008 mg/mL; 50mL/h = 0.4mg/h. Give 0.4-0.8 mg/h titrated to effect, or give 2/3 dose that caused reversal hourly.
<u>Renal failure</u>: No dosage adjustment.
<u>Caution</u>: Abrupt reversal of narcotic depression can cause HTN, tachycardia, N/V, tremulousness, seizures (especially with meperidine), cardiac arrest. Narcotic half-life may exceed that of naloxone. Large doses needed for pentazocine or propoxyphene.
<u>Incompatibility</u>: polyanions (heparin, albumin), alkali, bisulfite.


## Neostigmine
*See Anticholinesterases on page 175*


## Nesiritide [324] (*Natrecor*)
<u>Action</u>: Recombinant human B-type natriuretic peptide binds guanylate cyclase natriuretic peptide A/B receptors, promoting smooth muscle relaxation and dilation of arteries and veins. Dose-dependent decreases in left ventricular filling pressures and systemic arterial pressure in patients with heart failure. Not associated with ventricular ectopy compared with dobutamine. [325] Overall utility remains uncertain.
<u>Indication</u>: Acute decompensated heart failure with dyspnea at rest or minimal activity
<u>Kinetics</u>: Eliminated via liposomal proteolysis, proteolytic cleavage by endopeptidases, and renal filtration. T½=18 min
<u>IV</u>: Mix 1.5 mg into 250 mL D5W, NS, or ½ NS. Bolus 2 mcg/kg over 60 sec, then give 0.01 mcg/kg/min IV infusion. Dose may be titrated no more frequently than every 3 hours by bolusing 1 mcg/kg and increasing rate by 0.005 mcg/kg/min to a maximum of 0.03 mcg/kg/min. Little experience with use for more than 48 hours.
<u>Renal impairment</u>: No dosage adjustment.
<u>Hepatic dysfunction</u>: Avoid use if cirrhosis with ascites or significant sodium retention (non-renal, non-cardiac) due to blunting of natriuretic response.
<u>Adverse effects</u>: Hypotension, headache, nausea, back pain, ventricular arrhythmias.
<u>Contraindications</u>: Cardiogenic shock , hypotension.
<u>Caution</u>: Dose limiting hypotension may occur during therapy. Discontinue and institute supportive measures, then restart at 30% of the initial dose. Use caution in patients with significant valvular stenosis, pericarditis, pericardial tamponade, or low filling pressures.
<u>Incompatibility</u>: Heparin (including coated catheters), ethacrynate sodium, bumetanide, enalaprilat, hydralazine, and furosemide. Use solution within 24 hours of reconstitution.
<u>Pregnancy</u>: Category C

---

324 Colucci WS *et al*. Intravenous nesiritide, a natriuretic peptide, in the treatment of decompensated congestive heart failure. *NEJM* 2000; 343:246-253; de Lemos JA *et al*. B-type natriuretic peptide in cardiovascular disease. *Lancet*. 2003;362:316-22.

325 Burger AJ *et al*. Comparison of the effects of dobutamine and nesiritide (B-type natriuretic peptide) on ventricular ectopy in acutely decompensated ischemic versus nonischemic cardiomyopathy. Am J Cardiol. 2003;91:1370-2.

# Neuromuscular blockers [326]

Warning: In patients not already intubated, neuromuscular blockers should be used only by physicians skilled in advanced airway management including endotracheal intubation.

Action: Quaternary ammonium compounds that block motor response at neuromuscular junction (nicotinic acetylcholine receptor). Most are non-depolarizing agents, which block acetylcholine action without altering resting electrical potential. Succinylcholine is a depolarizing agent and has biphasic response: phase I produces tetany and twitching from depolarization and electrolyte shifts; phase II resemble non-depolarizing block. Sequentially affect eyes, face, neck THEN limbs, abdomen, chest THEN diaphragm. Ideally, ongoing blockade should be monitored by twitch response from an electrical nerve stimulator in addition to clinical assessment of voluntary muscle movements. Adequate tidal volumes with T-piece breathing may **not** predict ability to maintain airway if extubated.

Side-effects: **Histamine release:** Most with succinylcholine; less with vecuronium, rocuronium, and cisatracurium. **Cardiovascular:** Hypotension, tachycardia, bronchospasm, conduction abnormalities; seen to some degree in all agents, but least with vecuronium and newer agents (rocuronium, cisatracurium, and mivacurium). **Malignant hyperthermia:** Treat with dantrolene (see page 179) $\pm$ procainamide. **Muscarinic side effects:** Bradycardia, hypotension, salivation; blocked by pre-treatment with atropine.

Reversal: Nondepolarizing agents with cholinesterase inhibitors (neostigmine or pyridostigmine) plus atropine; IV calcium.

Caution/Interactions: Hyperkalemia may occur, especially with succinylcholine (exacerbated by digoxin). Neuromuscular blockade accentuated in presence of myasthenia gravis or myasthenic syndromes, hypothyroidism, dehydration, aminoglycosides; effects also potentiated by hypokalemia, hypocalcemia, hypermagnesemia, respiratory acidosis, metabolic alkalosis, hypothermia, and liver failure. Extended infusion may result in prolonged neuromuscular blockade, especially with steroidal agents (pancuronium and vecuronium); risk factors include renal failure and high-dose steroid use for associated asthma.[327] Syndrome often but not always associated with elevated CK levels. All chemically paralyzed patients should receive adequate sedation and analgesia, as well as eye protection and proper positioning to prevent pressure sores, nerve palsies, etc.

## Atracurium (*Tracrium*)

Indication: Paralysis in mechanically ventilated patient.
Dose: 0.4- 0.5 mg/kg IV bolus or 4-12 mcg/kg/min continuous infusion.
Kinetics: Onset 2-8 minutes, duration 25-35 minutes.
Advantages: No cardiovascular effects. Safe in renal dysfunction.
Disadvantages: Metabolite (laudanosine) accumulates in liver failure and may cause possible CNS effects. Histamine release at higher doses.

## Cisatracurium (*Nimbex*)

Indication: Paralysis in mechanically ventilated patient.
Dose: 0.1- 0.2mg/kg IV bolus or 2.5-3 mcg/kg/min continuous infusion.
Kinetics: Onset 2-8 minutes, duration 45-60 minutes.
Advantages: No cardiovascular effects or histamine release. Can be used with liver and renal dysfunction. Pregnancy category B.
Disadvantages: May cause prolonged neuromuscular blockade.

---

326 Murray MJ et al. Clinical practice guidelines for sustained neuromuscular blockade in the adult critically ill patient. Crit Care Med 2002; 30:142-56

327 Segredo V et al. Persistent paralysis in critically ill patients after long-term administration of vecuronium. NEJM 1992;327(8):524-8.

## Doxacurium (Nuromax)

Indication: Paralysis in mechanically ventilated patient.
Dose: Bolus 0.05 - 0.1 mg/kg or 0.3 - 0.5 mcg/kg/min continuous infusion.
Kinetics: Onset 5 minute. Duration 60-80 minutes.
Advantages: No cardiovascular effects or histamine release.
Disadvantages: Prolonged effect in renal dysfunction.

## Mivacurium (Mivacron)

Indication: Paralysis in mechanically ventilated patient.
Maintenance Dose: Initially 9-10 mcg/kg/min, then usually 6-7 mcg/kg/min continuous infusion.
Kinetics: Onset 2-6 minute, duration 10-20 minutes.
Advantages: No adverse hemodynamic effects.
Disadvantages: Histamine release; extended duration of action in both renal and hepatic failure. Little data to support use as continuous infusion in ICU.

## Pancuronium (Pavulon)

Indication: Paralysis in mechanically ventilated patient.
Dose: Bolus 0.06-0.1mg/kg; repeat incremental doses of 0.01 mg/kg q 25-60min or infuse 1-2 mcg/kg/min.
Kinetics: Onset 2-3 minutes, duration 90-100 minutes.
Disadvantage: Caution in renal failure because of reduced plasma clearance and doubling of half-life. Recovery of blockade may be slower in renal failure. Cardiovascular side effects.
Advantage: Inexpensive.

## Rocuronium (Zemuron)

Indications: May be used for intubation as well as paralysis in ventilated patient.
Dose: Intubation: 0.6-1.0 mg/kg IV. Maintenance: 0.1- 0.2 mg/kg as bolus or 10-12 mcg/kg/min continuous infusion.
Kinetics: Onset 60-90 sec, duration 30 minutes.
Advantages: No histamine release or cardiovascular effects. Safe in renal failure and liver disease. Pregnancy class B. Non-depolarizing alternative to succinylcholine for intubation.

## Succinylcholine

Indications: Intubation; sub-optimal for long-term paralysis of ventilated patient.
Dose: Intubation: 0.6-1.1 mg/kg IV. No maintenance bolus; infusion 0.5-10 mg/min (1 mg/mL).
Kinetics: Onset 1 minute, duration 4-6 min. Rapidly hydrolyzed in plasma.
Advantage: Rapid onset; doesn't cross placenta. Kidney-independent.
Disadvantages: Depolarization causes hyperkalemia (usual increase 0.5 mEq/L); avoid in predisposed patients, e.g. renal insufficiency, burns, crush injury. Prolonged paralysis with decreased hepatic production of cholinesterase. Vasopressor action may increase intracranial pressure. Avoid in stroke, 48 hr-6 mo after head or spinal cord injury (proliferation of postjunctional receptors may cause denervation hypersensitivity). Bradyarrhythmias (rare in adults; prophylax with atropine).

## Vecuronium (Norcuron)

Indications: Primarily used for paralysis of ventilated patient. May be used for intubation although onset slower compared to other agents.
Dose: Intubation: 0.08-0.10 mg/kg IV. Maintenance: 0.8-1.2 mcg/kg/min infusion.
Kinetics: Onset 60-90 sec, duration 25-30 minutes.
Advantages: No histamine release or related adverse hemodynamic effects.
Disadvantages: May cause prolonged neuromuscular blockade, especially in ESRD.

## Comparison summary of neuromuscular blockers

| | Cis-Atracurium | Doxa-curium | Miva-curium | Pancur-onium | Rocur-onium | Succinyl-choline | Vecur-onium |
|---|---|---|---|---|---|---|---|
| **Onset** | Intermed | Slow | Intermed | Intermed | Rapid | Ultrarapid | Rapid |
| **Duration** | Intermed | Long | Short | Long | Intermed | Ultrashort | Intermed |
| **Renal failure\*** | Yes | No | No | No | Yes | Yes | No |
| **Liver failure\*** | Yes | Yes | Yes | No | Yes | No | No |
| **Histamine release** | No | No | Yes | No | No | Yes | No |
| **Cardiovascular effects** | No | No | No | Yes | No | Yes | No |

\* May be used without dosage adjustment in these conditions

# Nicardipine IV *(Cardene)*

Action: Dihydropyridine calcium-channel blocker relaxes vascular >> cardiac smooth muscle. Used as parenteral antihypertensive as alternative to nitroprusside.
Kinetics: Onset 5-15 min, duration 3 hr. Rapid hepatic clearance.
IV: Mix 25 mg ampule in 240 mL fluid (0.1 mg/mL). Infuse 5 mg/h (50mL/h), titrate additional 2.5 mg/h q 5-15 min until desired BP or maximum 15 mg/h.
Transition to oral: Give PO nicardipine 1 hr before discontinuing infusion. 20 mg PO q 8 ≅ 0.5 mg/h; 30 mg PO q 8 ≅ 1.2 mg/h; 40 mg PO q 8 ≅ 2.2 mg/h.
Renal failure: No dosage adjustment.
Liver failure: Delayed clearance. May exacerbate portal hypertension.
Contraindication: Critical aortic valvular stenosis.
Caution: Causes reflex tachycardia, which may provoke/exacerbate myocardial ischemia. Negative inotrope in severe left ventricular dysfunction. Decreases GFR in renal dysfunction.
Interactions: Beta and calcium channel blockers have additive hypotensive effects. Levels increased by cimetidine. Increases cyclosporine levels.
Pregnancy: Class C. Embryocidal in certain animals.

# Nitrite

*See "Overdose" under the "Nitroprusside" section on page 202*

# Nitroglycerin

Action: Dose-dependent arterial and venous vasodilator. Increases coronary perfusion, decreases MVO$_2$, left ventricular filling pressure, pulmonary and systemic vascular resistance. Reduces infarct extent in acute MI. Improves cardiac output when combined with dobutamine in ischemic heart failure.
Kinetics: Plasma half-life 1-4 min.
IV: Mix 25 mg in 250 mL D5W or NS (100mcg/mL). Begin 10-20 mcg/min (6-12mL/h), titrate 10-20 mcg/min increments q 3-5min. Predominant hypotensive effect > 200 mcg/min.
Ointment: Antianginal onset 30 min. Begin 0.5 inch q 8h until desired effects achieved.
**Explosive** during cardioversion.
Renal failure: Half-life unchanged. No dosage adjustment.
Contraindication: Increased intracranial pressure or decreased cerebral perfusion; narrow-angle glaucoma; pre-load dependent states (constrictive pericarditis, pericardial tamponade, right ventricular infarct).
Side effects: Headache, N/V/abd discomfort, dizziness, dermatitis.
Note: Absorbed by plastic/PVC; usually mixed in glass bottle. If PVC tubing used, start at 25 mcg/min.

# Nitroprusside (Nipride)

<u>Action:</u> Arterial and venous vasodilator . Used for afterload reduction in acute heart failure, mitral regurgitation, aortic insufficiency, ventricular septal defect. Antihypertensive for most causes of severe hypertension including pheochromocytoma. Useful in aortic stenosis with decompensated heart failure in spite of prior adverse reports. [328] Free nitroso group (NO) inhibits excitation-contraction coupling of vascular, not visceral, smooth muscle. Reacts with hemoglobin to yield methemoglobin and unstable compound releasing cyanide. Cyanide converted (using thiosulfate) in liver and kidney to thiocyanate.

<u>Kinetics:</u> $T\frac{1}{2}$ < 10 min.

<u>IV:</u> Mix 50mg in 250mL D5W (200 mcg/mL). Range 0.5-10 mcg/kg/min. Titrate upwards to desired BP incrementally q 3-15 min, do not exceed 10 mcg/kg/min rate for >10 minutes. **Withdraw slowly** to avoid rebound vasoconstriction.

<u>Renal failure:</u> Half-life unchanged. No dosage adjustment. However, thiocyanate accumulates (removed by dialysis).

<u>Levels:</u> Blood cyanide not predictive of tissue levels or of toxicity. Follow **thiocyanate** daily after 24-48 hr infusion, especially if abnormal CNS function at baseline. Symptoms at 60 mcg/ml; "toxicity" at 100 mcg/ml. No problems usually when infused < 72h at less than 3 mcg/kg/min (normal kidneys) or less than 1 mcg/kg/min (anuric). Thiocyanate elimination $T\frac{1}{2}$ of 3 days (normals), 9 days (renal dysfunction). Keep **methemoglobin** < 10%.

<u>Toxicity:</u> Manifested clinically by tinnitus, blurred vision, confusion, psychosis, seizure, delirium, lactic acidosis, marrow suppression, pink color, electromechanical dissociation. Metabolic acidosis or failure to respond to adequate infusion may represent increased free cyanide. Infusion of **hydroxycobalamin** (not cyanocobalamin) 25 mg/h may reduce cyanide toxicity. Cyanide accumulates in liver disease; thiocyanate accumulates in renal dysfunction.

<u>Contraindications:</u> Severe liver disease (rhodanase deficiency), vitamin B12 deficiency, hypothyroidism (exacerbated by thiocyanate), aortic dissection, aortic coarctation, Leber congenital optic atrophy or tobacco amblyopia (absent rhodanase).

<u>Caution:</u> Hypovolemia, renal or liver disease, cerebrovascular disease.

<u>Overdose:</u> (1) Amyl nitrite (1 capsule over 15-30 sec); repeat q 3-5 minutes until sodium nitrite available (2) 3% sodium nitrite 4-6 mg/kg IV (0.2 mL/kg) over 2-4 minutes , may repeat 50% dose if response after 2 hr (3) Sodium thiosulfate 150-200 mg/kg (typically 50 mL of 25% solution) IV over 10min (4) Hemodialysis for severe thiocyanate toxicity (5) Methylene blue for methemoglobinemia

<u>Pregnancy:</u> Class C; considered $2^{nd}$-line in preeclampsia after hydralazine and labetalol.

# Norepinephrine (Levophed)

<u>Indications:</u> (1) Cardiogenic shock unresponsive to dopamine, dobutamine, or intraaortic balloon pump (2) Cardiogenic shock or pulseless electrical activity due to pulmonary embolism (3) Refractory hypotension in tricyclic overdose.

<u>Action:</u> Potent β-1 and α-agonist. No β-2 action (unlike epinephrine). β-1 prominent at low doses; α-1 predominates at higher doses. Vasoconstriction increases afterload and $M_VO_2$, decreases splanchnic perfusion and exacerbates peripheral ischemia, but spares cerebral and coronary circulation, which have fewer α-adrenergic receptors. Baroreceptor stimulation causes net balanced heart rate and cardiac output. Chronic use causes decreased circulatory volume related to vasoconstriction. Often used concurrently with low-dose dopamine. Compared with epinephrine: half as potent chronotrope and inotrope, equipotent vasoconstrictor, no vasodilator properties, less demand on $M_VO_2$, less arrhythmogenic. May exacerbate mitral and aortic regurgitation.

<u>Kinetics:</u> Rapid onset, duration 1-2 minutes.

<u>IV:</u> Mix 4,6,8 mg in 250mL D5W (not NS) = 16,24,32 mcg/mL. Initial 0.5-1mcg/min, max 30 mcg/min. Incompatible with alkali.

---

[328] Khot UN *et al.* Nitroprusside in critically ill patients with left ventricular dysfunction and aortic stenosis. *NEJM* 2003;348:1756-63.

**Groovy Drugs**

<u>Cautions</u>: Avoid extravasation; use long peripheral IV or central lines. BP tracing via peripheral arterial lines may be artifactually damped by vasoconstriction. Suspect volume depletion if hypotension develops, especially with chronic use. Correct hypocalcemia to preserve contractility.

<u>Extravasation</u>: See phentolamine page 204.

## Octreotide *(Sandostatin)*

<u>Action</u>: Synthetic somatostatin analogue. Suppresses release of gastrointestinal peptides including gastrin, VIP, insulin, glucagon, secretin, motilin. Also decreases splanchnic blood flow. Used IV to control bleeding from esophageal varices; also used SC for VIPomas & carcinoids, intractable diarrhea as in AIDS, chronic fistulae.

<u>Kinetics</u>: T½ 1.5-1.7h. Hepatic metabolism and renal excretion.

<u>IV</u>: Mix 1200 mcg in 250 mL D5W. **Variceal esophageal hemorrhage:** 25-50 mcg bolus, then 25-50 mcg/h × 5 days. [329]

<u>SC</u>: Begin 50 mcg SC qd, advance prn up to 600 mcg/day divided bid-qid.

<u>Interactions</u>: Reduces insulin requirements. Incompatible with insulin when mixed in TPN.

<u>Adverse effects</u>: Biliary sludge & stones, pancreatitis. Injection site pain. Nausea, vomiting, abdominal pain.

## Opiate analgesics [330]

| | Approximate equianalgesic | | Recommended starting dose | | | |
|---|---|---|---|---|---|---|
| | | | Adults >50kg | | Children/Adults 8 to 50 kg | |
| | IV / SC / IM | PO | IV / SC / IM | PO | IV / SC / IM | PO |
| **Opioid Agonists** | | | | | | |
| morphine | 10 mg q3-4h | †30 mg q3-4h †60 mg q3-4h | 10 mg q3-4h | 30 mg q3-4h | 0.1 mg/kg q3-4h | 0.3 mg/kg q3-4h |
| codeine | 75 mg q3-4h | 130 mg q3-4h | 60 mg q2h | 60 mg q3-4h | n/r | 1 mg/kg q3-4h |
| fentanyl | 0.1 mg q1h | n/a | 0.1 mg q1h | n/a | n/r | n/a |
| hydromorphone | 1.5 mg q3-4h | 7.5 mg q3-4h | 1.5 mg q3-4h | 6 mg q3-4h | 0.015 mg/kg q3-4h | 0.06 mg/kg q3-4h |
| hydrocodone | n/a | 30 mg q3-4h | n/a | 10 mg q3-4h | n/a | 0.2 mg/kg q3-4h |
| levorphanol | 2 mg q6-8h | 4 mg q6-8h | 2 mg q6-8h | 4 mg q6-8h | 0.02 mg/kg q6-8h | 0.04 mg/kg q6-8h |
| meperidine§ | 100 mg q3h | 300 mg q2-3h | 100 mg q3h | n/r | 0.75 mg/kg q2-3h | n/r |
| oxycodone | n/a | 30 mg q3-4h | n/a | 10 mg q3-4h | n/a | 0.2 mg/kg q3-4h |
| oxymorphone | 1 mg q3-4h | n/a | 1 mg q3-4h | n/a | n/r | n/r |
| **Opioid Agonist-Antagonist and Partial Agonist** | | | | | | |
| buprenorphine | 0.3-0.4 mg q6-8h | n/a | 0.4 mg q6-8h | n/a | 0.004 mg/kg q6-8h | n/a |
| butorphanol | 2 mg q3-4h | n/a | 2 mg q3-4h | n/a | n/a | n/a |
| nalbuphine | 10 mg q3-4h | n/a | 10 mg q3-4h | n/a | 0.1 mg/kg q3-4h | n/a |
| pentazocine | 60 mg q3-4h | 150 mg q3-4h | n/r | 50 mg q4-6h | n/r | n/r |

[329] Sung JJY et al. Octreotide infusion or emergency sclerotherapy for variceal haemorrhage. *Lancet* 1993; 342:637-41.

[330] Reprinted with permission from *The Pocket Deluxe Pharmacopoeia*, 2004 edition. Green S (ed).

* Approximate dosing, adapted from 1992 AHCPR guidelines, www.ahcpr.gov. All PO dosing is with immediate-release preparations. Individualize all dosing, especially in the elderly, children, and patients with chronic pain, opioid tolerance, or hepatic/renal insufficiency. Many recommend initially using lower than equivalent doses when switching between different opioids. Not available = "n/a". Not recommended = "n/r". Do not exceed 4g/day of acetaminophen or aspirin when using opioid combination formulations. Methadone is excluded due to poor consensus on equivalence.

† 30 mg with around the clock dosing, and 60 mg with a single dose or short-term dosing (i.e., the opioid-naïve).

§ Doses should be limited to <600 mg/24 hr and total duration of use <48 hr; not for chronic pain.

## Pamidronate *(Aredia)* [331]

Indications: Hypercalcemia, especially malignancy-related. Also used in osteoporosis (not FDA approved) and Paget's disease. Inhibits bone reabsorption via osteoclast inactivation.

IV: Dilute dose in 1000 mL NS or D5W and infuse over 2-24 hr. Dose based on serum calcium: for $[Ca^{++}]$ 12-13.5 mg/dL give 60-90 mg; for $[Ca^{++}]$ > 13.5 mg/dL give 90 mg.

Pharmacokinetics: Onset 1-2 days, peak action 6 days in malignancy. Excreted unchanged by kidney, but no dose adjustment in renal failure.

Toxicity: Fever in 20%; hypertension, thrombophlebitis, nausea.

Caution: "Overshoot" hypocalcemia (also low Mg, $PO_4$, $K^+$); may exacerbate pre-existing myelosuppression.

Pregnancy: Class C.

## Pancuronium

*See Neuromuscular blockers on page 198*

## Phenobarbital

Action: Barbiturate used in generalized and partial seizures.

Kinetics: Peak onset 30-60 minutes. Elimination 25% renal unchanged, 75% liver metabolites via urine. $T\frac{1}{2}$ 53-118 hr.

IV: 15-20 mg/kg load at 50-100 (ideally <60) mg/minute; if seizures persist may re-bolus 5-10 mg/kg to maximum of 30 mg/kg.

Maintenance: 60-250 mg/day PO (bioavailability 70-90%) divided bid-tid.

Levels: Therapeutic: 10-25 mcg/mL; acute therapy: 15 -40 mcg/mL; coma: >65 mcg/mL.

Renal failure: Give q 12-16 hr for CrCl < 10 mL/min. Supplement full dose after hemodialysis or hemofiltration; ½ dose after peritoneal dialysis.

Side effects: Respiratory depression, marked hypotension. Sedation, nystagmus and ataxia at toxic levels. Agitation and confusion in elderly and those with cognitive impairment. Maculopapular, morbilliform, scarlatiniform rashes 1-3%; erythema multiforme or Stevens-Johnson syndrome rarely. Chronic: folate and vit. D deficiency.

Drug interactions: Induces hepatic microsome oxidase. Decreases levels of phenytoin, warfarin, beta blockers, corticosteroids, contraceptives, quinidine, doxycycline, vitamin D. Increases levels of tricyclics. Displaces thyroxine from albumin. Causes production of toxic metabolites of chlorocarbon anesthetics and carbon tetrachloride.

## Phentolamine *(Regitine)*

Action: Nonspecific α-adrenergic antagonist used in excess adrenergic states, e.g. pheochromocytoma, clonidine withdrawal, MAO inhibitor drug interactions, cocaine toxicity. Also used to limit skin necrosis from extravasation of catecholamines.

Kinetics: Liver metabolism. Plasma $T\frac{1}{2}$ 19 min.

IV: Pheochromocytoma: 5mg IV/IM given 1-2 hr preoperatively, titrate for effect.

---

331 Gucalp R *et al.* Treatment of cancer-associated hypercalcemia. *Arch Int Med* 1994; 154(17):1935-44.

Sympathomimetic hypertensive crisis: 5-10 mg IV q 5 minutes to total of 20-30 mg. Administer prior to β-blocker to prevent unopposed α-mediated vasoconstriction.
<u>Extravasation of catecholamines</u>: Infiltrate area liberally with 5-10 mg/10-mL NS via 25g needle (should cause conspicuous hyperemia if used within 12 hr).
<u>Overdose</u>: Fluids, norepinephrine (**not** epinephrine).

# Phenylephrine (Neo-Synephrine)

<u>Indications</u>: Refractory hypotension or shock; spinal anesthesia or drug-related hypotension. Good anesthesia pressor in combination with cardiac irritants like cyclopropane or halothane.
<u>Action</u>: Postsynaptic alpha adrenergic agonist with virtually no beta activity. Vasoconstrictor as potent as norepinephrine but almost entirely without chronotropic or inotropic activity. Less demand on $M_VO_2$ compared to epinephrine or dopamine. Causes marked reflex bradycardia (prevented by atropine). Less arrhythmogenic than other catecholamines. Constricts coronary, cerebral, and pulmonary vessels. Exacerbates mitral and aortic regurgitation.
<u>Dose</u>: Bolus: 0.1-0.5 mg IV q 15 minutes. Continuous infusion: mix 10 mg in 250 mL NS or D5W, start at 100-180 mcg/min. Titrate down to maintenance dose, usually 40-60 mcg/min. Maximum infusion rate not specified by manufacturer (add 10 mg increments to infusion bag to maintain acceptable infusion rate).
<u>Caution</u>: MAO inhibitors, tricyclics, and oxytocic agents potentiate pressor effect; use vastly reduced doses of phenylephrine.

# Phenytoin (Dilantin)

<u>Indications</u>: First-line anticonvulsant for generalized, partial complex, or simple partial seizures. **Not** used in absence, myoclonic, or atonic seizures. Used also for arrhythmias of digitalis toxicity and after tetralogy repair. Enhances AV node conduction.
<u>Kinetics</u>: Maximal therapeutic effect within 20-25 minutes of IV infusion. T½ 6-24 hr initially, 20-60 hr at therapeutic levels.
<u>IV</u>: Load 10-15 mg/kg not faster than 50mg/min; if refractory seizures may give additional 5-10 mg/kg doses to total of 30 mg/kg. Maintenance 100 mg IV q 6-8 hr. Observe for hypotension (28-50% of patients) and arrhythmia (2%), especially with rapid infusion. **Fosphenytoin** (a water-soluble prodrug) is measured in phenytoin equivalents (PEs) but dosing is the same; may be administered more rapidly at 100-150 mg/min and causes less hypotension. However, no apparent difference in time to onset of clinical effect.
<u>PO</u>: Load 400 mg, then 300 mg q 2h x 2; then initial maintenance dose of 100 mg PO tid. Once stable may switch to once-daily dosing if no adverse symptoms. Increase doses in increments of 30-50 mg. Steady-state levels not reached until 7-10 days after dose change.
<u>Levels</u>: Therapeutic 10-20 mcg/mL, may use up to 30-40 mcg/mL in comatose patient with status epilepticus. Obtain level 2 hr after IV load. Measure **free** phenytoin levels (therapeutic 1-2 mcg/mL) in renal or liver failure, albumin< 2.8, warfarin, sulfonamides, salicylates, valproate.
<u>Renal failure</u>: T½ unchanged. No adjustment; however, the active drug (free phenytoin) is completely dialyzed, such that patients may seize with "normal" total phenytoin levels during or after dialysis. See "levels" above.
<u>Side effects</u>: Hypotension given IV (due to propylene glycol vehicle); folate, vitamin D and vitamin K antagonism; inhibition of insulin release, interstitial nephritis.
<u>Toxicity</u>: Ataxia, diplopia, slurred speech, stupor.
<u>Hypersensitivity</u>: Fever, lymphadenopathy, eosinophilia, blood dyscrasias, polyarteritis, Stevens-Johnson.
<u>Interactions</u>: **Decrease phenytoin levels**: barbiturates, carbamazepine, sucralfate, chronic ethanol, calcium antacids, folic acid. **Increase phenytoin levels**: amiodarone, chloramphenicol, chlordiazepoxide, cimetidine, diazepam, disulfiram, estrogens, acute ethanol ingestion, isoniazid, metronidazole, omeprazole, phenothiazines, salicylates,

sulfonamides, trimethoprim, trazodone, valproate. Free phenytoin increased in hyperbilirubinemia, hypoalbuminemia, uremia. Tricyclics lower seizure threshold. **Action altered by phenytoin:** Increases metabolism (decreases effectiveness) of multiple drugs including amiodarone, antibiotics, carbamazepine, digoxin, estrogens, oral contraceptives; also decreases effects of immunosuppressants, and neuromuscular blockers.

Pregnancy: Fetal hydantoin syndrome, neonatal coagulopathy; however, short-term use probably safe.

## Phosphorus [332]

PO: 1-2 g daily in 3 divided doses, increment as tolerated. Milk (skim 1 L = 1 g P). Neutra-Phos 4 × 1250 mg tabs = 1 g P + 28.5mEq Na + 28.5mEq K; Neutra-Phos-K 4 × 1450 mg tabs = 1 g P + 57mEq K.

IV: Reserve for patients who are symptomatic or unable to tolerate PO. Dispensed as 94 mg = 3 mmol phosphorus + 4.4 mEq Na or K per mL. Give 0.08-0.16mmol/kg in 50-500mL fluid over 6 hr; alternatively, administer the following in maintenance fluids in q 12 hr boluses infused over 6 hr. Subsequent dosing by serum levels.

| Serum PO₄ | Initial IV dose (mmol/kg ideal body weight per day) | |
|---|---|---|
| (mg/dL) | *Uncomplicated* | *Symptoms, chronic, or multifactorial* |
| 1.6-2.1 | 0.15 | 0.15-0.3 |
| 1.2-1.5 | 0.15-0.3 | 0.3 |
| 0.8-1.1 | 0.3 | 0.3-0.45 |
| < 0.8 | 0.45-0.6 | 0.6 |

Caution: May cause hypocalcemic tetany (especially if given rapidly), tissue calcification, and hyperkalemia. Large oral doses may cause diarrhea.

Interactions: Precipitates in fluids with calcium gluconate > 9.6 mEq/L.

## Physostigmine

See "Anticholinesterases" on page 175

## Pralidoxime (2-PAM, *Protopam*) [333]

Action: Quaternary ammonium reactivates acetylcholinesterase rendered inactive by organophosphate insecticides. Also directly detoxifies certain organophosphates. Used to reverse (respiratory) muscle paralysis. Possible use to reverse overdose of carbamate anticholinesterase drugs (e.g. neostigmine, pyridostigmine) but less effective and controversial. [334] Possible role in tetanus. Effectively reverses nicotinic toxicity (skeletal muscle, sympathetic ganglia); less effective against muscarinic effects but synergistic with atropine. Most effective given within 48 hr of exposure, indicated in all symptomatic exposures and those with RBC cholinesterase < 50% normal.

Kinetics: Onset 5-15 min IV, T½ 7-77 min. Renal excretion.

IV: 150 mg/kg (1-2 g) over 30 min. Repeat in 1 hr if muscle weakness continues or give 500 mg/h continuous infusion. Repeat q 6-12 hr for 24-48 hr. Pre-treat with atropine 2-4 mg IV. Reduce dose for renal insufficiency, elderly or frail. **Carbamate anticholinesterase toxicity:** After atropine as above, 1-2 g IV then 250 mg IV q 5 min until reversal. Max infusion rate is 200 mg/min.

Caution: May precipitate myasthenic crisis. Reduce in renal failure.

Interactions: Theophylline, aminophylline, succinylcholine, respiratory depressants.

Adverse effects: Rapid infusion may cause tachycardia, laryngospasm, neuromuscular blockade, hypertension (difficult to distinguish from organophosphate toxicity).

---

[332] Desai TK *et al.* Hypocalcemia and hypophosphatemia in acutely ill patients. *Crit Care Clin* 1987; 3(4):927-41. Solomon SM, Kirby DF. The refeeding syndrome: a review. *JPEN* 1990;14(1):90-7.

[333] Aaron CK, Howland MA. Insecticides: organophosphates and carbamates. In: *Goldfrank's Toxicologic Emergencies*, 6/e. Goldfrank LR, ed. Appleton & Lange: Stamford, CT, 1998.

[334] Kurtz PH. Pralidoxime in the treatment of carbamate intoxication. *Am J Emerg Med* 1990;8(1):68-70. Lifshitz M *et al.* Carbamate poisoning and oxime treatment in children. *Pediatrics* 1994;93(4):652-5.

# Procainamide

Indications: **(1)** Treatment of persistent, recurrent or intermittent ventricular fibrillation. **(2)** Treatment of wide-complex tachycardias of unclear etiology (in presence of normal ventricular function). **(3)** Pharmacologic conversion or suppression of supraventricular tachycardias (particularly atrial fibrillation or flutter) **(4)** Control of rapid ventricular rate via accessory pathway conduction in pre-excitation syndromes

Action: Class IA antiarrhythmic. Depresses conduction velocity and automaticity, prolongs refractoriness of atrial and ventricular myocardium and of accessory pathways while shortening refractoriness (via anticholinergic activity) of AV node. Mild anticholinergic without α-adrenergic blockade of quinidine. Negative inotropy in severe heart failure. Prolongs P-R and Q-T intervals.

Metabolism: Acetylated to NAPA (20% of dose in slow and 30% of dose in fast-acetylators). NAPA excreted in urine; accumulates in renal failure. PCA associated with lupus-like syndrome; infrequent in rapid-acetylators, in whom procainamide levels are lower. Plasma half-life 3-4 hr.

IV: 20 mg/min until arrhythmia stops **or** adverse effect (QRS prolonged 50%, QT prolonged > 35%, or hypotension) **or** maximum total dose of 17 mg/kg. May give at rates of up to 50 mg/min as tolerated during emergencies. **Maintenance:** Mix 1g in 100 mL D5W at 12 mL/h = 2 mg/min. Range 1-4 mg/min. May give 100 mg IV push Q5 minutes in refractory VF/VT. [335]

PO: Total 2-6 g/day, begin at 50 mg/day. First dose once renal half-life (3-4 hr) after last IV dose. Regular formulation q 3-4 hr; sustained release q 6 hr or q 12 hr (Procanbid ®) in equivalent total dose. If CrCl 10-50 mL/min give q 6-12 hr; CrCl < 10mL/h give q 8-24 hr, following levels. Peak levels at 90 min after oral dose.

Therapeutic levels: Procainamide 3-10 mcg/mL, sometimes higher. NAPA 10-30 mcg/mL.

Renal failure: Procainamide T½ 5-6 hr; NAPA T½ 42-70h (normal 6-8h). Adjust per levels.

Contraindications: Complete AV block (may produce asystole), *torsades* or long QT.

Interactions: Increased levels with cimetidine, β-blockers, amiodarone.

Caution: Myasthenia gravis, renal insufficiency, atrial fibrillation or flutter (may accelerate ventricular response), negative inotrope in high-doses (esp. severe LV dysfunction). Prolongs sinus node recovery time in sick-sinus syndrome, unpredictable effects in digitalis toxicity, prolongs QT (may predispose to *torsades*). Rarely causes agranulocytosis or lupus-like syndromes. Hypotension at supratherapeutic concentrations, especially during IV load.

# Propofol [336] *(Diprivan)*

Action: Water-insoluble sedative-hypnotic produces rapid unconsciousness with short duration of action. Crosses blood-brain barrier rapidly, then redistributed and eliminated. Formulated as lipid emulsion.

Indications: **(1)** Rapid IV sedation for procedures **(2)** Maintenance sedation of mechanically ventilated patient **(3)** 3rd line agent for status epilepticus.

Kinetics: Onset 1-2 min, duration 3-10 minutes. V$_d$= 60L/kg reflects water-insolubility and extensive tissue redistribution. Plasma T½ 5 min after 1 hr infusion, 7 min after 10 hr infusion. Eliminated by hepatic conjugation then renal excretion.

IV: Premixed 10mg/mL; may dilute to no less than 2 mg/mL with D5W to decrease pain at injection site. **Sedation for procedures:** Slow injection of 0.5 mg/kg over 3-5 min, or begin infusion of 100-150 mcg/kg/min (6-9 mg/kg/hr). Follow with maintenance infusion of 25-75 mcg/kg/min. **Sedation for mechanical ventilation:** 5 mcg/kg/min × 5 min then increase 5-10 mcg/kg/min q 5-10 min until desired sedation; max ~ 80 mcg/kg/min. **Status epilepticus:** 1-2 mg/kg initially, followed by 30-150 mcg/kg/min

---

335 Guidelines 2000 for cardiopulmonary resuscitation and emergency cardiovascular care. *Circulation* 2000; 102(Suppl I).

336 Jacobi J et al. Clinical practice guidelines for the sustained use of sedatives and analgesics in the critically ill adult. *Crit Care Med* 2002; 30:119-41.

(adjusted to EEG results).

<u>Renal failure/liver disease</u>: No dose adjustment necessary.

<u>Adverse effects</u>: Dose-related myocardial depression, hypotension (often severe), respiratory depression or apnea, bradycardia. Pain at injection reduced with lidocaine or large vein. Lipid emulsion supports microbial overgrowth[337]; use sterile technique and replace drug and tubing q 12 hr.

<u>Interactions</u>: Concurrent opioids potentiate cardiopulmonary depression.

# Protamine

<u>Action</u>: Polycation from salmon sperm forms inactive complex with heparin, thereafter probably metabolized and fibrinolysed with release of some heparin. Weak anticoagulant effect via platelet and fibrinogen action. Neutralizes heparin instantly, but duration of protamine effect often shorter than heparin.

<u>IV</u>: 1 mg neutralizes ~ 100 units estimated circulating heparin (calculate assuming heparin T½ of 60 min). Give IV over 10 minutes in doses not > 50 mg. If 30-60 min have elapsed since heparin dose, give 0.5 to 0.75 mg per 100 units heparin. Further reduce dose to 0.25 mg if >2 hr since heparin dose. Less effective in LMW heparin overdose but still used: 1mg protamine/1 mg enoxaparin, 1mg protamine/100 units dalteparin or tinzaparin. Excessive protamine probably causes mild anticoagulation.

<u>Warning</u>: Prior sensitization may occur with NPH insulin, protamine, vasectomy; predisposes to possible anaphylactoid reactions. Rebound heparin effect and bleeding may occur 0.5-18 hr after protamine administration. Too-rapid administration causes hypotension and anaphylactoid reaction.

<u>Incompatibility</u>: Penicillins and cephalosporins.

# Pyridostigmine
*See Anticholinesterases on page 175*

# Reteplase (rPA; *Retavase*)
*See Thrombolytic Agents on page 209*

# Rocuronium *(Zemuron)*
*See Neuromuscular Blockers on page 198*

# Sodium polystyrene sulfonate *(Kayexalate)*

<u>Action</u>: Cation-exchange resin exchanges $K^+$ for $Na^+$ in the gut. Treats severe hyperkalemia by removing K from body. Binds ~ 1 mEq $K^+$ per gram sodium polystyrene sulfonate. Onset 2-12 hr PO; 30-90 min per rectum.

<u>PO</u>: 15-60 g Kayexalate + 50-100 mL 70% sorbitol q 2-6 hr.

<u>PR</u>: 30-50 g Kayexalate + 50 mL 70% sorbitol + 100 mL water as retention enema q 6 hr followed by cleansing enema.

<u>Adverse effects</u>: Hypomagnesemia, hypocalcemia, alkalosis, overshoot hypokalemia. Sodium load may precipitate heart failure. May cause constipation or impaction if used without laxative. Rare reports colonic necrosis when administered PR in uremic patients

# Streptokinase
*See Thrombolytic Agents on page 209*

# Succinylcholine
*See Neuromuscular blockers on page 198*

---

SN Bennet et al. Postoperative infections traced to contamination of an intravenous anesthetic, propofol. *NEJM* 1995; 333(3):147-54.

## Tenecteplase (TNK-tPA; *TNKase*)
*See Thrombolytic Agents on page 209*

### Thiosulfate
*See "Overdosage" section under Nitroprusside on page 202*

# Thrombolytic Agents

<u>Action</u>:  Convert plasminogen to plasmin, which degrades fibrin clots.  Recombinant agents (tPA, rPA, TNK-tPA) have higher affinity for fibrin-bound plasminogen than streptokinase; thought to produce less generalized "lytic state" but effect of unclear clinical significance.  Recombinant agents also have less potential for allergic reactions.  Thrombolytics reduce mortality and preserve LV function in acute MI[338]; reduce disability in acute stroke [339] but no clear mortality benefit; and reduce clinical deterioration in sub-massive pulmonary embolism.[340]  Benefit in all indications offset by significant incidence of serious bleeding including intracranial hemorrhage (ICH); risk of ICH lowest with streptokinase without heparin.

| Indications | Contraindications |
|---|---|
| **Acute MI (AMI)**[341]<br>1) ST elevation (> 0.1 mV, ≥ 2 contiguous leads);  time to therapy ≤ 12 hr; and age < 75 **or** LBBB and history suggesting AMI (Class I) #<br>2) ST elevation and age > 75 (IIa) #<br>3) As per (1) but time to therapy 12-24 hr (IIb) #<br>4) As per (1) but BP > 180/110 and high-risk MI (IIb) #<br>**Note:**  Benefit greatest with early therapy (< 3 hr); anterior > inferior MI (unless posterior or RV involvement); diabetes; hypotension or tachycardia. | **Absolute:**<br>• Previous hemorrhagic stroke (ever)<br>• Stroke or cerebrovascular event within 1 year<br>• Known intracranial neoplasm<br>• Active internal bleeding (other than menses)<br>• Suspected aortic dissection<br>**Relative:**<br>• Ready availability of high-volume interventional cardiac cath lab<br>• BP > 180/110 or history of chronic severe hypertension<br>• Prior stroke or known intracranial pathology other than above<br>• Bleeding diathesis, or warfarin and INR > 1.7<br>• Recent trauma or GI/GU bleeding (2-4 wks)<br>• Traumatic or prolonged CPR (> 10 min)<br>• Recent major surgery (within 2-3 wks)<br>• Noncompressible vascular punctures<br>• Age > 75 or weight < 67 kg (increased bleeding risk)<br>• Pregnancy<br>• Active peptic ulcer |

338  GUSTO investigators.  The effects of tissue-plasminogen activator, streptokinase, or both on coronary-artery patency, ventricular function, and survival after acute myocardial infarction. *NEJM* 1993; 329:1615.

339  Kasner SE, Grotta JC.  Ischemic stroke.  *Neurol Clin N Am* 1998; 16(2): 355-372.

340  Konstantinides S *et al.* Heparin plus alteplase compared with heparin alone in patients with submassive pulmonary embolism. *NEJM* 2002; 347:1143-1150.

341  Ryan TJ *et al.* 1999 Update: ACC/AHA guidelines for the management of patients with acute myocardial infarction.  Executive summary and recommendations. *Circulation* 1999; 100:1016-30.

| Indications | Contraindications |
|---|---|
| **Acute Ischemic Stroke**[342]<br>Clinical diagnosis of ischemic stroke with:<br>• Clinically meaningful deficit<br>• Onset within 3 hr<br>• Age > 18 yrs<br>• Non-contrast CT without evidence of hemorrhage<br>**Notes:**<br>• tPA is only approved agent<br>• Heparin/antiplatelet agents should be withheld for 24 hr after treatment<br>• While uncontrolled hypertension is a contraindication to tPA, aggressive BP control (goal less than 180/105) with labetalol +/- nitroprusside is required *after* tPA administration | As per AMI, with following modifications:<br>• Stroke or head trauma within 3 months<br>• History of intracranial hemorrhage<br>• Rapidly improving symptoms<br>• Seizure at stroke onset<br>• CT evidence of hemorrhage<br>• CT evidence of large thrombotic stroke (> 1/3 of MCA territory)<br>• Symptoms suggestive of subarachnoid hemorrhage, even if CT normal<br>• Persistent BP > 185/110 despite "non-aggressive" treatment (e.g. labetalol up to 40 mg IV)<br>• Acute MI or post-MI pericarditis (within 3 mo)<br>• Glucose < 50 mg/dL<br>• Platelets < 100K<br>• Heparin within 48 hr and PTT > normal |
| **Venous Thromboembolism (PE)**<br>Relative indications: [343]<br>• Hypotension related to PE<br>• Severe hypoxemia<br>• Moderate-severe right ventricular dysfunction from PE<br>• Free-floating right ventricular clot<br>• Extensive deep vein thrombosis | Same as per AMI |

\# Level of evidence for AMI – Class I: evidence or general agreement that treatment is beneficial, useful and effective; Class IIa: Weight of evidence/opinion is in favor of usefulness/efficacy. Class IIb: Usefulness/efficacy less well-established

Adverse effects: Major hemorrhage, especially intracranial. **Increased risk with age > 65, body weight < 70 kg, and hypertension on presentation.** Risk of intracranial hemorrhage much higher in acute ischemic stroke compared to myocardial infarction.

Reversal for hemorrhage [344]: FFP, cryoprecipitate, ε-aminocaproic acid.

## Alteplase [345] (tPA; *Activase*)

<u>Action</u>: Recombinant human tissue plasminogen activator

<u>Kinetics</u>: Plasma half-life 5-10 min, prolonged in liver failure.

<u>IV</u>: **Acute MI:** Front-loaded "GUSTO" regimen: [346] 15 mg IV bolus followed by 0.75 mg/kg infusion over 30 min (maximum 50 mg) and then 0.50 mg/kg over 60 min (maximum 35 mg). Combine with aspirin (165-325 mg) and IV heparin for ≥ 48 hr to aPTT 50-70 sec (60 unit/kg IV bolus then 12 unit/kg/h; max 4000 unit bolus and 1000 unit/h for patients > 70 kg or 5000 unit bolus followed by 1000 unit/h infusion. *See page 189*). **Note:** "Double-bolus" dosing of tPA has been associated with a higher risk of intracranial hemorrhage and should not be used. **PE:** 100 mg infusion over 2 hr

342  Adams HP, Jr. *et al.* Guidelines for the early management of patients with ischemic stroke: A scientific statement from the Stroke Council of the American Stroke Association. *Stroke* 2003; 34:1056-83.

343  Goldhaber SZ. Echocardiography in the management of pulmonary embolism. *Ann Intern Med* 2002; 136:691-700.

344  Sane DC *et al.* Bleeding during thrombolytic therapy for acute myocardial infarction: mechanisms and management. *Ann Intern Med* 1989;111(12):1010-22.

345  The sixth (2000) ACCP guidelines for antithrombotic therapy for prevention and treatment of thrombosis. American College of Chest Physicians. *Chest* 2001; 119: 176-193S, 228-252S, 300-320S.

346  GUSTO investigators. The effects of tissue-plasminogen activator, streptokinase, or both on coronary-artery patency, ventricular function, and survival after acute myocardial infarction. *NEJM* 1993; 329:1615.

followed by standard heparin therapy after aPTT returns to twice normal. **Stroke:** [347] 0.9 mg/kg total dose (up to 90 mg), give 10% as bolus dose followed by 90% of the dose infused over 60 min. No anticoagulants or antiplatelet drugs for 24 hr.

## Reteplase (rPA; *Retavase*)

<u>Action:</u> Recombinant derivative of tissue plasminogen activator (tPA) with longer half-life. Simplified dosing regimen with equivalent efficacy and side-effect profile. May be useful for pre-hospital thrombolysis.

<u>Kinetics:</u> Half-life 13-16 min, prolonged in renal and liver failure.

<u>IV:</u> **Acute MI:** [348] 10 unit IV bolus given twice, 30 minutes apart. Combine with aspirin and probably with heparin, as for tPA above. **PE:** Same as for AMI; combine with heparin as per tPA above.

<u>Incompatibility:</u> Cannot be given in same line as heparin.

## Streptokinase [349] (SK)

<u>Action:</u> Natural plasminogen activator. Purified from Group C streptococcus.

<u>Kinetics:</u> Half-life of activator complex is 23 min. Unknown metabolism, cleared by liver; activator complex degraded in part by anti-streptococcal antibodies. Hyperfibrinolytic effect lasts several hours; thrombin time and fibrin-split products elevated ~24 hr. Loading dose required to overcome native anti-streptococcal antibodies. Patients with known allergy should receive t-PA, r-PA, or TNK-tPA.

<u>Contraindications:</u> As per table above; also recent previous SK use. **Ineffective if given within 5 days to 12 mo of prior streptokinase or streptococcal infection.**

<u>IV:</u> **Acute MI:** 1.5 million IU over 30-60 min. Combine with aspirin; heparin not warranted [350] unless high risk of systemic or venous thromboembolism (i.e. atrial fibrillation, anterior MI, heart failure). SC heparin may be given. **PE:** 250,000 IU over 30 min, then 100,000 IU over 24h (continue for 72 hr if concurrent DVT). **Stroke:** No data showing benefit.

<u>Renal failure:</u> No adjustment.

<u>Adverse reactions:</u> Anaphylaxis, rash, fever, hypotension, respiratory depression, back pain.

## Tenecteplase (TNK-tPA; *TNKase*)

<u>Action:</u> Mutant of wild-type tissue plasminogen activator with longer half-life; can be administered as single bolus. Less effect on systemic coagulation parameters *in vivo*; when compared to tPA has similar efficacy and major outcomes in MI.[351]

<u>Kinetics:</u> $T_{1/2}$ 20-24 minutes.

<u>IV:</u> **Acute MI:** Single IV bolus dose over 5 seconds based on body weight: < 60 kg, 30 mg; 60-69 kg, 35 mg; 70-79 kg, 40 mg; 80-89 kg, 45 mg; ≥ 90kg, 50 mg. Combine with ASA and heparin as per tPA above.

## Triiodothyronine (T3)

*See Liothyronine on page 196*

## Tirofiban (Aggrastat)

*See Glycoprotein IIb/IIIa inhibitors on page 187*

---

347 NINDS investigators. Tissue plasminogen activator for acute ischemic stroke. *NEJM* 1995;333:1581-7.

348 Bode C *et al.* Randomized comparison of coronary thrombolysis achieved with double-bolus reteplase and front-loaded, accelerated alteplase in patients with acute myocardial infarction. *Circulation* 1996; 94(5):891-8.

349 The sixth (2000) ACCP guidelines for antithrombotic therapy for prevention and treatment of thrombosis. Ibid.

350 ISIS-3 Investigators. A randomised comparison of streptokinase vs. tPA vs. anistreplase and of aspirin plus heparin vs. heparin alone among 41,299 cases of suspected acute myocardial infarction. *Lancet* 1992;339:753.

351 ASSENT-2 Investigators. Single-bolus tenecteplase compared with front-loaded alteplase in acute myocardial infarction. *Lancet* 1999; 354(9180): 716-722.

# Torsemide (Demadex)
*See Loop diuretics on page 181*

# Vasopressin
*See also Desmopressin on page 179*

<u>Action</u>: Antidiuretic hormone; potent direct vasoconstrictor independent of adrenergic mechanisms; procoagulant. Alternative vasopressor to epinephrine in cardiac arrest. Used in esophageal variceal hemorrhage to reduce portal pressure, hepatic flow, and as procoagulant. Used also in diabetes insipidus (DI) and as GI promotility agent.

<u>Kinetics</u>: Hepatic and renal metabolism. Renal excretion. $T\frac{1}{2}$10-20 min.

<u>IV</u>: Mix 100 units/100mL D5W or 0.1unit/min = 6 mL/h). **Cardiac arrest:** 40 units IV push, repeat if needed in 3 minutes. Follow with epinephrine if ineffective. Post-hoc data from randomized trial [352] suggests that in asystole, both vasopressin and vasopressin followed by epinephrine are superior to epinephrine alone for improving survival to hospital admission. **Upper GI hemorrhage:** 0.2 unit/min increased each hour by 0.2 units/min until bleeding controlled. Max 1-2 unit/min. Combine with nitroglycerin 40-400 mcg/min. **Diabetes insipidus:** 5-10 units SC q 8-12h.

<u>Side effects</u>: Myocardial ischemia via coronary vasoconstriction; water intoxication; skin necrosis if extravasated; abdominal cramps, sweating.

<u>Interactions</u>: Ganglionic blocking agents markedly increase vasopressor effects. Antidiuretic effect potentiated by carbamazepine, tricyclics, clofibrate, fludrocortisone, chlorpropamide. Antidiuretic effect antagonized by norepinephrine, lithium, alcohol, demeclocycline.

# Vecuronium
*See Neuromuscular blockers on page 198*

# Verapamil
<u>Action</u>: Slow calcium channel antagonist. Depresses SA node, slows AV node conduction (but not AV bypass tracts). Antihypertensive via cardiac and vascular smooth muscle relaxation. Used IV to interrupt reentrant rhythms involving AV node and to slow ventricular response to atrial fibrillation and flutter. Used PO to lower BP, suppress angina and supraventricular tachycardias..

<u>Kinetics</u>: Onset 3-5 min. Liver metabolism. $T\frac{1}{2}$ 2 hr acute, 4-12 hr chronic, extended in hepatic disease.

<u>IV</u>: Bolus 2.5-5 mg over 2-3 min; if tolerated, may repeat doses of 5-10 mg every 15-30 min to max of 20 mg. May infuse beginning at 0.005 mg/kg/min (typically 5-10 mg/h) for rate control.[353] Undesirable hypotension often responds to IV calcium (5-10 mL of 10% calcium chloride or 15-30 mL 10% calcium gluconate) over 5 min. Some physicians pre-treat with IV calcium. [354]

<u>Renal failure</u>: No adjustment.

<u>Liver failure</u>: Reduce dose by up to 50%.

<u>Contraindications</u>: Undiagnosed wide-complex tachycardia; Wolff-Parkinson-White syndrome; severe left ventricular dysfunction, sinus node dysfunction.

<u>Adverse reactions</u>: Hypotension; bradycardia or asystole when given IV, especially with concurrent β-blockers, digoxin, hypokalemia, or in sinus node dysfunction. May exacerbate heart failure.

<u>Interactions</u>: Digoxin clearance halved (reduce digoxin dose by 50%). Lithium interaction variable; carbamazepine, theophylline, cyclosporine levels increased;

---

[352] Wenzel V *et al.* A comparison of vasopressin and epinephrine for out-of-hospital cardiopulmonary resuscitation. *NEJM* 2004; 350:105-113.

[353] Barbarash RA *et al.* Verapamil infusions in the treatment of atrial tachyarrhythmias. *Crit Care Med* 1986;14(10):886-8. Iberti TJ *et al.* Use of constant-infusion verapamil for the treatment of postoperative supraventricular tachycardia. *Crit Care Med* 1986;14(4):283-4.

[354] Haft JI, Habbab MA. Treatment of atrial arrhythmias. Effectiveness of verapamil when preceded by calcium infusion. *Arch Intern Med* 1986;146(6):1085-9.

neuromuscular blockers potentiated; reports of vascular collapse with dantrolene. Cimetidine prolongs verapamil half-life. Phenytoin decreases verapamil effects.

Pregnancy: Category C.

# Warfarin [355] *(Coumadin)*

Action: Oral anticoagulant. Blocks vitamin-K-dependent activation of factors II, VII, IX, X, protein C, and S. Heterogeneous half-lives of clotting factors may cause transient hypercoagulability upon starting therapy, especially in partial factor C and S deficiency. Give concomitant heparin until INR is therapeutic for 2 days to overcome this phenomenon.

Kinetics: Hepatic metabolism, enterohepatic circulation, albumin-bound. Half-life 1-2 d, biological effect 2-7d.

Renal failure: No adjustment.

PO: Start 5 mg qd x 3-4 d (consider 2.5 mg in elderly, malnourished, liver disease, or patients at high risk for bleeding); adjust subsequent doses to achieve target PT or INR. Check INR daily until INR range reached and sustained 2 days, then 2-3 times weekly for 1-2 weeks, followed by less frequent monitoring until the INR stabilizes.

$$INR = \left[ \frac{Patient\ PT}{Control\ PT} \right]^{ISI}$$

Therapeutic endpoint: International Normalized Ratio (INR). The "ISI" (international sensitivity index) varies with batch of reagent. INR may overestimate *in vivo* anticoagulant effect during first few days of therapy (ideally should measure prothrombin antigen levels) but well suited for monitoring chronic therapy. *For specific indications, see table on page 214.*

Adverse effects: Major hemorrhage; risk increased if age > 65, stroke or GI bleeding history, renal insufficiency or anemia. Theoretical hypercoagulant effect during initiation of therapy. Skin necrosis via thrombosis of venules and capillaries of SC fat (usually seen in protein C and S deficiency on 3rd-8th day of therapy), systemic cholesterol microembolization, purple toe syndrome.

Overdose: *See tables pages 215-216.*

Pregnancy: Pregnancy Class X, especially in first trimester. Safe to nurse.

Drug interactions: *See table page 217.*

---

[355] Hirsh J *et al.* American Heart Association/American College of Cardiology Foundation guide to warfarin therapy. *J Am Coll Cardiol* 2003; 41:1633-52. Hirsh J *et al.* Oral anticoagulants: mechanism of action, clinical effectiveness, and optimal therapeutic range. *Chest* 2001; 119:8S-21S.

## Therapeutic goals for oral anticoagulation [356]

| Indication | INR * | Duration of Therapy |
|---|---|---|
| **Prophylaxis of venous thromboembolism (VTE)** after high-risk surgery † | 2-3 | ≥ 7-10 days |
| **Treatment of VTE/pulmonary embolus** | | |
| First episode, reversible/time-limited risk factor ‡ | 2-3 | ≥ 3 months |
| First episode, continuing risk factor § | 2-3 | 12 months - indefinite |
| First episode, idiopathic | 2-3 | ≥ 6 months |
| Prevention of recurrent VTE after idiopathic VTE | 2-3 | 2-4 years studied [357] |
| Recurrent, idiopathic or with clotting predisposition | 2-3 | 12 mo to indefinite |
| Isolated *symptomatic* calf vein thrombosis | 2-3 | 6-12 weeks |
| **Coronary heart disease** | | |
| Acute MI with increased embolic risk ‖ | 2-3 | 1-3 months |
| Acute MI with atrial fibrillation | 2-3 | Indefinite |
| Recurrent ischemic episodes following acute MI ¶ | 1.5 | Clinical judgment |
| Unstable angina with contraindication to aspirin | 2.5 | Several months |
| Primary prevention in men at high risk of cardiovascular events [358] # | 1.5 | Indefinite |
| **Valvular heart disease** | | |
| After thrombotic event or if LA diameter > 5.5 cm | 2-3 | Indefinite |
| **Atrial fibrillation** | | |
| Patients with ≥ 1 risk factor ** | 2-3 | Indefinite |
| Age ≥ 65 with diabetes or coronary disease ** | 2-3 | Indefinite |
| Elective cardioversion for atrial fibrillation > 48h | 2-3 | 3 weeks @ |
| **Acute spinal cord injury**, rehab phase | 2-3 | Not defined |
| **Postpartum** anticoagulation for VTE during pregnancy | 2-3 | At least 6 weeks |
| **Prosthetic heart valves**, mechanical | INR target and therapy duration vary based upon risk factors and valve type £ | |

* Aim for an INR in the middle of the INR range (e.g. 2.5 for a range of 2.0-3.0 and 3.0 for a range of 2.5-3.5).

† General surgery in very high risk patient, total hip/knee replacement, hip fracture surgery, gynecologic surgery

§ Cancer, anticardiolipin antibody, antithrombin III deficiency. Therapy duration unclear for 1st event associated with homozygous factor V Leiden (activated protein C resistance), homocystinemia, protein C or S deficiency, prothrombin gene mutation 20210, or multiple thrombophilias.

‖ Anterior AMI or AMI complicated by severe LV dysfunction, CHF, previous emboli, or echocardiographic evidence of mural thrombosis. Warfarin (target INR 2.5) is also an alternative when aspirin is contraindicated in patients with acute MI or unstable angina.

‡ Transient immobilization, trauma, surgery, or estrogen use.

¶ Plus aspirin 75-81 mg/day.

# Consider the addition of aspirin 75-81 mg/day.

356 Adapted from: *Chest suppl* 2001;119:129S,187S,203S,215S, 247S; *Am Fam Physician* 1999;59:635; *JACC* 1998;32:1486; *JACC* 2001;38:1266ii

357 Ridker PM *et al.* Long-term, low-intensity warfarin therapy for the prevention of recurrent venous thromboembolism. *NEJM* 2003: 348:1425-1434; Kearon C *et al.* Comparison of low-intensity warfarin therapy with conventional-intensity warfarin therapy for long-term prevention of recurrent venous thromboembolism. *NEJM* 2003; 349:631-639.

358 Thrombosis prevention trial: Randomised trial of low-intensity oral anticoagulation with warfarin and low-dose aspirin in the primary prevention of ischaemic heart disease in men at increased risk. *Lancet* 1998; 351:233-41.

** Risk factors:  age > 75, previous TIA/stroke or systemic embolism, reduced LV function, history of hypertension, rheumatic mitral valve disease, prosthetic heart valve.  Patients < 65 yo without heart disease can be treated with aspirin 325 mg/day or receive no treatment.  Patients < 65 yo with heart disease but no additional risk factors or patients ≥ 65 yo with no risk factors should receive aspirin 325 mg/day without warfarin.  The addition of aspirin 81-162 mg/day to warfarin is an option for patients ≥ 60 yo with diabetes or coronary disease.  A target INR of 3.0 (2.5-3.5) in combination with aspirin 81-100 mg/day is recommended for patients with caged ball or caged disc valves.
@ Begin 3 weeks before and continue for 4 weeks after sinus rhythm established
£ See www.americanheart.org and www.chestnet.org

**Warfarin Reversal:** Oral vitamin K at low dose effective for almost all situations: [359]

| INR | Serious bleeding? | Increased bleeding risk? @ | Urgent dental or surgical procedure? | Treatment * |
|---|---|---|---|---|
| 3.0 – 5.0 | No | - | No | Lower dose or omit 1 dose and resume therapy at lower dose when INR therapeutic. |
| 5.0 – 9.0 | No | No | No | Hold dose x 2 days and resume at lower dose when INR therapeutic **or** omit next dose and give Vit K 1.0-2.5 mg PO |
| 5.0 – 9.0 | No | Yes | No | Omit next dose and give Vit K 1.0-2.5 mg PO |
| 9 - 20 | No | - | - | Vit K 3 – 5 mg PO (INR reduction occurs in ~ 24 hr).  Monitor INR closely.  May repeat vit K if INR remains elevated. |
| Any | No | - | Yes | Vit K 2 – 5 mg PO # (INR reduction occurs in 24 hr) or 0.5 - 1 mg IV § |
| > 20 | No | - | - | FFP or prothrombin complex concentrate [360] or recombinant factor VIIa [361] +/- Vit K 10 mg slow IV infusion.§  Monitor INR closely.  May repeat Vit K q 12 |
| Any | Yes | - | - | p prn. |

@ Risk of bleeding is related to elevation of INR.  Other risk factors for bleeding include: recent major surgery or trauma; co-administration of antiplatelet agents; age > 65; history of GI bleeding or stroke; renal insufficiency; anemia.
* All patients with supratherapeutic INR should be carefully evaluated and monitored.  Consider inpatient admission if active bleeding or high risk of bleeding.
# If INR is still high after 24 hr, administer additional Vit K 1-2 mg PO.
§ Intravenous vitamin K generally effective and well-tolerated but carries small risk of anaphylaxis.  Should not prolong return to therapeutic anticoagulation. [362]

359 Hirsh J et al. American Heart Association/American College of Cardiology Foundation guide to warfarin therapy. J Am Coll Cardiol 2003; 41:1633-52;  Lubetsky A et al. Comparison of oral vs intravenous phytonadione (vitamin k1) in patients with excessive anticoagulation: A prospective randomized controlled study. Arch Intern Med 2003; 163:2469-2473.
360 Rapid reversal of oral anticoagulation with warfarin by a prothrombin complex concentrate (Beriplex): Efficacy and safety in 42 patients. Br J Haematol 2002; 116:619-24.
361 Deveras RA, Kessler CM. Reversal of warfarin-induced excessive anticoagulation with recombinant human factor VIIa concentrate. Ann Intern Med 2002; 137:884-8.
362 Shields RC et al. Efficacy and safety of intravenous phytonadione (vitamin k1) in patients on long-term oral anticoagulant therapy. Mayo Clin Proc 2001; 76:260-6.

## Reversal of Warfarin with Plasma or Prothrombin Complex Concentrate [363]

### 1) Choose target INR

| Clinical Scenario | Target INR |
|---|---|
| Moderate bleeding and high risk of thrombosis | 2.0 – 2.1 |
| Serious bleeding and moderate risk of thrombosis | 1.5 |
| Serious or life-threatening bleeding and low risk of thrombosis | 1.0 |

### 2) Convert target INR to % prothrombin complex (% complex found in normal plasma)

| Degree of anticoagulation | INR | % of normal plasma |
|---|---|---|
| Overanticoagulation | >5 | 5 |
| | 4.0 – 4.9 | 10 |
| Therapeutic range | 2.6 – 3.2 | 15 |
| | 2.2 – 2.5 | 20 |
| | 1.9 – 2.1 | 25 |
| Subtherapeutic range | 1.7 – 1.8 | 30 |
| | 1.4 – 1.6 | 40 |
| Complete reversal to normal | 1.0 | 100 |

### 3) Calculate dose of plasma or prothrombin complex concentrate (PCC):

Dose (mL of plasma or units of PCC) = (target % - current %) × (body weight in kg)

[363] Schulman S. Care of patients receiving long-term anticoagulant therapy. *N Engl J Med.* 2003;349:675-683.

# Warfarin – Selected Drug Interactions [364]

*Note: Assume possible drug interactions with any new medication. When stopping or starting a medication, the INR should be checked weekly for ≥ 2-3 weeks, especially with intensive anticoagulation (INR > 2.5).*

## Increased anticoagulant effect of warfarin and increased risk of bleeding

**• Monitor INR when agents below started, stopped, or dosage changed**

| | | | |
|---|---|---|---|
| Acetaminophen | efavirenz | itraconazole | propafenone |
| (≥2g/d for ≥3-4 d) | fenofibrate | ketoconazole | propoxyphene |
| allopurinol | fluconazole | leflunomide | quinidine |
| amiodarone* | fluoroquinolones | levamisole | quinine |
| amprenavir | fluorouracil | levothyroxine # | sertraline |
| cefazolin | fluoxetine | miconazole | tamoxifen |
| cefoxitin | flutamide | modafinil | tetracyclines |
| ceftriaxone | fluvoxamine | neomycin | thyroid hormones # |
| cisapride | fosphenytoin | olsalazine | tramadol |
| corticosteroids¶ | gemcitabine | omeprazole | valproate |
| cyclophosphamide | glucagon | penicillin, hi-dose IV | vitamin E |
| delavirdine | glyburide | pentoxifylline | tricyclics |
| | isoniazid | phenytoin (acute) | zileuton |

**• Consider alternative agents; monitor INR when started/stopped/dosage changed**

| | | | |
|---|---|---|---|
| cimetidine † | paroxetine | statins § | trazodone |
| macrolides ‡ | ranitidine | sulfonamides | zafirlukast |
| nalidixic acid | | St John's wort | |

**• Avoid unless benefit > risk; monitor INR when started/stopped/dosage changed**

| | | | |
|---|---|---|---|
| anabolic steroids | celecoxib | disulfiram | rofecoxib |
| androgens | clofibrate | gemfibrozil | sulfinpyrazone |
| aspirin ¶ | danazol | metronidazole | valdecoxib |

**• Avoid agents below; benefits do not justify risks**

| | | | |
|---|---|---|---|
| cefoperazone | danshen (Chinese herb) | fish oil | ginkgo |
| cefotetan | dong quai (Chinese herb) | garlic supplements | testosterone |

## Decreased anticoagulant effect of warfarin and ↑ risk of thrombosis

**• Monitor INR when agents below started, stopped, or dosage changed**

| | | | |
|---|---|---|---|
| aminoglutethimide | dicloxacillin | methimazole # | propylthiouracil # |
| azathioprine | efavirenz | nafcillin | rifabutin/rifampin |
| barbiturates | griseofulvin | panax ginseng | ritonavir |
| carbamazepine | mercaptopurine | phenytoin | St John's wort |
| coenzyme Q-10 | mesalamine | primidone | Trazodone |

**• Use alternative to agents below; or give at different times of day and monitor INR when agent started, stopped, dose/dosing schedule changed**

| | | |
|---|---|---|
| cholestyramine | colestipol (lower risk than cholestyramine) | sucralfate |

**• Avoid unless benefit > risk. Monitor INR when started, stopped, or changed**

| | | |
|---|---|---|
| oral contraceptives | phenobarbital | rifampin |

* Interaction may be delayed; monitor INR for several weeks after starting and several months after stopping amiodarone. May need to lower warfarin dose by 33% to 50%.
† Ranitidine, famotidine, nizatidine are alternatives.
‡ Azithromycin appears to have lower risk than clarithromycin or erythromycin.
§ Pravastatin appears to have lower risk of interaction.
# Increased response to warfarin therapy in hyperthyroidism or thyroid replacement

---

364 Reprinted from *The Pocket Pharmacopeia*, 2004 edition. Green S (ed). Table adapted from: www.coumadin.com; *Am Fam Phys* 1999;59:635; *Chest* 1998; 114: 447S, 448S; *Hansten and Horn's Drug Interactions Analysis and Management*.

## Zoledronate (*Zometa*) [365]

<u>Action:</u> Inhibits bone resorption via inhibition of osteoclast activity.

<u>Indication:</u> Hypercalcemia, especially malignancy-related.

<u>Kinetics:</u> Primarily eliminated via kidney; $T_{1/2}$=167 hours. 56% bound to plasma proteins

<u>IV:</u> 4 mg IV single dose IV infusion over > 15 min. Assure adequate hydration prior to drug administration. May repeat (4-8 mg) after 7 days if calcium does not return to normal.

<u>Renal dysfunction:</u> No specific dose reduction recommended; however, limited data exists for patients with creatinine > 3.0 mg/dL. Hold repeat doses if creatinine rises > 0.5 and 1 mg/dL from normal baseline or abnormal baseline, respectively.

<u>Interactions:</u> Additive renal toxicity when given with aminoglycosides and other nephrotoxic drugs. Risk of renal dysfunction increased in multiple myeloma, particularly when given with thalidomide

<u>Adverse effects:</u> Nephrotoxicity (including acute renal failure), fever, flu-like symptoms, nausea/vomiting, rash, chest pain.

<u>Incompatibility:</u> Calcium-containing infusion solutions (i.e. lactated Ringers)

<u>Pregnancy:</u> Category D

# *General Drug References*

*Cardiovascular Drug Therapy*, 2<sup>nd</sup> ed. Messerli FH (ed). Philadelphia: WB Saunders, 1996.

*Drug Facts and Comparisons*. Novak K (ed.) Facts and Comparisons, Wolters Kluwer Co.: St. Louis, MO, 2003.

*Drug Prescribing in Renal Failure.*, 4<sup>th</sup> ed. American College of Physicians-American Society of Internal Medicine: Philadelphia, PA, 1999.

*DRUGDEX® System*. Hutchison TA (ed). MICROMEDEX, Inc., Englewood, Colorado (2003 Edition).

*Goldfrank's toxicologic emergencies*, 7<sup>th</sup> ed. Goldfrank LR (ed). New York: McGraw-Hill Medical Pub. Division, 2002.

*Goodman and Gilman's Pharmacological Basis of Therapeutics*, 10<sup>th</sup> ed. Hardman JG (ed). New York: McGraw-Hill, 2001.

*Physicians Desk Reference.*. MICROMEDEX, Inc. Englewood, Colorado 2003 edition.

*Tarascon Pocket Pharmacopoeia*. Green S (ed). Tarascon Publishing: Lompoc, CA, 2004.

*UpToDate Online*. Rose B, Rush J. 2003 Edition.

---

[365] Major P *et al*. Zoledronic acid is superior to pamidronate in the treatment of hypercalcemia of malignancy: A pooled analysis of two randomized, controlled clinical trials. *J Clin Oncol* 2001; 19:558-567.

# Index

# Ordering From Tarascon Publishing

| INTERNET | FAX | PHONE | MAIL |
|---|---|---|---|
| Credit card orders at www.tarascon.com | Fax credit card orders toll free to 877.929.9926 | For phone orders or customer service, call 800.929.9926 | Mail order & check to: Tarascon Publishing, PO Box 517, Lompoc, CA 93438 |

| | Price/Copy by # of Copies Ordered | | | | | |
|---|---|---|---|---|---|---|
| | PHONE | | | | MAIL | |
| **TARASCON POCKET PHARMACOPOEIA®** | 1-9 | 10-49 | 50-99 | ≥100 | # Ordered | Price |
| Classic Shirt-Pocket Edition | $9.95 | $8.95 | $7.95 | $6.95 | | $ |
| Deluxe Labcoat Pocket Edition | $17.95 | $15.25 | $13.45 | $12.55 | | $ |
| PDA software on CD-ROM, 12-month subscription* | $29.95 | $25.46 | $23.96 | $22.46 | | $ |
| PDA software on CD-ROM, 3-month subscription* | $8.97 | $7.62 | $7.18 | $6.73 | | $ |
| **OTHER POCKETBOOKS & MAGNIFIER** | 1-9 | 10-49 | 50-99 | ≥100 | | |
| Tarascon Internal Medicine & Critical Care Pocketbook | $14.95 | $13.45 | $11.94 | $10.44 | | $ |
| Tarascon Adult Emergency Pocketbook | $14.95 | $13.45 | $11.94 | $10.44 | | $ |
| Tarascon Pocket Orthopaedica® | $14.95 | $13.45 | $11.94 | $10.44 | | $ |
| Tarascon Primary Care Pocketbook | $14.95 | $13.45 | $11.94 | $10.44 | | $ |
| Tarascon Pediatric Emergency Pocketbook | $11.95 | $9.90 | $8.95 | $8.35 | | $ |
| How to be a Truly Excellent Junior Medical Student | $9.95 | $8.25 | $7.45 | $6.95 | | $ |
| Sheet magnifier – fits in any book to make reading easier! | $1.00 | $0.89 | $0.78 | $0.66 | | $ |
| | | | | | Subtotal | $ |
| | | | | California Sales Tax (7.75%) | | $ |

*Palm OS or Pocket PC. download the software directly from www.tarascon.com for an approximately 10% discount!

**SALES TAX - California only**

| CHOOSE SHIPPING METHOD: cost based on subtotal → | ≤$10 | $10-29 | $30-75 | $76-300 | | |
|---|---|---|---|---|---|---|
| ☐ Standard shipping | $1.00 | $2.50 | $6.00 | $8.00 | Shipping | $ |
| ☐ UPS 2-day air (no post office boxes) | $12.00 | $14.00 | $16.00 | $18.00 | TOTAL | $ |

| Name | ☐ VISA ☐ Mastercard ☐ AmEx ☐ Discover | Card number |
|---|---|---|
| Address | Expiration date | CID# (if available) | Signature |
| City / State / Zip | E-mail and phone | |